Health and Well-Being Considerations in the Design of Indoor Environments

Roberto A. González-Lezcano
Universidad CEU San Pablo, Spain

IGI Global
PUBLISHER of TIMELY KNOWLEDGE

A volume in the Advances in Civil and Industrial Engineering (ACIE) Book Series

Published in the United States of America by
IGI Global
Engineering Science Reference (an imprint of IGI Global)
701 E. Chocolate Avenue
Hershey PA, USA 17033
Tel: 717-533-8845
Fax: 717-533-8661
E-mail: cust@igi-global.com
Web site: http://www.igi-global.com

Library of Congress Cataloging-in-Publication Data

Names: González-Lezcano, Roberto Alonso, 1971- editor.
Title: Health and well-being considerations in the design of indoor environments / Roberto Alonso Gonzalez-Lezcano, editor.
Description: Hershey, PA : Engineering Science Reference, [2021] | Includes bibliographical references and index. | Summary: "The chapters in this book will address issues concerning Indoor Environmental Quality (IEQ), which are described more simply as the conditions inside the building and cover issues such as air quality, access to daylight and views, pleasant acoustic conditions and occupant control over lighting and thermal comfort"-- Provided by publisher.
Identifiers: LCCN 2021012376 (print) | LCCN 2021012377 (ebook) | ISBN 9781799872795 (h/c) | ISBN 9781799872801 (s/c) | ISBN 9781799872818 (eISBN)
Subjects: LCSH: Buildings--Environmental engineering.
Classification: LCC TH6021 .H424 2021 (print) | LCC TH6021 (ebook) | DDC 696--dc23
LC record available at https://lccn.loc.gov/2021012376
LC ebook record available at https://lccn.loc.gov/2021012377

This book is published in the IGI Global book series Advances in Civil and Industrial Engineering (ACIE) (ISSN: 2326-6139; eISSN: 2326-6155)

British Cataloguing in Publication Data
A Cataloguing in Publication record for this book is available from the British Library.

All work contributed to this book is new, previously-unpublished material. The views expressed in this book are those of the authors, but not necessarily of the publisher.

For electronic access to this publication, please contact: eresources@igi-global.com.

Advances in Civil and Industrial Engineering (ACIE) Book Series

Ioan Constantin Dima
University Valahia of Târgovişte, Romania

ISSN:2326-6139
EISSN:2326-6155

Mission

Private and public sector infrastructures begin to age, or require change in the face of developing technologies, the fields of civil and industrial engineering have become increasingly important as a method to mitigate and manage these changes. As governments and the public at large begin to grapple with climate change and growing populations, civil engineering has become more interdisciplinary and the need for publications that discuss the rapid changes and advancements in the field have become more in-demand. Additionally, private corporations and companies are facing similar changes and challenges, with the pressure for new and innovative methods being placed on those involved in industrial engineering.

The **Advances in Civil and Industrial Engineering (ACIE) Book Series** aims to present research and methodology that will provide solutions and discussions to meet such needs. The latest methodologies, applications, tools, and analysis will be published through the books included in **ACIE** in order to keep the available research in civil and industrial engineering as current and timely as possible.

Coverage

- Construction Engineering
- Production Planning and Control
- Materials Management
- Hydraulic Engineering
- Transportation Engineering
- Operations Research
- Earthquake engineering
- Structural Engineering
- Engineering Economics
- Coastal Engineering

IGI Global is currently accepting manuscripts for publication within this series. To submit a proposal for a volume in this series, please contact our Acquisition Editors at Acquisitions@igi-global.com or visit: http://www.igi-global.com/publish/.

The Advances in Civil and Industrial Engineering (ACIE) Book Series (ISSN 2326-6139) is published by IGI Global, 701 E. Chocolate Avenue, Hershey, PA 17033-1240, USA, www.igi-global.com. This series is composed of titles available for purchase individually; each title is edited to be contextually exclusive from any other title within the series. For pricing and ordering information please visit http://www.igi-global.com/book-series/advances-civil-industrial-engineering/73673. Postmaster: Send all address changes to above address.

Titles in this Series

For a list of additional titles in this series, please visit:
http://www.igi-global.com/book-series/advances-civil-industrial-engineering/73673.

Visibilities and Invisibilities in Smart Cities Emerging Research and Opprtunities
H. Patricia McKenna (AmbientEase, Canada)
Engineering Science Reference • © 2021 • 289pp • H/C (ISBN: 9781799838500) • US $195.00

Transforming Urban Nightlife and the Development of Smart Public Spaces
Hisham Abusaada (Housing and Building National Research Center (HBRC), Egypt) Abeer Elshater (Ain Shams University, Egypt) and Dennis Rodwell (Independent Researcher, UK)
Information Science Reference • © 2021 • 290pp • H/C (ISBN: 9781799870043) • US $195.00

Handbook of Research on Driving Transformational Change in the Digital Built Environment
Jason Underwood (University of Salford, UK) and Mark Shelbourn (Birmingham City University, UK)
Engineering Science Reference • © 2021 • 569pp • H/C (ISBN: 9781799866008) • US $295.00

Structural Dynamics and Static Nonlinear Analysis From Theory to Application
Mourad Belgasmia (Setif 1 University, Algeria)
Engineering Science Reference • © 2021 • 347pp • H/C (ISBN: 9781799843993) • US $195.00

Handbook of Research on Developing Smart Cities Based on Digital Twins
Matteo Del Giudice (Politecnico di Torino, Italy) and Anna Osello (Politecnico di Torino, Italy)
Engineering Science Reference • © 2021 • 674pp • H/C (ISBN: 9781799870913) • US $295.00

Data-Driven Optimization of Manufacturing Processes
Kanak Kalita (Vel Tech Rangarajan Dr. Sagunthala R&D Institute of Science and Technology, India) Ranjan Kumar Ghadai (Sikkim Manipal Institute of Technology, Sikkim Manipal University, Majhitar, India) and Xiao-Zhi Gao (University of Eastern Finland, Finland)
Engineering Science Reference • © 2021 • 298pp • H/C (ISBN: 9781799872061) • US $225.00

Developing and Monitoring Smart Environments for Intelligent Cities
Zaigham Mahmood (University of Northampton, UK & Shijiazhuang Tiedao University, China)
Engineering Science Reference • © 2021 • 367pp • H/C (ISBN: 9781799850625) • US $215.00

Applications and Challenges of Maintenance and Safety Engineering in Industry 4.0
Alberto Martinetti (University of Twente, The Netherlands) Micaela Demichela (Politecnico di Torino, Italy) and Sarbjeet Singh (Luleå University of Technology, Sweden)
Engineering Science Reference • © 2020 • 321pp • H/C (ISBN: 9781799839040) • US $265.00

IGI Global
PUBLISHER of TIMELY KNOWLEDGE

701 East Chocolate Avenue, Hershey, PA 17033, USA
Tel: 717-533-8845 x100 • Fax: 717-533-8661
E-Mail: cust@igi-global.com • www.igi-global.com

Editorial Advisory Board

Table of Contents

Detailed Table of Contents

This study is based on the analysis of the facades of tobacco drying sheds located in the regions of Cáceres and Toledo in Spain as an example of bioclimatic production architecture. Using modular and permeable façade designs, it is possible to generate an interior space with specific hygrothermal conditions. The drying sheds are the places where the tobacco plant is cured with the air penetrating through the holes on their facades, and the tobacco dries under certain conditions of humidity and temperature. The design of these patterns based on a module, such as the brick, not only affects the composition but also determines the permeability characteristics, conditioning the interior space hygrothermally. Analysing the conceptual relationship, textures, patterns, and construction methods of the dryers with contemporary architecture, numerous examples can be found in other buildings in which modular patterns are used in the composition of the facades similar to those used in the dryers.

Tactic and strategic management and policing of atmospheric pollution in México, specifically by particulate material (PM) from mobile sources (internal combustion powered vehicles), critically requires state-of-the-science technologies due to the problem's complexity including its public health dimension. The authors consider that proper decision making on the problem would benefit from permanent revision on currently employed PM monitoring and measurement systems and also the effort to improve them. These later currently offer information on O(10^0) ultraviolet-visible-infrared (UV-VIS-IR) spectral bands at O(10^0) spatial resolutions and O(10^1) in [min^-1] temporal resolutions. In contrast, they propose the novel use of acousto-optic tunable filter (AOTF) spectrometry to study PM in atmospheric suspension, capable of offering information on O(10^2) UV, VIS, or IR spectral bands at similar or better spatial and temporal resolutions. The potential of AOTF spectrometry towards PM assessment is clear and the objective is to explore its usefulness.

When designing for wellbeing, noise is usually not properly accounted for (if at all) during the design phase of a building. However, noise is often rated as the number one cause of dissatisfaction in offices; it negatively affects patients and staff in hospitals, prevents quality learning and teaching in schools, and bests poor service as the most irksome complaint for restaurants users. The question that arises is then, "How can we design to avoid the negative effects of noise on the end-users to enable wellbeing in indoor spaces?"

The extraction of building materials from their resources through harvesting, preservation, and utilization has become a significant segment of human contribution to the global ecosystem since the industrial revolution. Bamboo is the world's fastest-growing woody plant, and bamboo grows multiple times quicker than most species. Housing is one of the focused demands for bamboo, and as a result of the current scarcity of home units, the demand for bamboo is increasing. Bamboo building construction is portrayed by a basic edge approach like that applied in traditional building design and construction. Applying bamboo as an environmentally friendly material is seen as a movement towards creating a sustainable environment and reducing greenhouse emissions. The need to employ government policy in addressing the production and application of bamboo is reported, and the challenges of bamboo in the global market are highlighted in this chapter.

The world population is expected to be 9.3 billion by 2050, with a high increase in the urban population. It is worth considering that 71.7% of the surface of the earth covered by water, but only 3% of this water can be used as drinking water. In cities, buildings are recognized as one of the largest users of freshwater resources in construction and operation. The water use impact is different in some countries because some use conventional water treatments while other ones rely on advanced desalination. Climate change and population growth are clearly putting pressure on the world's water supply, so the first environmental assessment plan for buildings was launched in 1990 by the BRE in the United Kingdom where the water category is included in its environmental assessment.

University studies for the architecture degree in Spain give very little weight to considerations related to the design of a healthy interior environment. The low number of subjects related to interior comfort criteria may cause the student to underestimate the importance of environmental design of closed spaces in favor of aesthetic or merely functional aspects. However, there is a direct relationship between formal design decisions and environmental conditions in buildings, and future architects must understand those connections in order to make designs that combine efficiency and high aesthetic value. In this chapter, several pedagogical strategies are presented to get architecture students to learn and internalize the link between design and interior conditions, aiming at the acquisition of an adequate environmental awareness.

The aim of this study is to create a checklist of roof garden design criteria. This scope of work includes an encompassing review of international standards studies such as German Landscape Research, Development, and Construction Society; the American Society for Testing and Materials; the U.S. Green Building Counci; and Green Roofs for Healthy Cities, whereas the generated checklist was evaluated in the Marmara Forum Mall. As a result of the study, an answer was sought to the question, "What are the prerequisites for a roof garden serving the needs of users in today's conditions?" whereas on-site detection, observation, and photography were used as working methods. As a result, in considering the evaluation of the checklist on a scale of the Marmara Forum Mall, climatic data, activities with its hard structure, promenade areas, and designs of plantlife and water elements in soft structure are moderately sufficient, whereas it was determined there is no problem in the roof furniture design and maintenance.

Heating and cooling consume a high amount of energy, which is today mainly provided by fossil fuels. To save fossil resources and simultaneously reduce pollutants and CO2, heating and cooling energy consumption should be reduced. Geothermal energy is a clean, inexhaustible source of energy that is available all year round because it does not depend on the weather. Nevertheless, the use of tempered subsoil air has been used as a traditional air conditioning strategy; however, nowadays, its use has been questioned by the discovery of the leaks of radon gas from the ground. The investigation searches a heat exchange system with the subsoil which prevents the introduction of radon gas into living spaces. The system that is exposed increases the performance of aerothermal heat pumps by means of thermal exchange with tempered air in the sanitary chamber. This exchange is more favorable than air at the outside temperature, increasing the COP of the machine. This system complies with the regulations for protection against radon, protecting the building from this radioactive gas.

The older segments of the adult population in cities experience problems conditioned by the climate of each place. Since the 2003 heat wave which caused 70,000 heat deaths, the dramatic consequences of climate change and rising temperatures in Europe have led to the elderly being most at risk. Insufficient adaptability and economic resources among them also lead to repercussions on architecture, causing energy poverty issues as a result of a real consumption needed which is very different from the actual consumption. The demands of these people are determined by environmental stress, which differ greatly throughout the year. In addition, illnesses influence the daily health and the decrease in sensory capacity of the elderly, making them more vulnerable to constant changes. Faced with this problem, the main aim of this research is to analyse the degree of comfort and well-being of the elderly due to the environmental changes that occur in Andalusian rural homes in order to include some considerations in the design of indoor environments.

At present, the implementation of the concepts of tellurism and sacred geometry in the schools of architecture is neither obvious nor simple. It starts with the historical heritage of patterns that are shaped and molded according to professorships that have worked independently in territories at different scales within building and urbanism. Moreover, they share the same premise of the occupation of space and creation. In this study, the authors focus on the intrinsic value of the land, its energy, and how this affects not only the overall design of the building, but also the interior of a healthy dwelling. The psychological, psychosomatic, and symptomatic effects on the human being are related to the intrinsic use of a dwelling, as well as to the building's placement on the land. The work method in this investigation has implemented a comparative case study carried out in El Pardo and Carabanchel.

Developing useful objects for a functional reeducation of senior citizens persons about the basic activities of daily living must be conceptualized considering theories, techniques, and approaches in methodology, based on ecologically bearable structures, economically viable, and socially equitable. Consequently, the present chapter has the objective to state the criteria and strategies of a sustainable design, from a detailed study of applicability of 1) user-product interaction, observation, understanding, dimensional relationship, and evaluation; 2) creative process, identification, ideation, definition, prototypes, evaluation, and structuration; 3) technical specifications, structure, sustainability, ergonomics, aesthetics, and evaluation; 4) manufacture method, sustainability, production method, life cycle, capital assets, official

Preface

Indoor residential environments have a direct influence on human health, both in developed and developing countries. Significant levels of indoor pollution can make housing unsafe and can negatively impact on human health. Housing, therefore, is a key health factor for people all over the world, and various parameters such as air quality, ventilation, hygrothermal comfort, lighting, physical environment, building efficiency, and others can contribute to healthy architecture and the conditions that can result from the poor application of these parameters.

Health and Well-Being Considerations in the Design of Indoor Environments addresses issues concerning indoor environmental quality (IEQ), including air quality and ventilation, access to daylight and views, acoustic conditions, and control over lighting and thermal comfort, as well as the impact that this environment can have on human health and mental well-being. The book also investigates the functional aspects of interior design such as whether the layout provides easy access to tools and sufficient space for occupants. It also considers energy demand and building energy losses due to such issues as air renovations and enclosure infiltrations. Covering topics such as sustainable design, pollution, building materials, and lighting, this book is an effective resource for students, professors, academicians, researchers, architects, designers, planners, engineers, interior designers, building managers, construction companies, and other industry professionals looking to increase building occupant satisfaction by considering all aspects of IEQ.

This book will address a topic of great relevance today, taking into account that in developed countries, most of the time is spent indoors and, depending on each person, the presence in the home ranges from 60% to 90% of the day, and 30% of that time is spent sleeping. Taking into account these data, indoor residential environments have a direct influence on human health. Added to this in developing countries, significant levels of indoor pollution make housing unsafe, with a impact on the health of inhabitants. Housing is therefore a key health factor for people all over the world and various parameters such as air quality, ventilation, hygrothermal comfort, lighting, physical environment, building efficiency and others can contribute to healthy architecture, and the conditions that can result from the poor application of these parameters.

In this book we look for a range of innovative research and evidence-based policy ideas that demonstrate the importance of housing research and policy for health and well-being.

This research book will update the current state of knowledge on the subject, since the authors of the chapters will all be researchers and professors from prestigious universities. It will not be a theoretical book, but will be based on where current research is taking us in terms of energy saving.

CHAPTER 1: PERMEABILITY IN BIOCLIMATIC MODULAR FACADES – SPANISH SHEDS

This study is based on the analysis of the facades of tobacco drying sheds located in the regions of Cáceres and Toledo in Spain, as an example of bioclimatic production architecture. Using modular and permeable façade designs, it is possible to generate an interior space with specific hygrothermal conditions. The drying sheds are the places where the tobacco plant is cured, with the air penetrating through the holes on their facades, and the tobacco dries under certain conditions of humidity and temperature. The design of these patterns based on a module, such as the brick, not only affects the composition, but also determines the permeability characteristics, conditioning the interior space hygrothermally. Analysing the conceptual relationship, textures, patterns and construction methods of the dryers with contemporary architecture, numerous examples can be found in other buildings in which modular patterns are used in the composition of the facades similar to those used in the dryers.

CHAPTER 2: A NOVEL METHODOLOGY TO STUDY PARTICULATE MATERIAL/AEROSOL POLLUTION VIA REAL-TIME HYPERSPECTRAL ACOUSTO-OPTIC INTELLIGENT SPECTROMETRY

Tactic and strategic management and policing of atmospheric pollution in México, specifically by Particulate Material -PM- from mobile sources (internal combustion powered vehicles), critically requires state-of-the-science technologies, due to the problem's complexity; including its public health dimension. We consider that proper decision-making on the problem would benefit from permanent revision on currently employed PM monitoring and measurement systems and also the effort to improve them. These later currently offer information on O(10^0) Ultraviolet-Visible-Infrared (UV-VIS-IR) spectral bands at O(10^0) spatial resolutions, and O(10^1) in [min^-1] temporal resolutions. In contrast, we propose the novel use of Acousto-Optic Tunable Filter (AOTF) Spectrometry to study PM in atmospheric suspension, capable of offering information on O(10^2) UV, VIS, or IR spectral bands at similar or better spatial and temporal resolutions. The potential of AOTF Spectrometry towards PM assessment is clear and our objective is to explore its usefulness.

CHAPTER 3: ACOUSTIC DESIGN OF ORDINARY SPACES – OFFICES, SCHOOLS, HEALTHCARE FACILITIES, RESTAURANTS, AND RETAIL

When designing for wellbeing, noise is usually not properly accounted for (if at all) during the design phase of a building. However, noise is often rated as the number one cause of dissatisfaction in offices; it negatively affects patients and staff in hospitals; it prevents quality learning and teaching in schools as well as noise bests poor service as the most irksome complaint for restaurants users. The question that arises is then… how can we design to avoid the negative effects of noise on the end-users thus enabling wellbeing in indoor spaces?

CHAPTER 4: BAMBOO UTILIZATION AS A SUSTAINABLE BUILDING MATERIAL – BAMBOO IN BUILDINGS

The extraction of building materials from their resources through harvesting, preservation, and utilization has become a significant segment of human contribution to the global ecosystem, since the coming of the industrial revolution. Bamboo is the world's fastest-growing woody plant and bamboo grows multiple times quicker than most different species. Housing is one of the focused demands for bamboo and as a result of the current scarcity of home units; the demand for bamboo is in increasing in order. Bamboo building construction is portrayed by a basic edge approach like that applied in traditional building design and construction. Applying bamboo as an environmentally friendly material is seen as a movement towards creating a sustainable environment and reducing greenhouse emissions. The need to employ government policy in addressing the production and application of bamboo is reported and challenges of bamboo in the global market highlighted in this chapter.

CHAPTER 5: BEYOND THE WATER ENVIRONMENTAL MANAGEMENT IN THE OPERATIONAL BUILDING PHASE FOR ITS APPLICATION TO THE PERUVIAN CONTEXT

World population is expected to be 9.3 billion by 2050, with a high increase in the urban population considering that the availability on the surface of the earth is full of water by 71.7%, but that only 3% of this water can be used as drinking water. In cities, buildings are recognized as one of the largest users of freshwater resources in construction and operation. The water use impact is different in some countries because ones use conventional water treatments, while other ones rely on advanced desalination. Climate change and population growth are clearly putting pressure on the world's water supply, so the first environmental assessment plan for buildings was launched in 1990 by the BRE in the United Kingdom where the water category is included in its environmental assessment.

CHAPTER 6: ENVIRONMENTAL AWARENESS – AN IMPROVEMENT STRATEGY IN THE EDUCATION OF ARCHITECTS

Felix Aramburu

University studies for the architecture degree in Spain give very little weight to considerations related to the design of a healthy interior environment. The low number of subjects related to interior comfort criteria may cause the student to underestimate the importance of environmental design of closed spaces in favor of aesthetic or merely functional aspects. However, there is a direct relationship between formal design decisions and environmental conditions in buildings, and future architects must understand those connections in order to make designs that combine efficiency and high aesthetic value. In this chapter, several pedagogical strategies are presented to get architecture students to learn and internalize the link between design and interior conditions, aiming at the acquisition of an adequate environmental awareness.

CHAPTER 7: EVALUATION OF THE ROOF GARDEN DESIGN CRITERIA IN THE EXAMPLE OF ISTANBUL MARMARA FORUM MALL

The aim of this study is to create a checklist of roof garden design criteria. This scope of work includes an encompassing review of international standards studies such as; German Landscape Research, Development and Construction Society, the American Society for Testing and Materials, the U.S. Green Building Council, and Green Roofs for Healthy Cities, whereas the generated checklist was evaluated in the Marmara Forum Mall. As a result of the study, an answer was sought to the question, "What are the prerequisites for a roof garden serving the needs of users in today's conditions?" whereas on-site detection, observation and photography were used as working methods. As a result, in considering the evaluation of the checklist on a scale of the Marmara Forum Mall, climatic data, activities with its hard structure, promenade areas and designs of plantlife and water elements in soft structure are moderately sufficient, whereas it was determined there is no problem in the roof furniture design and maintenance.

CHAPTER 8: GROUND AIR TEMPERATURE CONTROL FOR HEAT PUMP EXCHANGE – APTAE SYSTEM: JUSTIFICATION OF HS6 (RADON PROTECTION)

Heating and cooling consume a high amount of energy, which is today mainly provided by fossil fuels. To save fossil resources and simultaneously reduce pollutants and CO2, heating and cooling energy consumption should be reduced. Geothermal energy is a clean, inexhaustible source of energy that is available all year round because it does not depend on the weather. Nevertheless, the use of tempered subsoil air has been used as a traditional air conditioning strategy, however nowadays, its use has been questioned by the discovery of the leaks of radon gas from the ground. The investigation search a heat exchange system with the subsoil which prevents the introduction of radon gas into living spaces. The system that is exposed, increases the performance of aerothermal heat pumps by means of thermal exchange with tempered air in the sanitary chamber. This exchange is more favorable than air at the outside temperature, increasing the COP of the machine. This system complies with the regulations for protection against radon, protecting the building from this radioactive gas.

CHAPTER 9: HEALTH AND WELL-BEING – CONSIDERATIONS IN THE DESIGN OF INDOOR ENVIRONMENTS FOR THE ELDERLY

The older segments of the adult population in cities experience problems conditioned by the climate of each place. Since the 2003 heat wave which caused 70,000 heat deaths, the dramatic consequences of climate change and rising temperatures in Europe have led to the elderly being most at risk. Insufficient adaptability and economic resources among them also lead to repercussions on architecture, causing energy poverty issues as a result of a real consumption needed which is very different from the actual consumption. The demands of these people are determined by environmental stress, which differ greatly throughout the year. In addition, illnesses influence the daily health and the decrease in sensory capacity of the elderly, making them more vulnerable to constant changes. Faced with this problem, the main aim of this research is to analyse the degree of comfort and well-being of the elderly due to the environmental changes that occur in Andalusian rural homes in order to include some considerations in the design of indoor environments.

CHAPTER 10: INTEGRATION OF TELLURISM AND SACRED GEOMETRY IN PROFESSIONAL TRAINING – INNOVATION, HEALTHY ARCHITECTURE, LANDSCAPE

At present, the implementation of the concepts of tellurism and Sacred Geometry in the Schools of Architecture is neither obvious nor simple. It starts with the historical heritage of patterns that are shaped and molded according to professorships that have worked independently in territories at different scales within building and urbanism. Moreover, they share the same premise of the occupation of space and creation. In this study we will focus on the intrinsic value of the land, its energy and how this affects not only the overall design of the building, but also the interior of a healthy dwelling. The psychological, psychosomatic, and symptomatic effects on the human being are related to the intrinsic use of a dwelling, as well as to the building's placement on the land. The work method in this investigation has implemented a comparative case study carried out in El Pardo and Carabanchel.

CHAPTER 11: SUSTAINABLE DESIGN FOR A FUNCTIONAL REEDUCATION OF SENIOR CITIZENS ABOUT THE BASIC ACTIVITIES OF DAILY LIVING

Developing useful objects for a functional reeducation of senior citizens persons about the basic activities of daily living must be conceptualized considering theories, techniques and approaches in methodology, based on ecologically bearable structures, economically viable and socially equitable. Consequently, the present chapter has the objective to state the criteria and strategies of a sustainable design, from a detailed study of applicability of a) user-product interaction; observation, understanding, dimensional relationship and evaluation; b) creative process, identification, ideation, definition, prototypes, evaluation and structuration; c) technical specifications, structure, sustainability, ergonomics, aesthetics and evaluation; d) manufacture method, sustainability, production method, life cycle, capital assets, official norms and optimization. A contextual and conceptual analysis is proposed for the beginning, development and conclusion of the projects so as to reestablish the relationship between natural processes and human activity.

CHAPTER 12: INDOOR LIGHTING WORKPLACES – TOWARDS NEW INDOOR LIGHTING

When I was invited to write a chapter in this book about interior lighting, I thought at first I would call it Towards new Indoor lighting workplaces but when I was collecting information for its development, I was surprised because without realizing the Abstract I sent had simply titled Towards new Indoor lighting. I realized that my subconscious had made me put the title that comes closer and closer to the reality that we are living. Cuttle asks himself at the beginning of one of his articles these questions, what is the situation of professionals working in lighting? Can we see the stages of our development, and are we at the beginning of a new and innovative stage? I think the answer to the first question is that this is an exciting ongoing process of study and innovation. This article is a search for an affirmative answer to the second question you pose.

The chapters will address issues concerning Indoor Environmental Quality (IEQ), which are described more simply as the conditions inside the building. It includes air quality, but also access to daylight and views, pleasant acoustic conditions and occupant control over lighting and thermal comfort. They will also include the functional aspects of the space, such as whether the layout provides easy access to tools and people when needed and whether there is sufficient space for the occupants. Building managers and operators can increase building occupant satisfaction by considering all aspects of IEQ rather than focusing on temperature or air quality alone.

Within these objectives, housing ventilation becomes a challenging goal to solve as it is directly related to occupant health and wellbeing. The biggest challenge is its strong connection to energy demand as a big share of building energy losses are due to air renovations and enclosure infiltrations.

In this book, we look for a range of innovative research and evidence-based policy ideas that demonstrate the importance of housing research and policy for health and wellbeing.

Roberto A. González-Lezcano
Universidad CEU San Pablo, Spain

Chapter 1
Permeability in Bioclimatic Modular Facades:
Spanish Sheds

Tamar Awad
https://orcid.org/0000-0001-9119-504X
ICAI Comillas University, Spain

ABSTRACT

This study is based on the analysis of the facades of tobacco drying sheds located in the regions of Cáceres and Toledo in Spain as an example of bioclimatic production architecture. Using modular and permeable façade designs, it is possible to generate an interior space with specific hygrothermal conditions. The drying sheds are the places where the tobacco plant is cured with the air penetrating through the holes on their facades, and the tobacco dries under certain conditions of humidity and temperature. The design of these patterns based on a module, such as the brick, not only affects the composition but also determines the permeability characteristics, conditioning the interior space hygrothermally. Analysing the conceptual relationship, textures, patterns, and construction methods of the dryers with contemporary architecture, numerous examples can be found in other buildings in which modular patterns are used in the composition of the facades similar to those used in the dryers.

INTRODUCTION

This article is a continuation of the thesis that the author presented in 2015 with the title "Tobacco industrial architecture in Peninsular Spain: dryers and factories" by E.T.S.A.M. Polytechnical University of Madrid. (Awad, 2015).

This study is based on the analysis of the facades of tobacco drying sheds located in the regions of Cáceres and Toledo, as an example of bioclimatic production architecture.

Using modular and permeable façade designs, it is possible to generate an interior space with specific hygrothermal conditions.

DOI: 10.4018/978-1-7998-7279-5.ch001

The drying sheds are the places where the tobacco plant is cured, with the air penetrating through the holes on their facades, and the tobacco dries under certain conditions of humidity and temperature.

The design of these patterns based on a module, such as the brick, not only affects the composition, but also determines the permeability characteristics, conditioning the interior space hygrothermally.

Analyzing the conceptual relationship, textures, patterns, and construction methods of the dryers with contemporary architecture, numerous examples can be found in other buildings in which modular patterns are used in the composition of the facades similar to those used in the dryers.

The study analyses the specific climatic conditioning systems of the drying rooms, which can be used as a reference for other constructions.

Therefore, it aims to achieve the adaptation of the construction and formal system to other uses, from a double perspective:

- Architecture for climate adaptation to the environment.
- Architecture as a generator of specific climatic conditions, in the interior.

The conditions generated by the patterns on the facades of the drying sheds are constructively adaptable to other uses.

The utility of these shade-houses is basically: to provide shade, ventilation and an enclosed but permeable space.

The patterns are a useful form of enclosure for spaces where ventilation is required while ensuring a certain degree of safety.

Although it must be considered that the degree of ventilation required depending on the use of the building is different, with 40% being necessary for homes while 15% is enough for a tobacco shed.

The tobacco sheds are a bioclimatic production building.

From this analysis, it can be concluded that modular pattern facades generate very specific climate conditioning systems, which can be used as a resource for other constructions.

Drying sheds' hygrotermal and environmental conditions are analyzed in this chapter to compare them with the values of human comfort and find suitable relationships and parameters.

All the drying sheds that have been analyzed are constructed with brick. This implies a consideration of "zero degree" for both the construction and the composition of the architectural process. The detailing - entails making all the accumulative processes explicit as the brick walls are left exposed.

This minimal component allows a wide range of options that are never random but based on the logic of the way in which it is combined. The "sincerity" in the exposition of material, displaying them in their very nature and showing how they are really used, is a basic characteristic of industrial architecture, and it is even more expressive in these types of buildings.

The walls of the drying sheds undergo a permeability assessment in order to determine the degree of ventilation and orientation, the lattice pattern used and the overall volume.

This specific conditioning system can serve as a resource for other buildings, and consequently, it could be transferred to other uses within a two-pronged approach:

Drying sheds' main purposes / aims deal with how to provide shade, ventilation, and a covered space as well as permeability.

BACKGROUND

Interest and Opportunity

The factors of interest of this study are:

- To collect part of the industrial heritage, which could be considered as industrial archaeology.
- To provide information on the functioning of the drying sheds, the internal organization of production.
- The architecture of production reflects the advances of industrialization, anticipating the use of materials and types of structures, and condenses the complex relationships between product, people, and space into a specific typology. (Cliff, 1979).
- Industrial architecture consists of a concrete and practical architectural program for a specific use, with very particular characteristics of scale. It is possible to establish the relationship between human scale versus machine scale.
- The interest of the examples analyzed lies in the possibility of reuse and adaptation to other uses of the drying sheds as examples of bioclimatic production construction.
- In the case of the drying sheds, the advanced deterioration and abandonment they are suffering means that valuable examples of industrial production architecture are being lost, which on the other hand lack cataloguing, graphic documentation, plans and protection.

MAIN FOCUS OF THE CHAPTER

Case Study

The environment in which they are inserted constitutes the territorial context, so that industrial heritage cannot be considered as an isolated element without analyzing the relationship with the environment in which it was generated, especially when industry is a direct consequence of society's use of the natural environment. It is not possible to preserve, interpret and value industrial heritage without proposing a defense strategy for the landscape.

The tobacco drying sheds studied are in the agricultural and rural environment of the Tiétar, Alagón and Jerte valleys in the north of the province of Cáceres, as well as in the Talavera de la Reina area in Toledo. Others are located in the urban centers of some municipalities, as a result of their growth, as is the case of those studied in Calera and Chozas, in the region of Toledo.

The module used in the construction of the facades of the examples is brick.

The location of the tobacco drying sheds on which the research focuses corresponds to the north of Cáceres. The microclimate of the Tiétar, Alagón and Jerte valleys contributes to the optimum quality of the harvests, especially of the Virginia and Burley tobacco varieties (fermentable and processable).

The introduction of tobacco cultivation in the Iberian Peninsula began in 1919.

Tobacco was one of the plants brought to agriculture by the native Indians of America, - there is evidence of its consumption as early as the conquest of Mexico in 1519. With seeds from the Yucatan, tobacco cultivation and production began in Santo Domingo around 1531, and quickly spread to Trinidad. Com-

mercial production began in Cuba in 1580 and marketed it in Venezuela practically at the same time as in Cuba. (García de Paredes, 2008).

In 2005, Spain was the third largest tobacco-growing country in the European Community - behind Italy and Greece - with 40,991 tons contracted for the 2005 harvest. And Extremadura, with 85% of the production, was the Spanish region where the largest crop was concentrated.

Despite the growing industrialization of the sector, the harvesting, collection, drying and curing of tobacco is a laborious process that requires some 2,200 hours of work per hectare, more than any other type of farming. The progressive cutback of European subsidies to this sector means the slow death of villages such as Talayuela (Cáceres), and the consequent deterioration of these examples of agricultural production architecture.

According to Goodmen (1994), tobacco is a plant in the *Nicotiana* genus and the Solanaceae (nightshade) family. Its main characteristic is that it is a perennial plant, with a generally simple stem, 1 to 3 meters high, large oval-lanceolate or elliptical leaves, perfectly isolated, with abundant veins and 10 to 60 centimeters long, with numerous cream-colored flowers.

When the plant reaches the appropriate maturity, it is cut and transferred to the drying room where it will remain for 45 to 60 days, until curing is complete.

A few hours after cutting the plants, the leaves are introduced into the drying room, at which time they contain almost 90% water in relation to their total weight. During the curing process, the moisture content of the leaves is reduced to 15-20%. During this process their chemical composition also changes, and the leaf's color changes to brown, orange or golden, depending on the type of tobacco and the curing process.

These significant moisture transformations take place inside these buildings, allowing external climatic conditions to enter through the openings in the façades.

There are currently two different types of tobacco in the Spanish tobacco industry, especially in the curing phase:

- Dark or Burley tobacco: this type of tobacco is cured or air-dried, in the drying sheds with modular facades such as those studied in this article.
- Blond, yellow, Virginia or Bright tobacco: this is light tobacco, cured in an artificial atmosphere, with heat input, they cannot be dried in the dryers studied, as they require temperature, humidity, and ventilation control.

The work of Bermejo, (1976) has been used to understand the difference between tobacco types.

Flue-cured tobacco, also known as Bright, yellow or Virginia type, was authorized in 1941-42 in the areas of Cáceres and Granada, allowing 10,000 plants to be grown by each of the growers who wished to carry out trials. In Cáceres, the first trials were carried out in 1952, on the Las Lomas cultivation area, in Talayuela.

The main difference between black and blond tobaccos lies in the drying process: black tobaccos are air-dried in ventilated interiors, as in the drying sheds of the examples. The leaves or plants are hung whole and the process takes 1 to 3 months. Blond tobaccos require controlled atmosphere dryers with automatic ventilation. They are cured by leaves and take 5 to 7 days.

The Drying Shed

This is the building where the first stage of tobacco production, curing or drying, takes place. It is an example of agricultural architecture of bioclimatic production, which is influenced by the territory in which it is located. These constructions have a great interest, and they are presented as unique and identifiable elements in the areas to which they belong.

The problem is that with the decrease in European Union subsidies for tobacco cultivation, many of the drying sheds have been abandoned or transformed into warehouses, without respecting their singular configuration and their specific characteristics of permeable façades.

Although there are many drying sheds in Spain, this study focuses on those built with brick masonry and those located within the study area, already specified in the introduction to this article.

The most complete research work on Spanish drying sheds is Puente and García Serrano (1998).

Main Characteristics of a Drying Shed

All premises used for tobacco curing must meet certain requirements, which according to the indications for tobacco growing and curing in Spain (Madrid, 1948) are as follows:

1. regulated ventilation system allowing the outside conditions to enter the interior of the room
2. airtight sealing, in order to be able to isolate the product when the outside atmospheric conditions are not appropriate
3. c) Flexibility of hanging devices, depending on the collection system used.
4. d) The possibility of using artificial heat.

In the book entitled "The curing of leaf tobacco" (National Tobacco Growing and Fermentation Service, 1952), it is stated that the buildings must meet the following conditions for the drying and curing of the product:

1. Adjustable ventilation, so that at the different stages of drying and curing, the temperature and humidity are appropriate.
2. Heating system, depending on the type of tobacco to be obtained.
3. Tobacco hanging devices adapted to the harvesting system and the characteristics of the tobacco variety.

According to the manual "Build drying sheds and you will improve your tobacco" published by the National Tobacco Growing and Fermentation Service, S.N.C.F.T. (1962), the avoidable losses of kilos of tobacco could be solved:

Building premises with the capacity proportional to the number of plants grown.

Hanging the crop with the appropriate compactness for its characteristics and the development of the plant.

By regulating the installations and ventilation devices so that the product dries under the appropriate temperature and humidity conditions at each stage of the process.

Among the conditions that air drying sheds must comply with are the following:

The enclosures must have a height of 5 meters so that the space in the room can be used when hanging the tobacco.

They are also to be built "with a double wall formed by two brick walls, or an outer wall and an inner wall with an air chamber 10 to 15 centimeters thick, building pillars with two posts to support the frames or knives".

Openings or windows will be opened in all facades and in large numbers, so that ventilation reaches the entire volume of the premises.

Module Used: Brick

The module used in the construction of the façades of the examples analysed is brick.

"Architecture starts when you carefully put two bricks together. There it begins." Mies van der Rohe's words.

Choosing brick as the determining element and feature for the elaboration of a building implies the consideration of a "degree zero" or basic of the whole constructive and compositional system. This module, or minimum element, due to its dimensions, allows an enormous freedom of combinations and generation of patterns. Leaving the brick exposed allows all the structural processes of a hand-laid piece to be made explicit.

The origin of the composition of any masonry façade lies in the brick module and is therefore a modular building process.

The use of the "vara" as a unit of measurement, and its subdivisions into three feet and four quarters or spans, suggests bricks one foot long and one quarter wide.

The Castilian vara was used as a unit of measurement until 1796, when the meter was used as an international unit, and its use became compulsory from 1889. The vara became a bar with a length of 835 mm and 9 tenths.

This leaves a brick approximately 28 cm long, 19 cm wide and 3.5 cm thick. The brick of these measurements has two dimensions in proportion to the bed, but not directly to each other, not fulfilling the ratio of 1 to 2 between its edges, which makes it impossible to arrange the bricks in the factory alternatively, making any type of rigging, which implies the situation of bricks in both directions, null and void.

According to Adell (1986),the common brick has the following dimensions: 28 cm long, 14 cm wide and 4.5 cm thick, with proportions of 1 to 2 in its bed, which allows for stretcher bond construction.

Although the proportions of length and width are double each other, the thickness is not one quarter of the length. This means that the arrangement of the courses with a soldier or sailor brick position, does not coincide in height with a given number of brick courses, with their corresponding joints.

The Parts of a Brick

Its shape is that of a rectangular prism, in which its different dimensions are called "soga" or length, "tizón" or width and thickness, with the "soga" being the largest dimension. Likewise, the different faces of the brick are called 'tabla' or bed, 'canto' or stretcher and 'testa' or header (the 'tabla' being the largest). As can be seen in figure 1, the "soga" is twice as long as the "tizón" or, more precisely, two "tizones" and a joint, which allows them to be combined freely. The thickness, on the other hand, may not be modulated.

There are different formats of bricks, generally of a size that allows them to be handled with one hand.

In Spain, the metric format stands out, in which the dimensions are: 24 x 11,5 x 5,25 / 7 / 3,5 centimeters (each dimension is twice the immediately smaller one, plus 1 cm of the joint) and the Catalan format with dimensions 29 x 14 x 5,2 / 7,5 / 6 centimeters, and the more common ones which measure 25 x 12 x 5 centimeters.

Currently, due to their great demand, given their low cost on site, sizes of 50 x 24 x 5 centimeters are also used.

Figure 1. Parts of a brick. Drawing of the author.

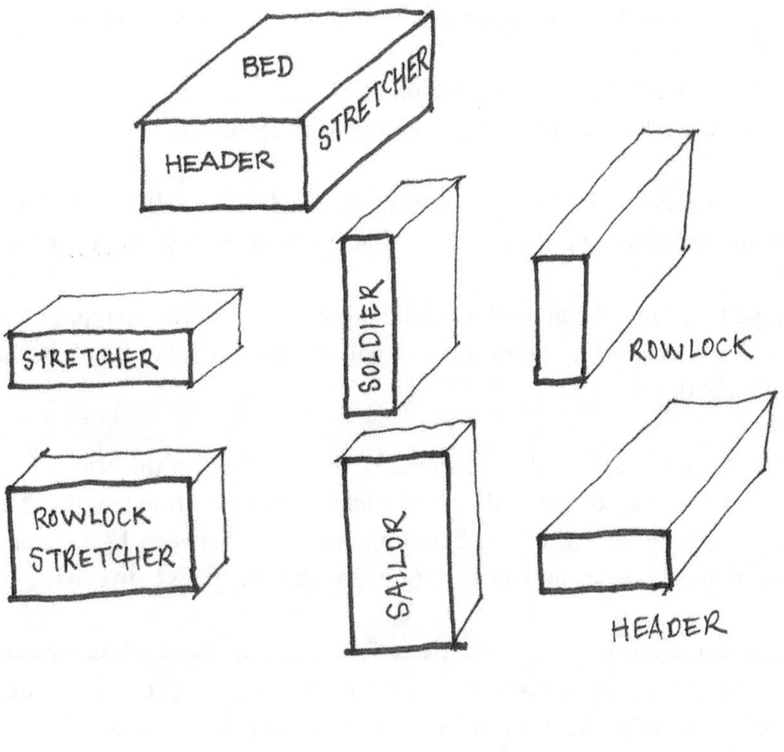

The size of the brick has been related to the size of the palm of the hand, as the needs of manufacture and installation make it advisable, with measurements ranging around a foot or a span.

There are countless variations in the exact dimensions of bricks, depending on the country and region.

For geometrical reasons, the ideal piece would be one in which the formula is fulfilled:

$$l = 2w + j = 4t + 3j$$

Where: l = length, w = width, t= thickness, j = joint
This is a proportion: 2, 4, 8.
According to their shape, bricks are classified as follows:

- Cored bricks are all those with perforations in the bed that occupy more than 10% of the surface of the slab. Very popular for the execution of brick facades.
- Solid bricks, those with less than 10% of perforations in the bed. Some models have recesses in the bed and in the header for the construction of walls without joints.
- Curved brick, is that which has a curved profile, so that when a course of brick is laid, generally with a trammel method, "sardinel", it forms a curved line. The name comes from the templates used by stonemasons to work the stones, which are used to give the brick the aforementioned shape.
- Hollow bricks are those that have perforations on the stretcher or on the header that reduce the volume of material used in them. They are used for partition walls that will not be subject to special loads. They can be of various types:
- "Rasilla": its thickness and its length are much greater than its width. Their usual dimensions are 24 x 11,5 x 2,5 centimeters.
- Single hollow brick: it has a row of perforations on the header
- Double hollow brick: it has two rows of perforations on the header

Bonding is the law of brickwork or arrangement of the bricks in a wall, stipulating from the dimensions of the wall to the junctions and the joints, so that the wall rises evenly over the entire height of the building.

The work of Lloyd (1925) has been used by many professors to show the types of bonding

Some types of brickwork used in the examples analysed are: stretcher bond, header bond, soldier and rowlock stretcher bond.

- Stretcher bond: the sides of the wall are formed by the stretchers of the brick, it is half a foot thick
- Header bond form the sides of the wall and its thickness is 1 foot (the length). It is widely used in walls that support structural loads (load-bearing) and can be between 12.5 cm and 24 cm thick.
- "Palomero" bond: it is like the tambourine rigging, but leaving gaps between the horizontal pieces.

The material most commonly used as an enclosure for factory drying sheds is ceramic brick and solid brick; and concrete block in drying sheds with a metal or reinforced concrete structure. T

The insulating behaviour of perforated brick is good, with a thermal conductivity coefficient of 0.65 Kcal/m h °C, and the double cavity of 0.42 Kcal/m h °C, coinciding with that of concrete block.

According to the works of García arroyo (1973), for a 12 cm thick perforated brick wall, the heat transmission coefficient will be 2.6 Kcal/m2 h °C and 2.06 Kcal/m2 h °C for a double hollow brick wall.

Types of Brickwork

Stretcher Bond is the most commonly used bond, a pattern is made only using stretchers, with the joins on each course centred above and below by half a brick. This type of bonding is not particularly strong. It can be seen in the Figure 2.

A variation is **the raking stretcher bond**. The overlap between bricks is a third or a quarter of a brick, instead of half a brick.

English Bond: This is a pattern formed by laying alternate courses of stretchers and headers. The joins between the stretchers are centered on the headers in the course below. This is one of the strongest bonds but requires more facing bricks than other bonds. It can be seen in the Figure 2.

English Garden Wall: This is similar to the English bond but with one course of headers for every three courses of stretcher. The headers are centered on the headers in course below. This gives quick lateral spread of load and uses fewer facings than an English bond.

English Cross Bond: This alternates courses of stretchers and headers, with the alternating stretcher course being offset by half a brick. The stretchers are centered on the joins between the stretchers below them, so that the alternating stretcher courses are aligned. Staggering stretchers enables patterns to be picked out in different texture or coloured bricks.

Flemish Bond: This is formed by laying headers and stretchers alternately in each course. The headers of each course are centered on the stretchers of the course below. This bond is strong and often used for walls which are two bricks thick.

Flemish Garden Wall or Sussex Bond: This variant of Flemish bond uses one header to three stretchers in each course. The header is centered over the stretcher in the middle of a group of three in the course below. It can be seen in the Figure 2.

Monk Bond is a variant of Flemish bond involves two stretchers between the headers in each course. The headers are centered over the join between the two stretchers in the course below.

Header Bond: This bond features courses of headers offset by half a brick. It is like the stretcher bond but with headers instead of stretchers.

Climatic Conditions

The article examines the climatic conditions involved in the construction of these buildings, such as their location, orientation and dimensions.

Of the stages of tobacco cultivation, curing (yellowing, leaf and vein drying), it is the last stage that concerns the curing rooms or drying rooms.

When the plant reaches the appropriate maturity, it is cut and transferred to the 'tobacco drying shed' where it will remain for 45 to 60 days until curing is complete.

A few hours after cutting the plants, the leaves are introduced into the drying room, at which time they contain almost 90% water in relation to their total weight. In the curing process, the moisture level can be reduced to 15 to 20%.

The curing process in the drying sheds takes place from mid-October to mid-November.

The main difference between dark and blond tobaccos lies in this drying process: dark tobaccos are air-cured in ventilated interiors, as in the drying sheds of the examples.

It will be established that the situation is conditioned by the direction of the dominant winds in the region, so that the longitudinal axis of the premises will be placed perpendicular to the dominant wind direction with the intention of helping cross ventilation, and that as much air as possible penetrates through the openings in the façades, crossing the interior space and exiting through the opposite façade. In cases where the wind direction is variable, and a predominant direction cannot be established, the longitudinal axis of the building should coincide with the north-south axis, so that the sunlight on the side façades is equivalent.

Figure 2. Types of brick bonds.

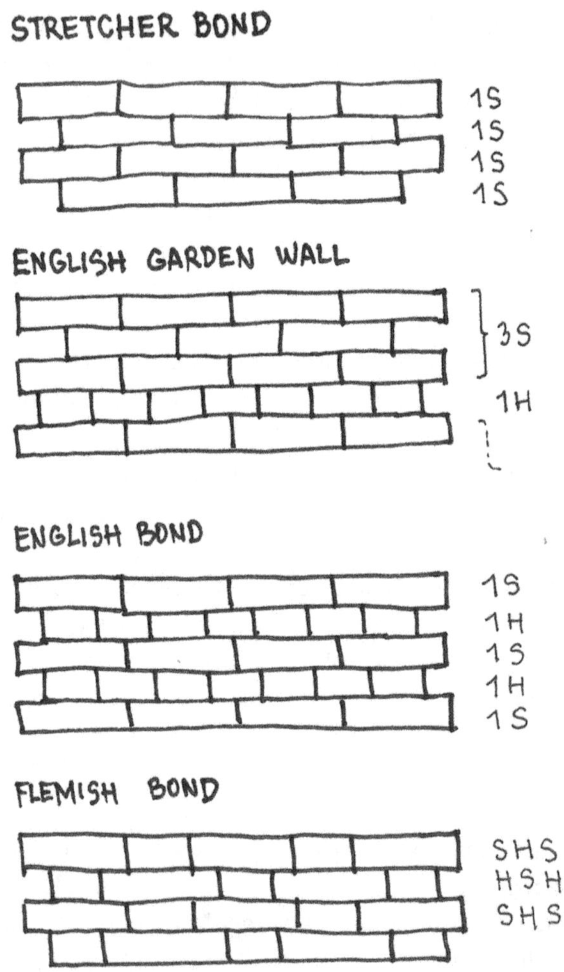

In order to decide on the ideal size of these constructions, several factors must be taken into account, such as: budget, type of structure, height or planned ventilation spaces.

It will be concluded that the width is the most important dimension of a dryer, and that it is influenced by two factors: the type of roof structure, in order to achieve open spaces and larger spans, which allow free circulation, and secondly, the ventilation capacity of the interior of the dryer, taking into account that the width should not be excessive so that the passage of air through the interior elements is possible. The recommended width is between 7.50 and 8.00 metres.

As the drying sheds are modular constructions, they can be exported to other buildings with other uses and other dimensions. The length depends on the number of times the porticoes are repeated or the number of modules in total.

The dimension of a module is the distance between porticoes, or the span between columns. In brick masonry walls, it is recommended that the distance between supports does not exceed 4 metres. Another important factor to consider is the bracing of these frames in the longitudinal direction.

In order to dimension the height, it must be taken into account that these structures must withstand the wind loads and the internal loads, the hanging of the tobacco plants, and must also have a ventilation space at the bottom, from the last hanging floor to the drying room floor, of at least 0.80 metres, reaching up to 1.50 metres in order to be able to water and humidify the drying room environment without damaging the plants.

Each hanging floor has a height of 1.70 metres on average.

For 2 hanging floors we are between 4.20 and 4.90 metres from the ground to the underside of the roof slab, and between 5.90 and 6.60 m for 3 hanging floors.

In order to study the hygrothermal conditions of the interior of these buildings, the AEMET Normal Climate data of the areas studied are included, together with climograms of human comfort based on Olgyay (1998). In this way, it is possible to know in which months it would be optimal to use these spaces for people instead of drying plants.

A study of the permeability of the façades of three drying sheds is carried out, by surveying the plans of all their façades and calculating: the percentage of openings compared to the solid part, the floor area, the total volume, the height, depth and length, the total façade area, and the percentage of openings in longitudinal and transversal façades, and the areas of the lattice pattern module are also analysed.

The area of openings in the façade remains constant in a dryer regardless of its height, as this percentage is related to the volume of plants inside, and not to the proportions of the dryer.

In 1970, the National Tobacco Cultivation and Fermentation Service acquired the farm called "La Cañalera" in Talayuela, with a cultivable area of 15 hectares of irrigated land, to set up an Experimental Station there, which would become the experimental centre for new techniques. It was set up in 1972.

Climatic Study

Case 1: Climograms of Talayuela

Study of the climatic data of the drying shed located in Talayuela (Cáceres).

The maximum temperatures (Max T) and minimum temperatures (Min T) and the maximum relative humidity (MaxRH) and minimum relative humidity (MinRH) during all months are analysed in Table 1.

As the climogram of human comfort in Talayuela shows in figure 4, the months of human comfort with ventilation would be June, July and August in the afternoons, and September and October in the mornings.

Overlaying climograms of human comfort and tobacco growing and drying in Talayuela, as can be seen in Figure 5, the hygrothermal conditions of the months of June and July at night, and those of September, October and part of November, are the most suitable for human comfort and for tobacco drying.

The drying process under ambient hygrothermal conditions, and without the need to modify either the temperature or the relative humidity, could be carried out in two periods: in June and July or in September and October.

On the other hand, by modifying one of the two variables, we would cover a wider range of months.

By maintaining the ambient temperature and modifying the relative humidity, drying could be carried out in July and August.

Figure 3. Drying shed in Talayuela (Cáceres). Photograph by the author. July 2011

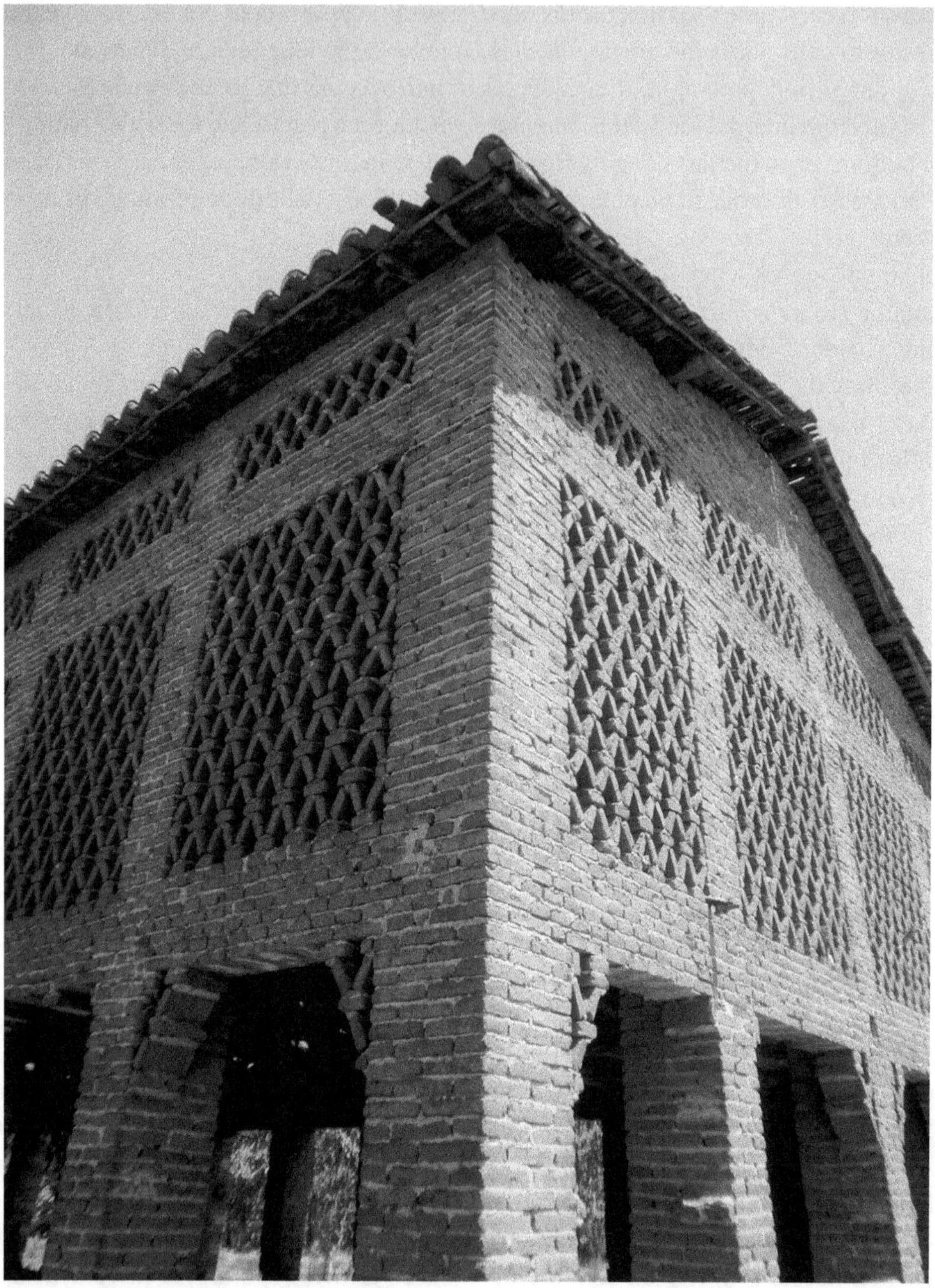

By maintaining the relative humidity of the environment and increasing the temperature, we could dry tobacco in June, July, August, September and October.

In the month of August, we will need to increase the relative humidity in the drying room.

Table 1. AEMET climatological data for Talayuela (Cáceres)

Month	JN	JL	A	S	O	N	D	J	F	M	A	MY
Max T	30	37	33	30	24	18	12	11	13	16	19	23
Min T	15	20	18	17	14	12	3	4	4	7	9	12
MaxRH	72	78	58	76	89	73	88	95	71	60	84	68
MinRH	22	21	31	44	57	54	65	67	49	40	72	24

Case 2: Talavera Climograms

As the Table 2 shows, the climatic data of the drying shed located in Talavera de la Reina (Toledo), based on Weather Data from AEMET, The maximum temperatures (Max T) and minimum temperatures (Min

Figure 4. Climograma del confort humano en Talayuela drawing by the author.

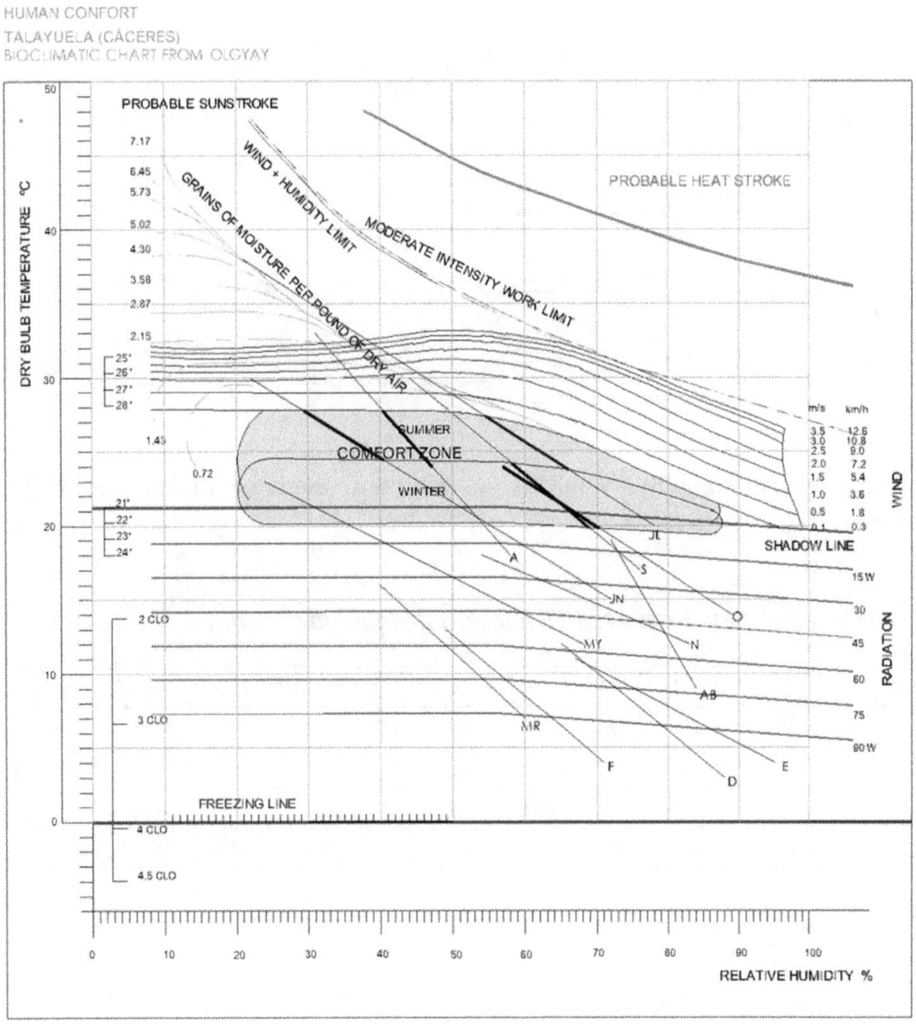

Figure 5. Overlaying climogramme of human comfort and tobacco cultivation and drying in Talayuela drawing by the author.

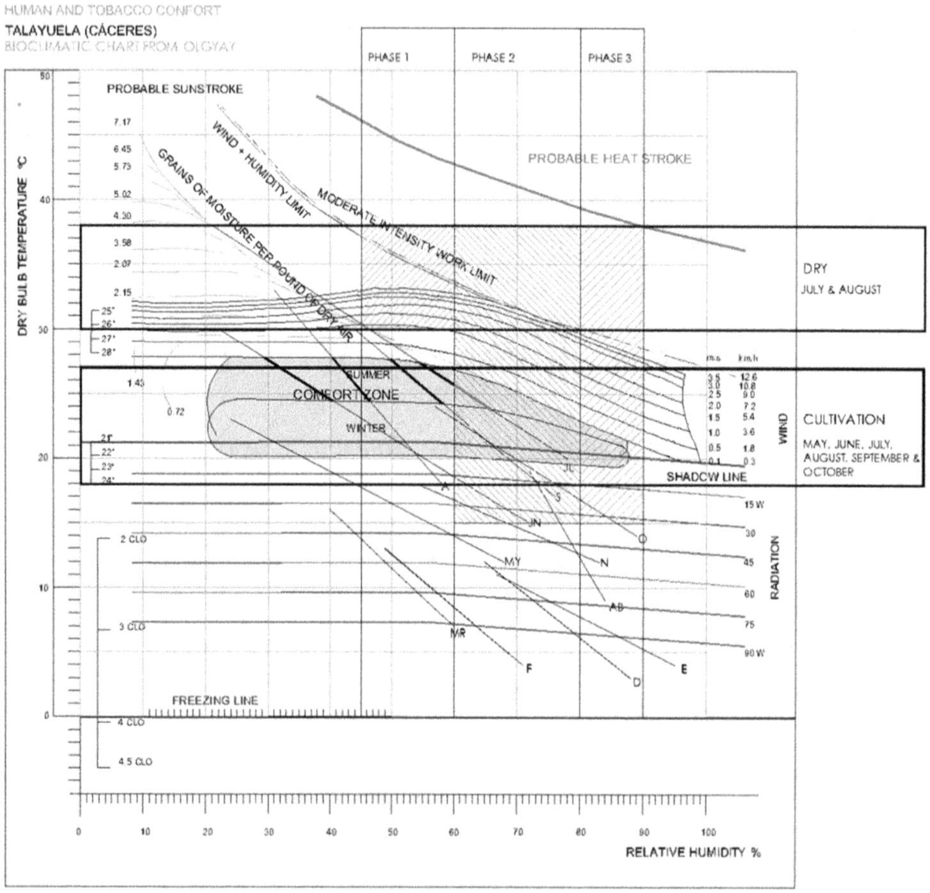

T), the maximum relative humidity (MaxRH) and minimum relative humidity (MinRH) are analysed during all months.

Table 2. Normal weather data from AEMET talavera de la reina (Toledo)

Month	JN	JL	A	S	O	N	D	J	F	M	A	MY
Max T	18	33	32	27	20	14	10	10	12	16	19	22
Min T	15	19	18	15	10	5	2	2	2	5	7	11
Max RH	74	60	58	58	87	94	87	72	84	78	62	58
Min RH	32	28	26	30	65	62	66	49	33	42	32	30

As can be interpreted from Figure 6, CLIMOGRAM OF HUMAN COMFORT IN TALAVERA, the months of human comfort with ventilation would be June, July and August in the afternoons, and September and October in the mornings.

The drying process under ambient hygrothermal conditions, and without the need to modify either the temperature or the relative humidity, could be carried out in two periods: in June or in October.

On the other hand, by modifying one of the two variables, we would cover a wider range of months.

Figure 6. Climogram of human comfort in Talavera drawing by the author.

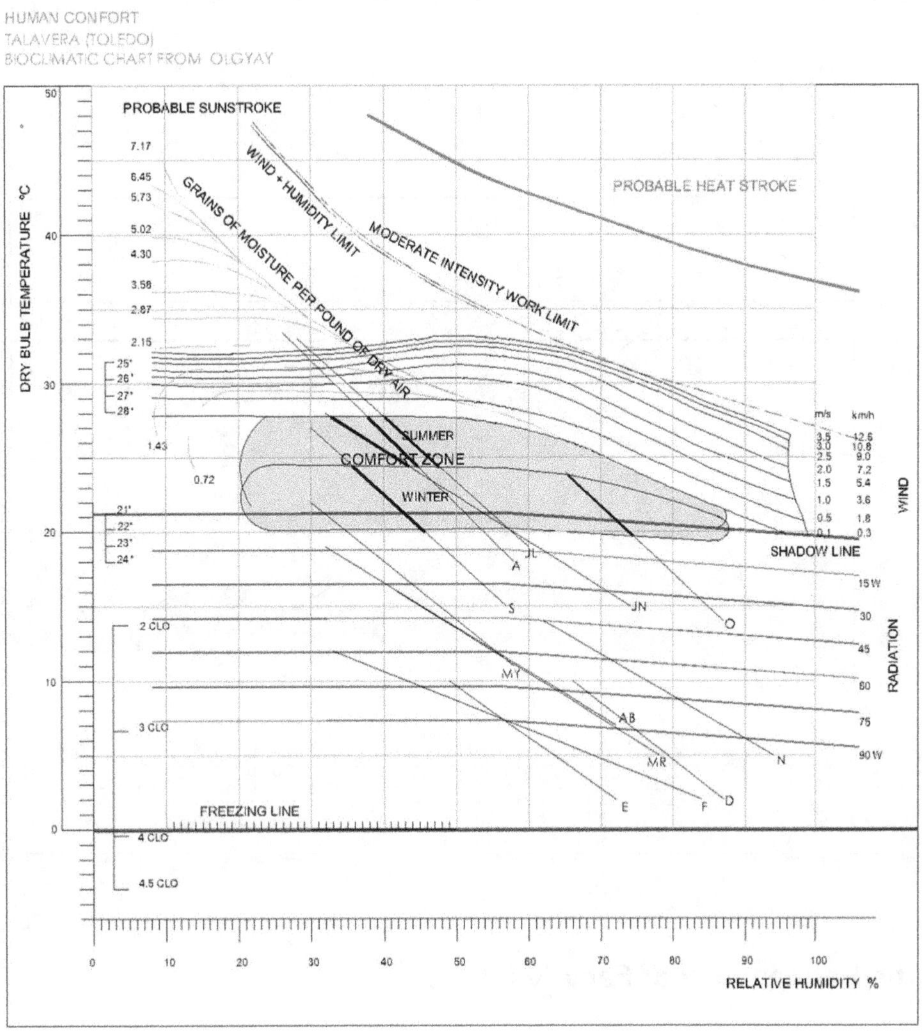

By maintaining the ambient temperature and modifying the relative humidity, drying could be carried out in July and August.

By maintaining the relative humidity of the environment and increasing the temperature, we could dry tobacco in June and October.

In July and August, we will need to increase the relative humidity in the drying room.

Overlaying climograms of human comfort and tobacco growing and drying in Talavera and overlaying the data for tobacco drying and for human comfort, as shown in figure 7, the hygrothermal conditions in October are the most suitable for both human comfort and tobacco drying.

Figure 7. overlaying climograms of human comfort and tobacco growing and drying in Talavera drawing by the author.

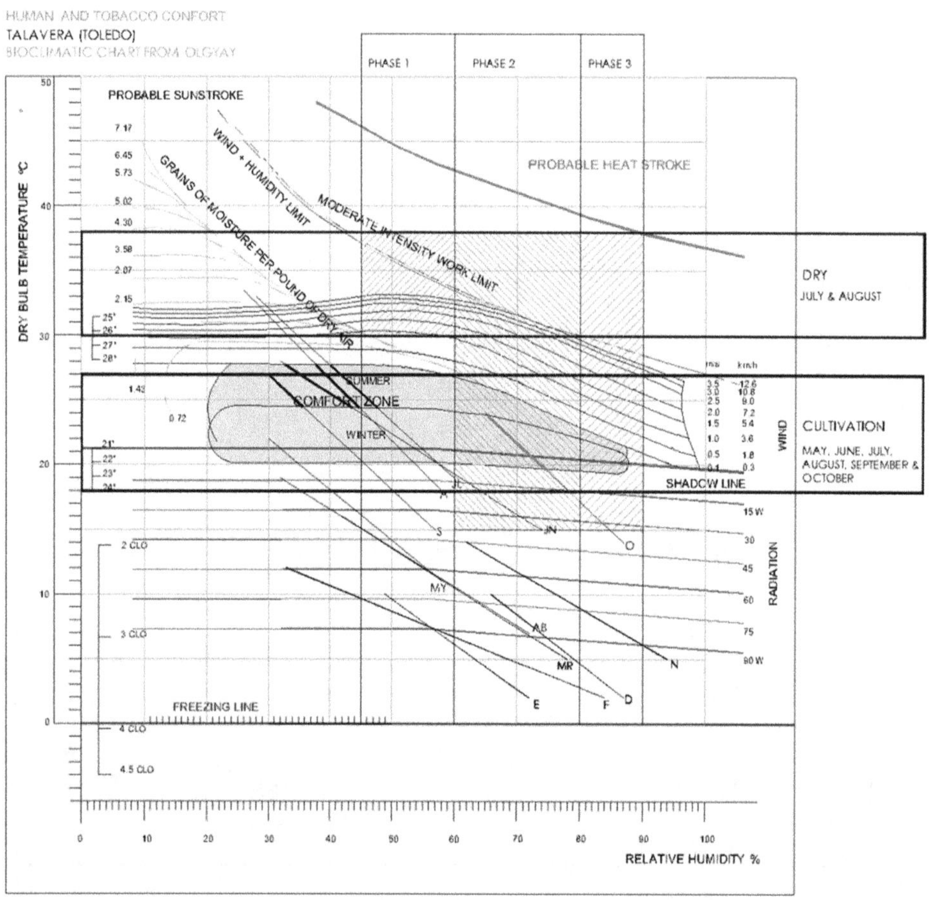

Study of the Permeability of Façades

In order to study permeability, it is necessary to analyse the data in table 3, which includes: floor area, volume, area of openings in the façade, total façade area and permeability as a percentage.

It can be concluded from the case studies that while 40% ventilation is required in dwellings, in the three examples of drying sheds analysed, we find different degrees of permeability: the first corresponds to 10%, the second to 15% and the last to 20%.

Table 3. Analysis of permeability in façades.

Location of the Drying Shed	Floor area (m2)	Volume (m3)	Gap area (m2)	Facade area (m2)	Permeability
Talayuela Cáceres	382	2440	100	676	15%
Calera y Chozas -Talavera Toledo	380	2740	68	689	10%
Puente del Arzobispo Cáceres	251	1882	100	536	20%

For this reason, the larger the volume of the drying shed, the lower the permeability of its façade, although this may also be due to design criteria in the lattice pattern, with the dovecote rigging being much less permeable than those that form a pattern with inclined-edged soldier bricks.

Other elements that can influence permeability are natural climatic factors: such as prevailing winds, proximity to streams, greater or lesser exposure to sunlight.

It is important to consider the proximity of rivers, in order to provide water for the cultivated fields.

The study of prevailing winds also becomes fundamental to achieve adequate ventilation and air-drying of the leaf.

Figure 8. Drying sheds in Talayuela photograph by the author. 2009

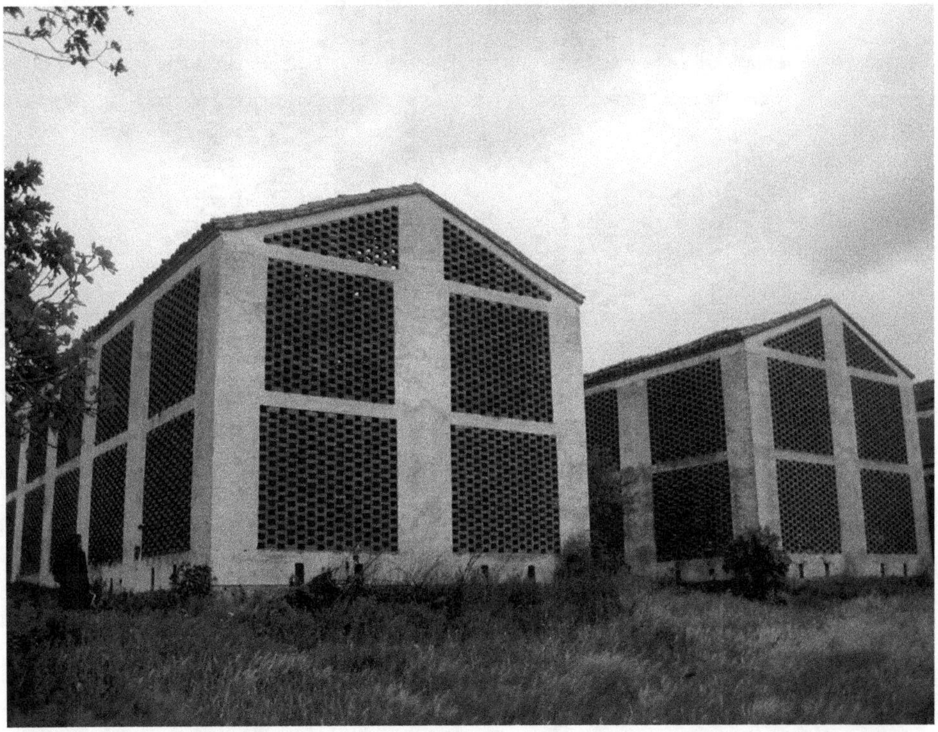

Case 1 Drying Shed in Talayuela (Cáceres).

The construction of the lattice pattern on the façade uses the "palomero" rigging as can be seen in Figure 8.

The total floor area of the dryer is 382 square metres and the total volume is 2,440 cubic metres.

The dimensions of the dryer are: Height 7.30 m, width 7.30 m and length 52.50 m.

The total surface area of the façade is 676 m2, the total surface area of openings in the façades is 100.60 m2, which represents a15% of permeability.

The total area of a longitudinal façade is 292 m2, while the total area of openings in a longitudinal façade is 44 m2, representing 15% permeability.

The total area of a transversal façade is 46 m2, and the total area of openings in a transversal façade is 5.5 m2, representing 12% permeability in these façades.

The lattice pattern module has a total area of 4.82 m2 and a void area of 1.53 m2, which would be 32% permeability.

This analysis can be seen in Figure 9 in the drawings made by the author.

Figure 9. Drying sheds in Talayuela drawing by the author. 2009

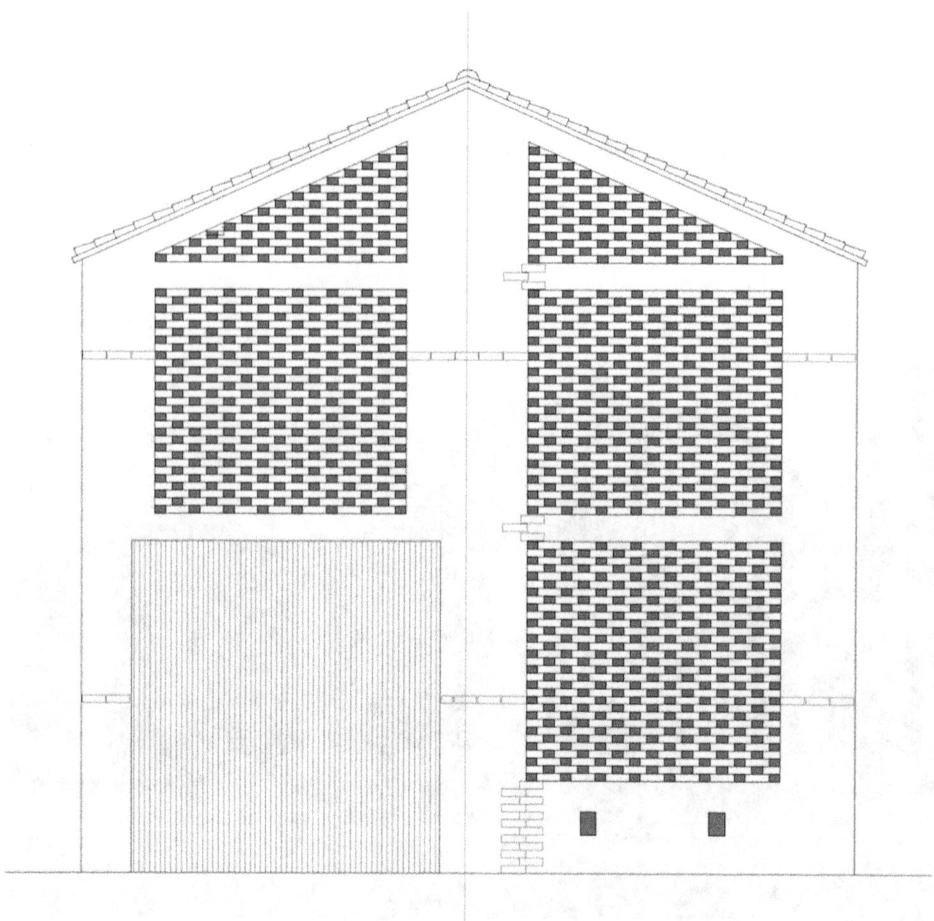

Case 2 Drying Shed in Calera y Chozas - Talavera (Toledo).

This drying shed has three bays separated by rows of pillars: a central nave and two side aisles. The elevation shows the basilica structure, with the two side aisles lower than the central nave and with the roof sloping outwards. As it can be seen in figure 12, the central nave, with a gabled roof, rises above the two side aisles in order to illuminate the interior.

The construction of the lattice pattern on the façade uses the "palomero" style, as can be seen in image 10.

The openings in the lower part are at a height of more than 30 cm from ground level, specifically 80 cm.

This dryer has a floor area of 381 m2, the total volume is 2,739 m3. The dimensions of this dryer are length 45.50 m, total height 8.50 m and width 8.50 m.

With regard to the façades, they have a total surface area of 689 m2, while the total surface area of openings in the façades is 68 m2, which represents only 10%.

Analysing the façades separately, and considering them symmetrical,

The total area of a longitudinal façade is 284 m2.

The total area of openings in the longitudinal façade is 28.7 m2.

The total area of a transversal façade is: 60 m2

And the total area of openings in the transversal façade is: 5,25 m2

If we study the minimum generating module of the façade, which is repeated throughout the dryer, the total area is 14.46 m2, while the area of openings is 1.41 m2, which represents a permeability of 10% in the module.

This analysis can be seen in figure 11 in the drawings made by the author.

Case 3 Drying Shed in Puente del Arzobispo (Toledo)

The courses of the façade of this drying shed are laid out in a sheared pattern. As can be seen in Figure 12.

The total floor area is 251 m2, and the total volume is 1882 m3.

The dimensions of the dryer are as follows: Height of 8.64 m, length of 34.50 m, width of 7.20 m and 15 m.

Width of 7.20 m and 15.50 m if the porch is included.

The total façade area is 536 m2, while the total area of openings in the façades is 103 m2, which represents 20% permeability.

The total area of the longitudinal façade is 218 m2, and the total area of openings in the longitudinal façade is 45 m2, which represents 21% permeability.

The total area of the transversal façade is 55 m2 and the total area of openings in the transversal façade is 6.5 m2, giving a permeability of 12%.

The Lattice Pattern Module has a total area of 4.63 m2 and an area of openings: 2.05 m2, which would be 44% permeability, as shown in figure13.

Case 4 Drying Shed in Calera y Chozas (Toledo)

This is a drying shed built in a street in Calera y Chozas.

It has only one exterior façade, facing west.

Figure 10. Drying shed in Calera y Chozas. Photograph by the author. 2009

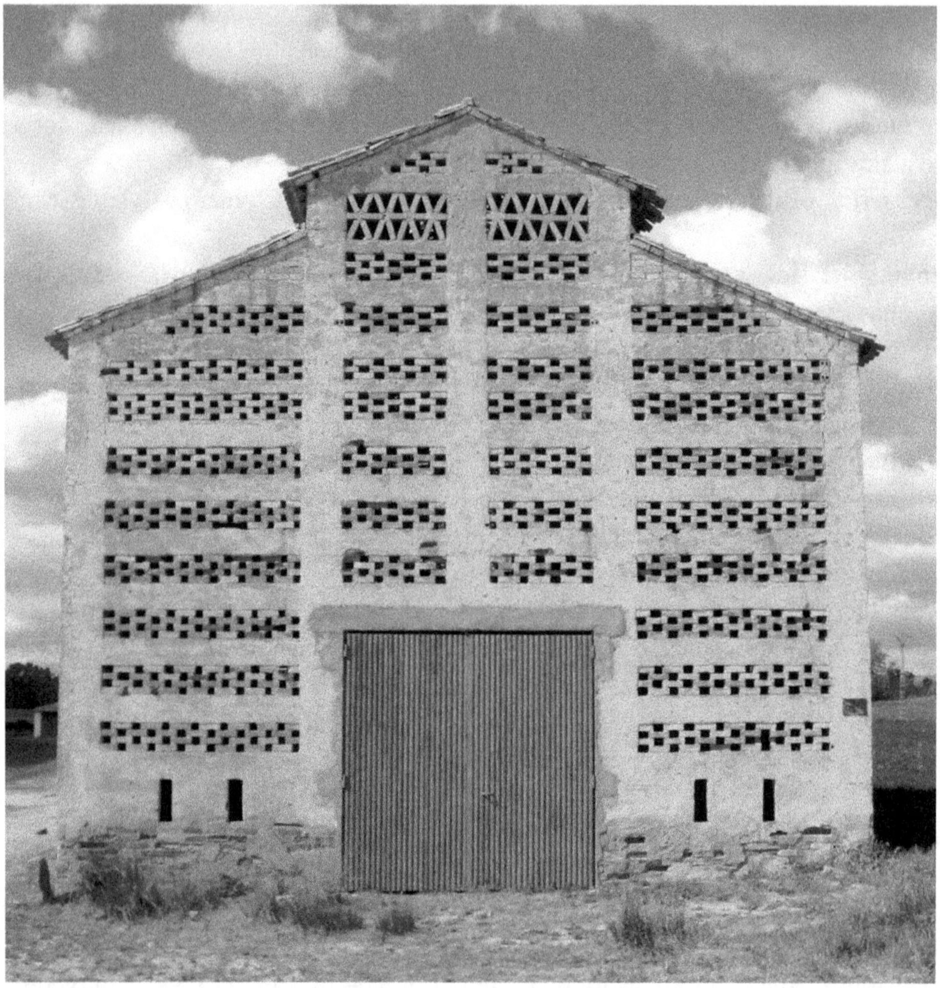

As can be seen in figures14 and 15, simple hollow bricks or "rasilla" are used on the upper part of the façade, rope bonding is used on the lower part of the façade and flattened bricks are used on the openings.

The height of the drying room is 7.10 metres.

The permeability of the façade is 20%.

As can be seen in the photographic documentation, figures 16 and 17, the latticework patterns of the drying shed façades are an example of the enormous richness and variety of this type of unprotected **construction.**

Examples in Other Buildings

Despite its ancient origins, the varied texture, color and shape of brick causes architects to continuously explore new and unexpected applications that harness this versatile material for the evolving needs.

Examples of buildings with other uses that employ modular patterns on their façades are analysed and compared with the rigs used in the drying sheds.

Figure 11. Transversal façade of the tobacco drying shed in Calera y Chozas. drawing by the author. 2009.

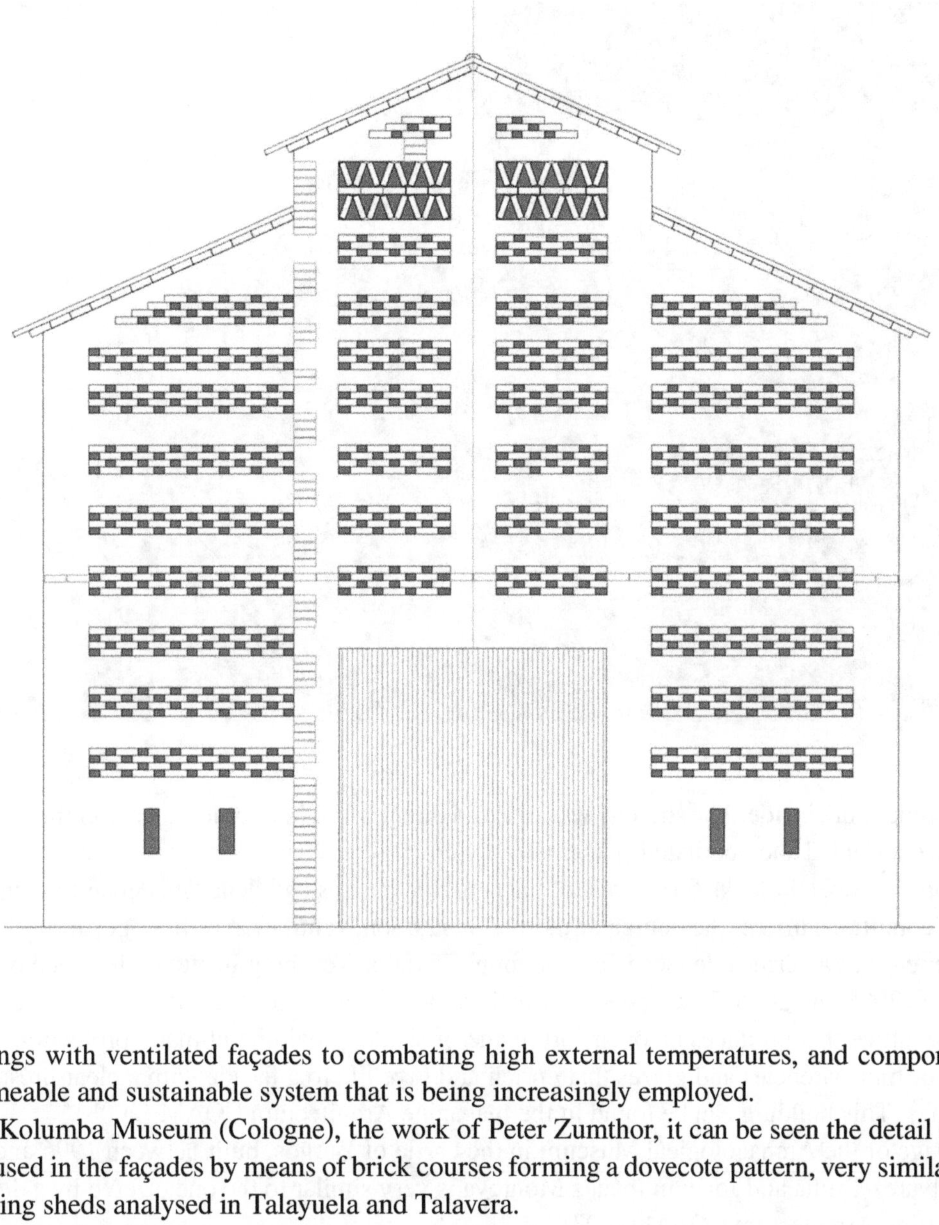

Buildings with ventilated façades to combating high external temperatures, and components of a semi-permeable and sustainable system that is being increasingly employed.

In the Kolumba Museum (Cologne), the work of Peter Zumthor, it can be seen the detail of the latticework used in the façades by means of brick courses forming a dovecote pattern, very similar to those of the drying sheds analysed in Talayuela and Talavera.

Ngamwongwan House built by Junsekino Architecture & Design, in Bangkok, Thailand explores the common brick, this house embraces a tropical lifestyle with a brick screen façade and two-layer brick walls that let in natural light. Bricks in the façade were rotated to stand proud of the envelope and create a vertical pattern.

The Dominius Winery (California, U.S.A.) built between 1995-1998 by the architects Herzog & De Meuron, that can be consulted at AV Monographs magazine number 77(1999) "Herzog & De Meuron". In this project, the façade is made up of blocks of stones placed inside a regular mesh, reminiscent of the permeability achieved in the drying sheds. In this case, the climate of the area, which has significant temperature fluctuations between day and night, required the building to find a solution to maintain a

Figure 12. Drying shed in Puente del Arzobispo (Toledo). Photograph by the author.

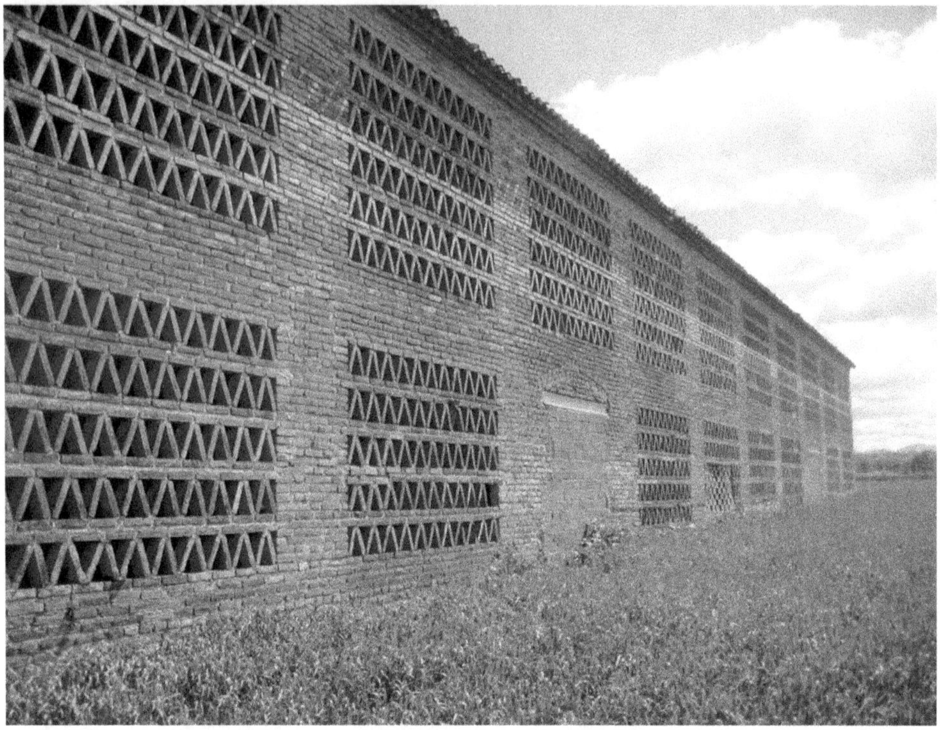

constant temperature inside. The strategy was to avoid direct sunlight in order to protect the wine barrels and to create a shaded and ventilated space.

The stone and metal blocks form walls of varying thicknesses and densities depending on the environmental conditions inside: the degree of thermal insulation, ventilation or light permeability.

Another case of a permeable façade can be found Badajoz Teaching Institute, designed by Gonzalo Moure in the 2003 and 2005. The west side, which is the one that faces the city centre, is resolved with a terracotta lattice that produces an openwork plane of shade, providing climatic protection and creating a play of transparencies and glazes that enrich and give life to a façade with a clear presence in its surroundings. This building can be found in the magazine Arquitectura COAM (2008).

The image of the Archaeological Museum in the castle of Burgos, built between 1996 and 2003 by Maryan Álvarez-Builla and Joaquín Ibáñez Montoya is very similar to the one offered by a drying shed from the inside Arquitectura COAM (2003).

TR House located in Barcelona, Spain, built in 2014 by PMMT arquitectura, the facades are wrapped with a green vitrified ceramic skin, that camouflages the house with its verdant surroundings.

NDC House in Ho Chi Minh City, Vietnam, made in 2016 by Tropical Space Architecture firm is another example of bioclimatic building.

WG·M·Cube made by MVRDV in Beijing, China in 2018, while some areas of the surface were required to have blind facades to accommodate the stores behind, other stores are able to use diffuse light to their advantage, and here the ceramic tiles are used in a checkerboard pattern.

Figure 13. Drying sheds in Talayuela drawing by the author. 2009

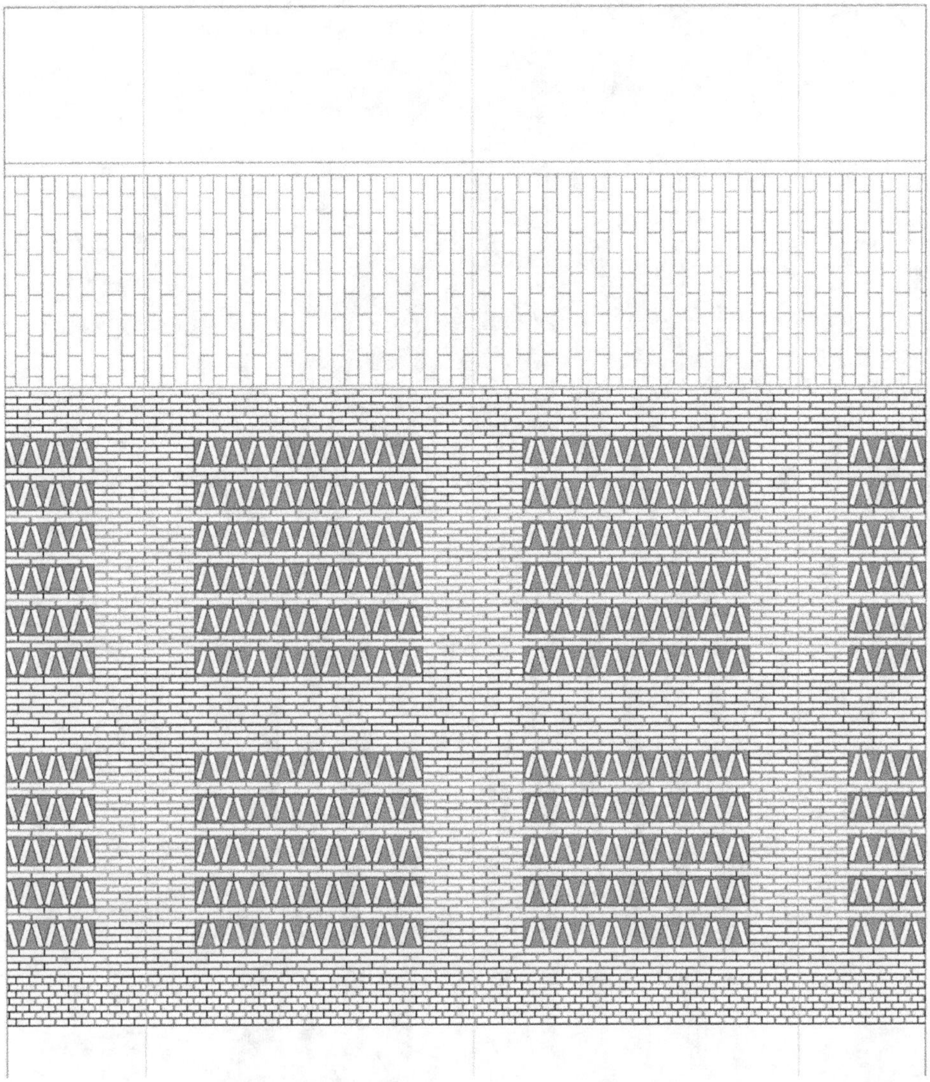

The New Crematory in Riehen, Switzerland, built in 2017 by Architekturbüro Bernhard Maurer shows a brick skin. The brick is a hand-made and hand-laid material. The latter stretches around the building and opens to light and air, defining a porous border that is open and closed at the same time.

The Lantern designed by VTN Architects uses a perforated terracotta façade. The terracotta blocks were traditionally used in Vietnam before air-conditioning. Designed for tropical climates, they allow for passive ventilation and shade from harsh sunlight. The blocks are both functional and inexpensive. Furthermore, the bespoke fixing system allowed for a quick and simple assembly.

Saint Peter House built by Proyecto Cafeína + Estudio Tecalli in San Pedro Cholula, Mexico, integrates regional materiality elements like the red brick allowing expressive geometry due to the modular repetition.

Figure 14. Case 4 drying shed in Calera y Chozas (Toledo).

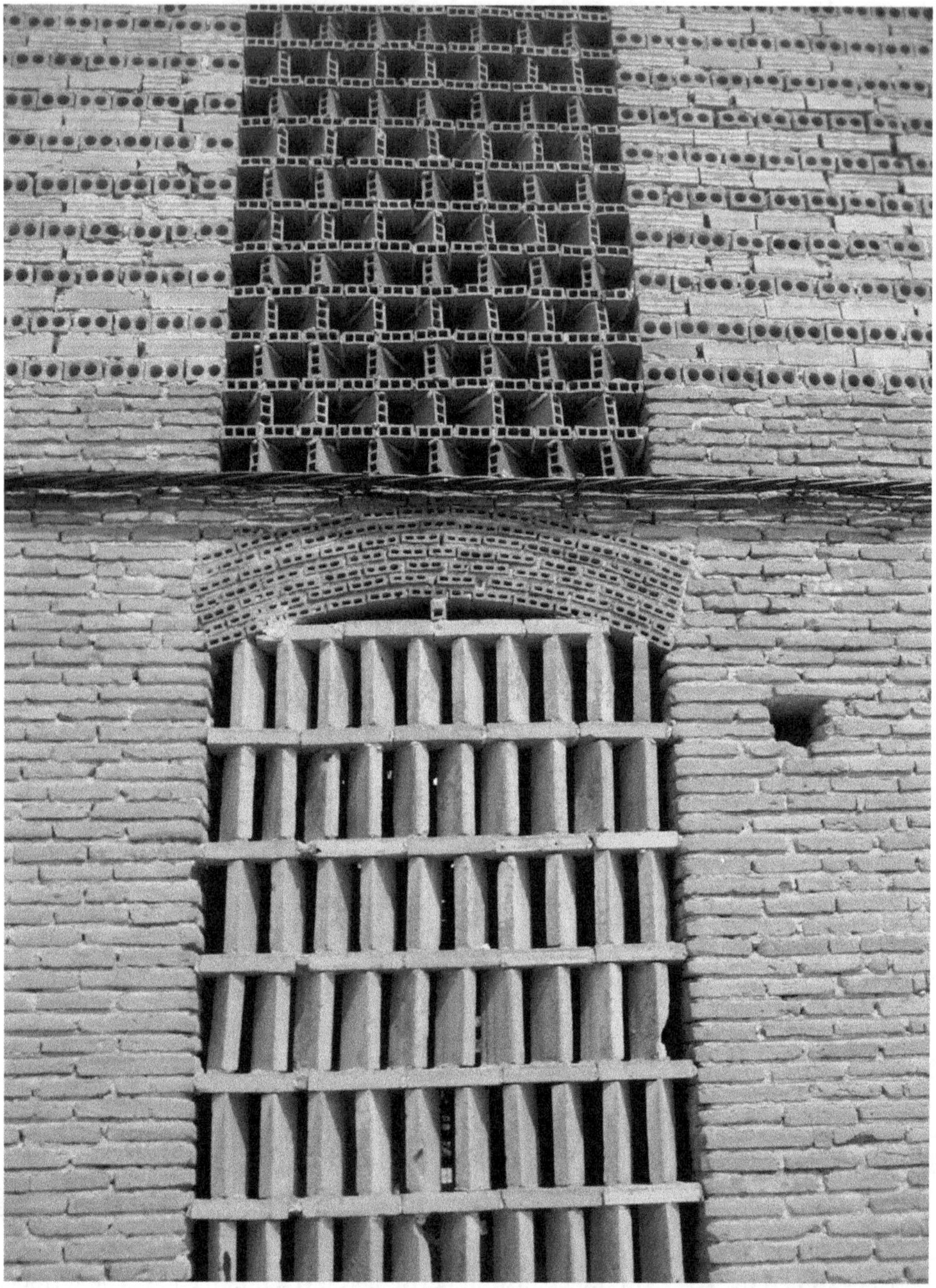

Catalinas Houses by Agustín Lozada, in Argentina is an austere and detail less design, that reduces construction costs.

Dos Plátanos School built by Murmuro Portugal Sintra in 2017, is an example of natural ventilation is the requisite to create a permeable brick facade that allows air to flow for the natural ventilation of the building, illuminates, protects the windows and hides the necessary ventilation grids.

Figure 15. Case 4 drying shed in Calera y Chozas (Toledo) drawing by the author. 2009

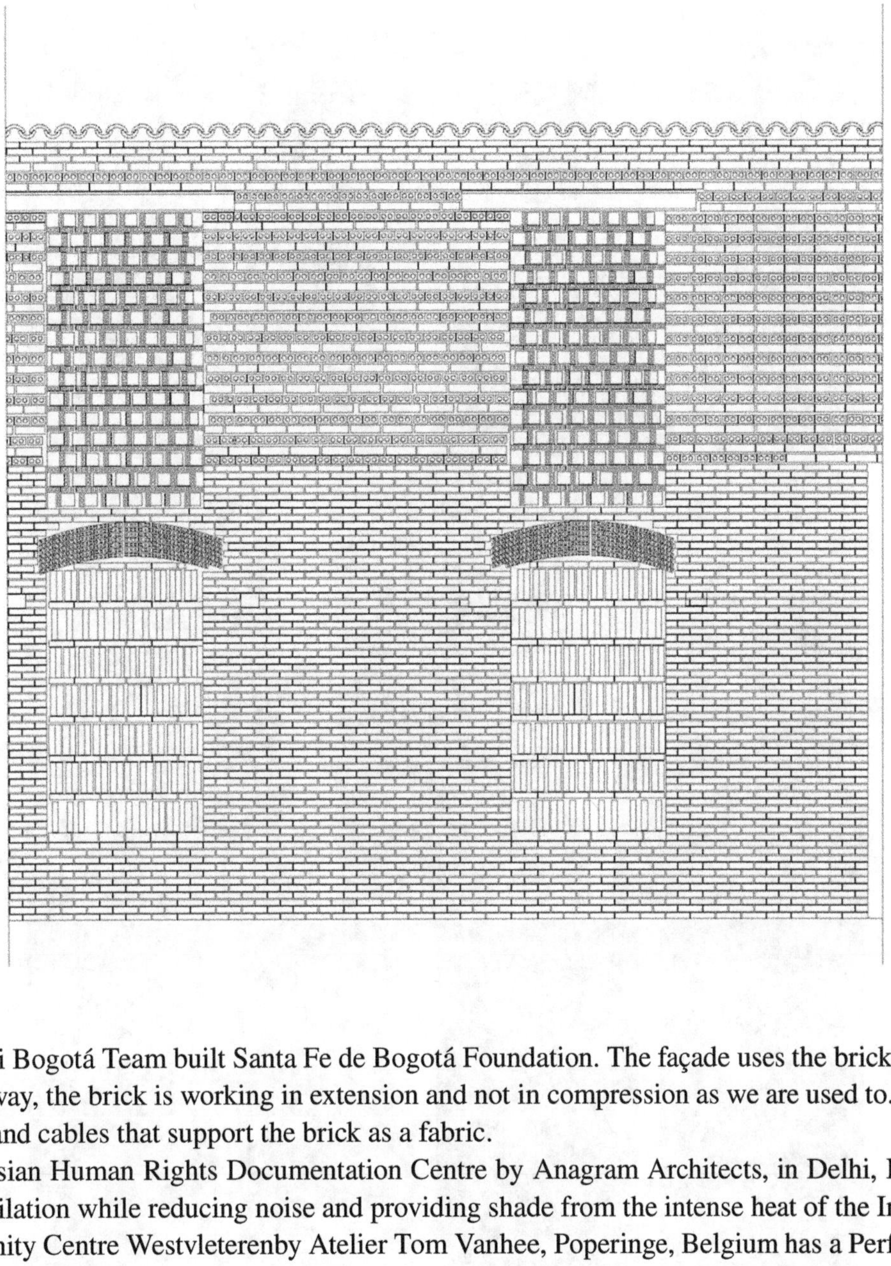

Mazzanti Bogotá Team built Santa Fe de Bogotá Foundation. The façade uses the brick in the most innovative way, the brick is working in extension and not in compression as we are used to. It uses metallic parts and cables that support the brick as a fabric.

South Asian Human Rights Documentation Centre by Anagram Architects, in Delhi, India allows natural ventilation while reducing noise and providing shade from the intense heat of the Indian sun.

Community Centre Westvleterenby Atelier Tom Vanhee, Poperinge, Belgium has a Perforated Grid façade.

ABC Building built by WISE Architecture, in Seoul, South Korea. Bricks were laid with slight gaps for certain parts of the façade, allowing light and air to filter through.

Angdong Hospital by Rural Urban Framework, in Baojing, China, uses recycled traditional brick provide the necessary thermal comfort.

This 8- Storey Apartment Block Feature in Tehran, Iran, was built by Mohsen Kazemianfard in 2018 using angular screens of perforated bricks. the porous brick façade brings in light into the interior space,

Figure 16. Photographs taken by the author.

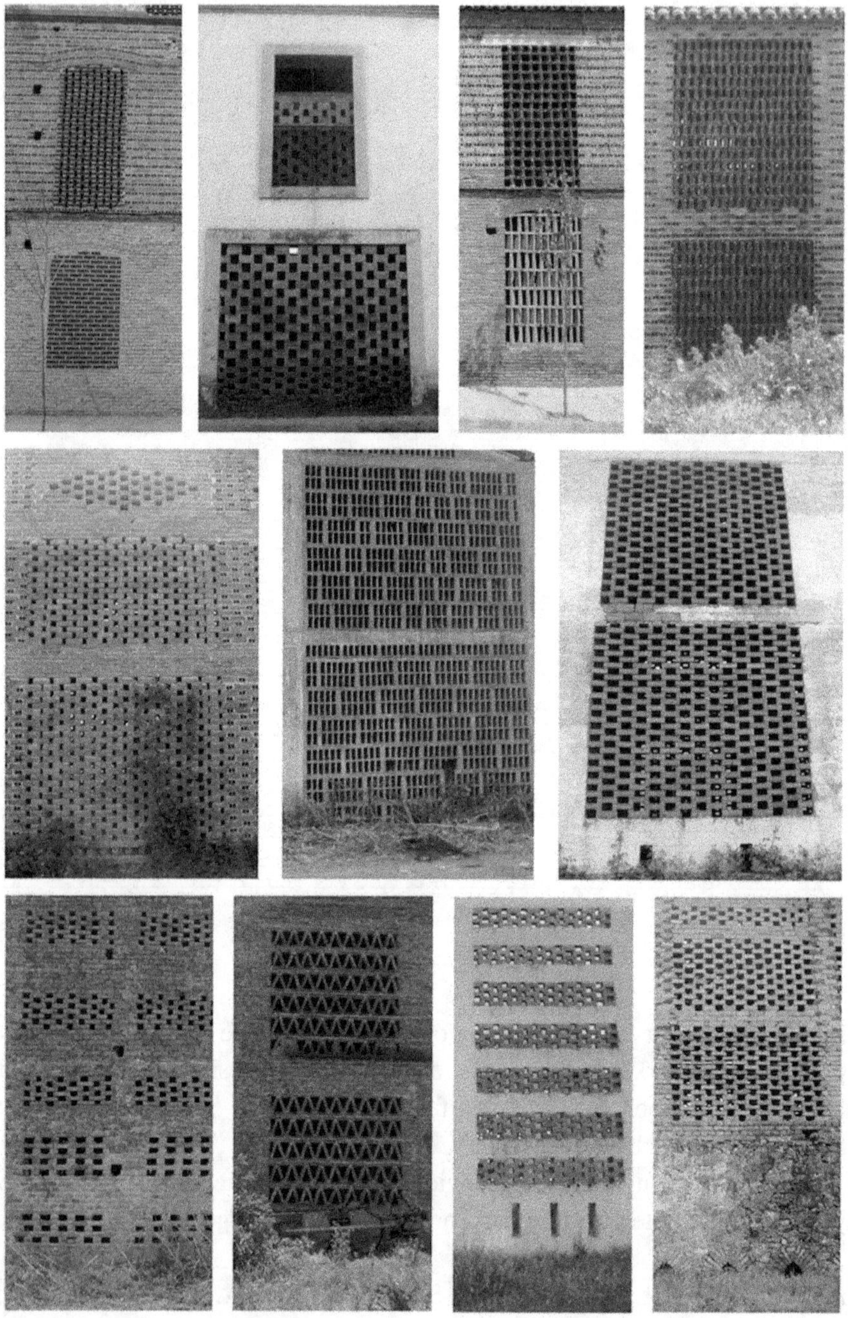

Figure 17. Photographs taken by the author.

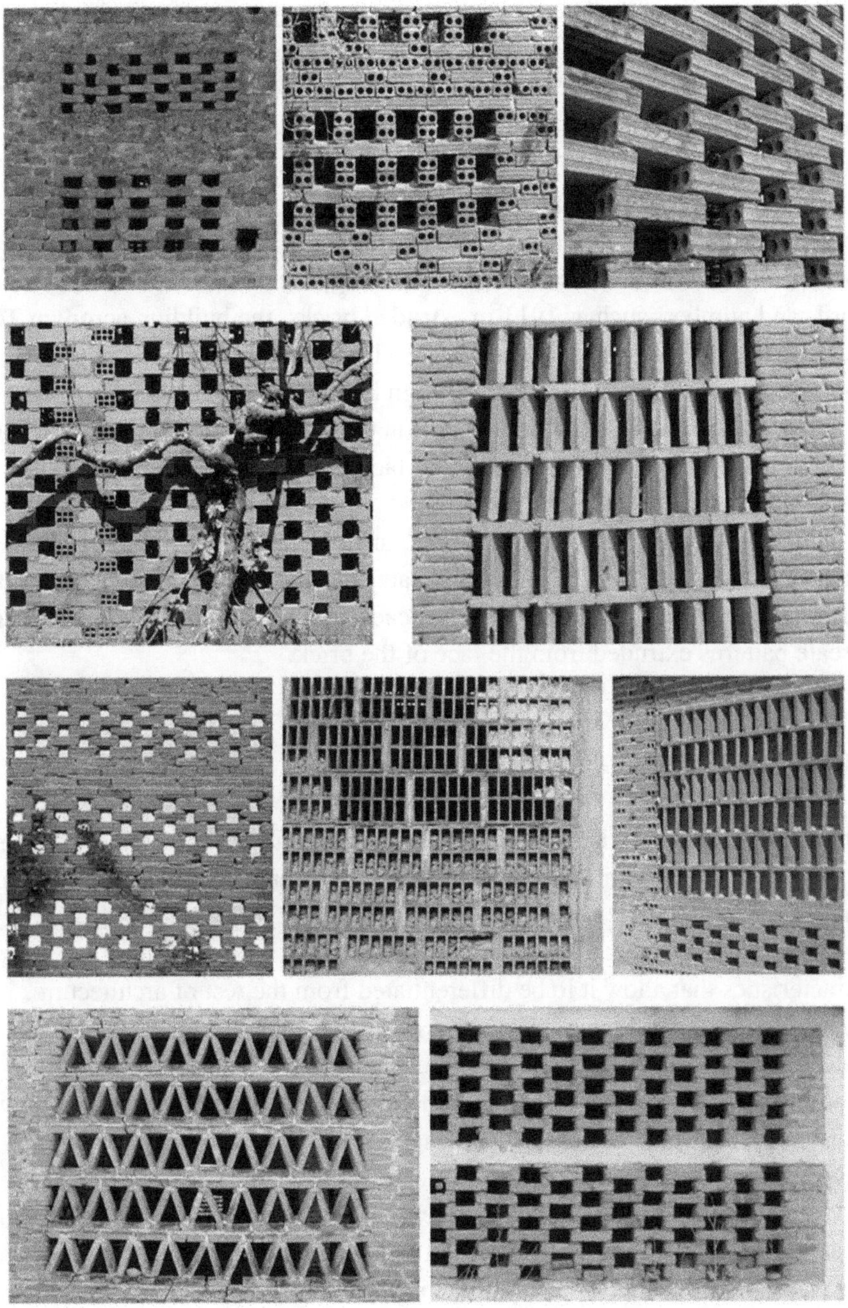

creating this beautiful effect of light and shadow. The permeable façade not only brightens up space but also creates this warm feeling inside the structure which is very comforting.

Gramalote Market Square built by Niro Arquitectura + OAUo in 2017, in Colombia. The permeability allows continuous ventilation as well as security and visual control, thanks to an arrayed brick framework on the façades

A permeable brick envelope clads Natura Futura's mixed-use building in Ecuador (Montalvo) 2020.

Chapel of the Capuchin Mothers in Tlalpan, Mexico City, designed by Luis Barragan between 1952 and 1955 is an example of the architectural use of filtered natural light, filtered through louvres.

Central Canteen of Tsinghua University in Beijing by SUP Atelier + School of Architecture Tsinghua University. The masonry external walls have an artistic significance as well as a functional purpose. bricks form words and numbers such as 1911 in extruded bricks, the building acronym TCCH in solid, monolithic bricks and GHUA in overhung and concave bricks.

New Delhi-based design studio Zero Energy Design Lab has completed a girls' hostel building with a perforated concrete facade and an exterior staircase in Gurugram, India. used hollow concrete blocks in a red-brick colour for the exterior. The ventilated facade is a solution of coating and protection of exterior walls.

38 Housing Units by Avenier Cornejo Architectes, in Clichy, France. Setting a new standard for integrating landscape with the suburbs, the building creates morphological diversity through its form and envelope. Brick was chosen for the north and west façades, where vibrant colors and elegant detailing were used to create patterns extruded from the face of the brick.

CONCLUSION

This research focuses on the analysis of the construction characteristics of the drying sheds, as it is a typology with sufficient entity, with a certain formal category, and an example of bioclimatic production architecture.

Industrial architecture must be recognised as a separate genre within the heritage as a whole, due to its specific characteristics that allow it to be differentiated from the rest of architecture.

This architectural typology refers us to a world of great symbolic relevance because industry has become the material expression of the idea of progress.

Production architecture creates a new language in accordance with the advances of industrialisation, anticipating materials and structures, and condensing in a specific typology the complex relationships established between men, product and space.

Drying sheds are a cultural expression that condenses innumerable symbolic, artistic, historical and functional values. Regardless of their state of conservation, they are particularly important as a vehicle for transmitting ways of seeing and understanding local life: the intangible heritage.

These singular isolated buildings or industrial complexes were widely implanted in the territory, and possess a series of technological, architectural, sociological and landscape values, which make them a document of the first magnitude to know: the evolution and implantation of construction techniques (materials and structures), the processes of typological innovation (spatial arrangement in plan and height) and the economic structure and technical procedures used.

The landscape in which they are inserted constitutes their territorial context, so it would be wrong to consider these buildings as isolated elements, without analysing the relationship with the environment in which they were generated, especially when industry is a direct consequence of society's use of the natural environment.

From the analysis of the overlapping of the climograms, it can be determined that the environmental hygrothermal conditions of the months of June and July at night, and those of September and October, are the most suitable both for human comfort and for drying tobacco, and any human activity can be carried out inside the drying sheds studied under optimum conditions.

The examples of drying sheds analysed are all masonry, because choosing brick as the determining element and feature in the design of a building implies, in a certain way, the consideration of a "degree zero" of the whole constructive and compositional apparatus of architecture.

This minimal element, which allows for enormously open, but not absolutely random, freedoms, defines its own combinatory logic.

Leaving the brick exposed means making explicit all the cumulative processes of a piece of manual manipulation.

The demand for sincerity so characteristic of industrial architecture in the exhibition of materials, displaying them in their own nature and in the real way they are used, is evident in this type of construction.

From the study on permeability, we can conclude that while 40% ventilation is required for dwellings, in the three examples of drying sheds analysed, we find different degrees of permeability: from 10% to 20%, with this ventilation being permanent in most cases.

It can be determined that the larger the volume of the dryer, the lower the permeability of its façade. Although this factor may also be due to design criteria in the pattern of the lattice, being much permeable those that form a triangular pattern.

Other factors that may influence the choice of the degree of permeability are the natural climatic elements: such as prevailing winds, proximity to streams, and greater or lesser exposure to sunlight.

There is an initiative promoted by the Junta de Extremadura for the reuse of drying sheds, which has two objectives: on the one hand, to promote an element that has earned a place in the memories of many regions and therefore a space in the regional ethnology of Extremadura, and on the other, to try to provide solutions - as far as possible, viable - for the future of these constructions, being aware that some of them have already been converted into warehouses, second homes, paprika drying sheds and rural houses.

These drying sheds could be converted into buildings for public use (agricultural and livestock centre, heliciculture centre, gastronomic school, tobacco museum), or converted into facilities for leisure and sporting activities.

The proposals that could be made related to the drying activity are: drying of flowers, spices, firewood, tiles, and biomass crops as an alternative fuel.

From the study we obtain the conditions of this specific climatic conditioning system, which can be used as a resource for other constructions.

Therefore, the constructive and formal system of the drying sheds could be transferred to other uses, from a double perspective:

Analysing the conceptual relationship, textures, patterns and construction methods of the drying sheds with historical and contemporary architecture, it can be found similar solutions to those used in the constructions studied in other buildings.

This type of façade or lattice patterns can be transferred to other architectures, as they are aesthetically and constructively adaptable.

The use of this buildings is fundamentally to provide shade, ventilation and a covered but permeable space on the façades.

REFERENCES

Argiles & María. (1986). *Arquitectura de ladrillos del siglo XIX: técnica y forma.* Academic Press.

Arroyo, G. A. (1973). Estudio analógico de la transmisión de calor en los muros tradicionales y ligeros. Instituto E. Torroja.

Cliff, T. (1979). *Industria y paisaje.* Madrid I.E.A.L.

Delgado & Martín, E. (1892). La renta de tabacos. Academic Press.

García de Paredes Andújar, J. (2008). *El cultivo del tabaco Virginia en España.* CETARSA

Garner, W. W. (1951). *The production of tobacco.* Academic Press.

GRETA (Grupo de Estudios del Tabaco). (2002). *El consumo de tabaco en España en el siglo XVIII.* Cuadernos de Investigación Histórica nº 19.

Hernández, B. M. (1976). El cultivo del tabaco en la provincia de Cáceres: variedades de los tipos Burley y Flue-cured. Editorial Confederación Española de Cajas de Ahorros.

Herzog & De Meuron. (1999). *AV Monographs Magazine, 77.*

Instituto Nacional de Colonización. (1963). *Construye secaderos y mejorarás tu tabaco.* Publicaciones del Instituto Nacional de Colonización.

Jordan, G. (1994). *Tobacco in History: The cultures of dependence.* Academic Press.

Lloyd, N. (1925). *A History of English Brickwork.* The Antique Collectors' Club Ltd.

Madrid. (1948). *Cartilla para el cultivo y curado del tabaco en España.* Academic Press.

Martínez, P., Luís, M., Serrano, G., & Patricio, Á. (1998). *Los secaderos de tabaco en la provincia de Granada.* Universidad EUAT de Granada.

Olgyay, V. (1998). Arquitectura y Clima. Manual de diseño bioclimático para Arquitectos y Urbanistas. Gustavo Gili.

Parada & Tamar. (2015). *Tobacco industrial architecture in Peninsular Spain: dryers and factories.* E.T.S.A.M. Polytechnical University of Madrid.

Plumridge, A., & Meulenkamp, W. (1993). *Brickwork: Architecture and Design.* Harry N Abrams.

S.N.C.F.T. (1952). *El secado de la hoja de tabaco.* Author.

S.N.C.F.T. (1962). *Construye secaderos y mejorarás tu tabaco.* Author.

Thomas, K. (1996). *Masonry walls: Specification and design.* Academic Press.

KEY TERMS AND DEFINITIONS

Bioclimatic: Relating to the interrelation of climate or environment and activities of living organisms.

Bonding: Is the arrangement of bricks in a structure.

Brick: A rectangular element or block made of ceramic used for building walls.

Drying Sheds: Bioclimatic constructions where the drying process takes place) are an example of bioclimatic industrial architecture, there is a close relationship between drying sheds and the surroundings in which they are located.

English Bond: This is a pattern formed by laying alternate courses of stretchers and headers. The joins between the stretchers are centered on the headers in the course below.

Flemish Bond: This is formed by laying headers and stretchers alternately in each course. The headers of each course are centered on the stretchers of the course below.

Header Bond: This bond features courses of headers offset by half a brick. It is like the stretcher bond but with headers instead of stretchers.

Industrial Architecture: Buildings constructed to facilitate the needs of industry, types and styles that mix functionality and design, conceived around the specialized systems, processes, equipment, and worker safety considerations of manufacturing.

Masonry: Art, craft, and practice of building in the traditional style done with bricks.

Modular Facade: Enclosure made from the repetition of a module, or minimum element.

Pattern: Model to be used as a sample to produce a larger element or a mosaic, repeating the module several times.

Permeability: The ability of a wall to allow air to go through it.

Stretcher Bond: Is the most commonly used bond, a pattern is made only using stretchers, with the joins on each course centred above and below by half a brick.

Tobacco: Is a plant of the genus *Nicotiana* that produces leaves which are smoked.

Chapter 2
A Novel Methodology to Study Particulate Material/Aerosol Pollution via Real-Time Hyperspectral Acousto-Optic Intelligent Spectrometry

José Amílcar Rizzo Sierra
Universidad de Querétaro, Mexico

Ely Karina Anaya Rivera
Universidad de Querétaro, Mexico

Gastón Sanglier Contreras
https://orcid.org/0000-0002-8981-5622
Universidad CEU San Pablo, Spain

César Isaza
Universidad de Querétaro, Mexico

Jonny Paul Zavala de Paz
Universidad Politécnica de Querétaro, Mexico

ABSTRACT

Tactic and strategic management and policing of atmospheric pollution in México, specifically by particulate material (PM) from mobile sources (internal combustion powered vehicles), critically requires state-of-the-science technologies due to the problem's complexity including its public health dimension. The authors consider that proper decision making on the problem would benefit from permanent revision on currently employed PM monitoring and measurement systems and also the effort to improve them. These later currently offer information on O(10^0) ultraviolet-visible-infrared (UV-VIS-IR) spectral bands at O(10^0) spatial resolutions and O(10^1) in [min^-1] temporal resolutions. In contrast, they propose the novel use of acousto-optic tunable filter (AOTF) spectrometry to study PM in atmospheric suspension, capable of offering information on O(10^2) UV, VIS, or IR spectral bands at similar or better spatial and temporal resolutions. The potential of AOTF spectrometry towards PM assessment is clear and the objective is to explore its usefulness.

DOI: 10.4018/978-1-7998-7279-5.ch002

INTRODUCTION

Particulate material (PM) in atmospheric suspension monitoring is crucial in big cities (i. e., Megalopolis and sub-urban areas), regarding both tactical and strategic environmental and epidemiological governmental policing. One of the main causes of PM pollution is the use of internal combustion vehicles operating in high densities over constrained vehicular traffic networks (Molina et al., 2019). Even though the push for alternative automotive vehicular power plants is strong, with hybrid electric-internal combustion vehicles leading the front, it is clear that we will have to deal with the impact of internal combustion as one of the most important automotive energy sources for decades still to come. Thus, *Universidad Politécnica de Querétaro* (UPQ) and associate institutions to this research proposal have the call to assist within their capacities to the management of subjects related to PM pollution, and its effects on human health and society. The main PM monitoring methods used in México are based on Beta radiation attenuation instrumentation, in order to measure its concentration (Molina et al., 2019; Red Automática de Monitoreo Atmosférico de la ZMVT, 2019). These instruments are reliable and accurate, but their sampling frequency is hourly at best, and in most cases the logistics required for deployment and implementation better functions at ground level or close to it. Moreover, they only assess PM2.5 and PM10 concentration, not being able to assess on critical information such as PM physico-chemical speciation/reactivity and epidemiological relevance. On the other hand, there is instrumentation that in some cases can give information closer to real time, and at different levels above ground on PM concentration, such as the Moderate Resolution Imaging Spectroradiometer (MODIS), mounted on the Terra-Earth Observing System-EOS satellite (Just et al., 2015), solar spectrometers/photometers (Volkova et al., 2018), and Light Imaging Detection and Ranging -LIDAR- devices (Hair et al., 2008). These instruments measure particulate material parameters by aerosol optical depth (AOD) in the atmosphere via the physical principle of comparative radiance/irradiance at different atmospheric column heights respect to ground level. Within this context, a more general denomination for PM in atmospheric suspension would be aerosols in atmospheric suspension, since it considers its nature of molecular agglomerates beyond their current material physical state. Atmospheric Aerosol Optical Depth measured in satellites such as the one carrying MODIS and other means represent the fundamentals of global climatological monitoring systems such as the World Climate Research Program (Holben et al., 2001; Van Donkelaar et al., 2010); and have also recently been used specifically for PM-aerosol monitoring in México City, as reported by (Just et al., 2015). Unfortunately, measurements in these systems are limited to a few spectral bands for each available spatial resolution. For example: bands 1 through 7 and 20 (MODIS bands and spectral ranges, 2019), that is, O(10^0) spectral bands are used at 10 and 3 km (at *nadir*) spatial resolution above ground, and a 12 min^-1 temporal resolution for atmospheric aerosol study by MODIS (MODIS aerosol product information, 2019a; MODIS aerosol product information, 2019b).

In contrast, we propose here to use acousto-optic tunable filtering -AOTF- spectrometry to measure Aerosol Optical Depths by comparative irradiance within open atmospheric or enclosed laboratory atmospheric columns exposed to combustion engine exhaust gases, to have another type of instrumentation to not only measure PM concentration but also provide significatively more information on suspended aerosols via hyper-spectral (i. e., O(10^2)) bands in the visible range and/or infrared and closer to real time temporal resolutions. It is important to point out here that our research team has so far successfully employed AOTF hyper-spectroscopy to propose a segmentation technique for image analysis/processing (Isaza et al., 2019), and also to study automotive plastic parts color characterization (Rizzo Sierra et al., 2019). This has been accomplished using México's current only operational visible range AOTF hyper-spectrometer at *Universidad Politécnica de Querétaro*. An scheme of the physical functioning of an acousto-optic tunable filter image acquisition system is presented in Figure 1.

Figure 1. Simplified schematics of the functioning principle of an AOTF-based image acquisition system. Light from the object of interest gets selected in narrow wavelength bandwidths by the TeO_2 crystal while its refraction index changes according to the acoustic wave propagating through it. The control of the former wave is performed via the computer interfaced RF generator signal sent over the transducer. Schematics in figure as shown in (Rizzo Sierra et al., 2019).

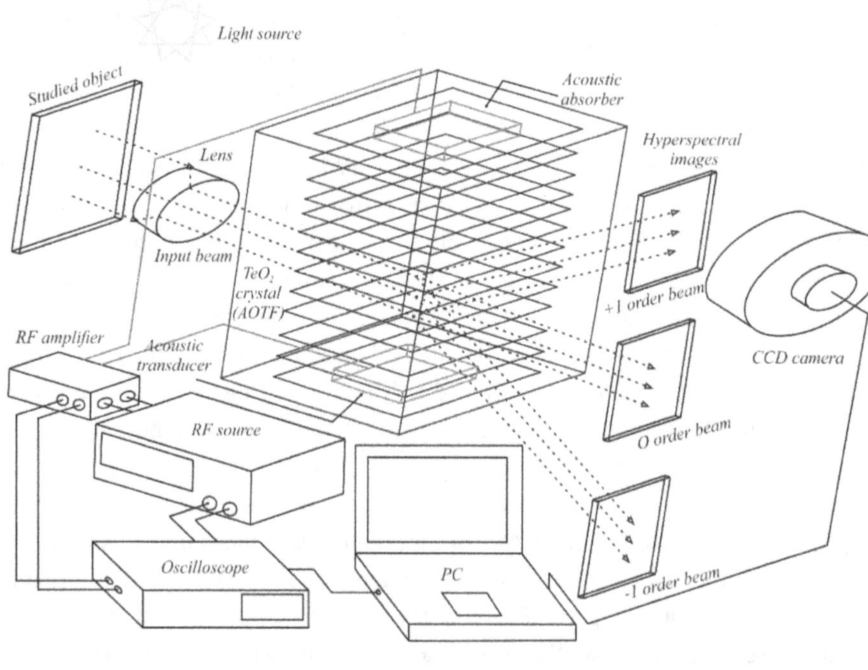

TECHNICAL HYPOTHESIS

We can hypothesize that the amount of information gathered from suspended PM-aerosols by AOTF spectrometry will have benefits such as advancing our understanding of speciation, atmospheric dispersion dynamics, physico-chemical atmospheric processing, and epidemiologically relevant mechanisms regarding suspended PM-aerosols from internal combustion engines and other sources. Moreover, it will also enable the development of alternative accurate, closer to real time sampling capable, and logistically more flexible instruments for monitoring PM-aerosols in open or closed urban or rural environments. On the other hand, information about the concentration of suspended aerosols at specific locations (latitudinal and longitudinal coordinates) will be publicly available by means of specially developed computational tools running on social networks serving as communication platforms. This will contribute into users gaining conscience of the PM-aerosol pollution problem with its implications, effects, and prevention strategies. We believe these proposed systems could contribute towards present and future generations of the general public, developing conscience dealing with the air pollution issue.

PROPOSED METHODOLOGY

The scientific methodology proposed to this project is straightforwardly divided into three main parts:

1. System setup and configuration to study PM-aerosols from internal combustion engines in open or confined air columns. It implies:
    a. Design, configuration, purchase, and setup of the AOTF system components. The working principle to be used is comparative irradiance between cross sections (normal to) and limiting the air column of interest due to the presence of PM-aerosols in it. The final AOTF system and its enclosure must be embedded in order to be usable in both indoors and outdoors conditions.
    b. Design, configuration, and setup of enclosed air column chambers for indoors and outdoors testing, potentially usable as standard (pattern/calibration) experimental setups.
2. System testing, firstly in confined air columns using closed chambers exposed to combustion engines exhaust gases. It implies:
    a. Testing with gasoline engines.
    b. Testing with diesel engines.
    c. Testing with liquefied petroleum gas (LPG), and natural gas engines.
3. Development of a methodology for the system's calibration as a whole. It implies:
    a. Assessing traceability of the proposed methodology with other measurement methodologies.
    b. Use of artificial intelligence (AI) with machine learning (ML) algorithms to attain self-calibration of the proposed system.

EXPECTED RESULTS

1. Development of analytical and instrumental methods to complement current comparative irradiance spectrometry applied to climatology and atmospheric pollution study. The previous to be used in determining Aerosol Optical Depth (AOD) or related parameters by means of AOTF assisted spectrometry.
2. Improvement of the data collection capabilities of instruments currently measuring AOD or similar parameters. Current instruments such as MODIS gather information on O(10^0) spectral bands. Instead, AOTF assisted spectrometry could gather information on O(10^2) spectral bands at choosable ranges such as ultraviolet, visible and infrared. It is important to notice that this informational aspect of AOTF spectrometry has been demonstrated in several instances, such as within the context of automotive parts (auto-parts) color characterization (Rizzo Sierra et al., 2019). Cf. Figure 2.

Figure 2. This figure presents a comparison between experimental results for light reflectance on a plastic auto-part, gray in visually perceivable color. Datasets compared were provided by a Colorimeter setup operated by Centro Nacional de Metrología (CENAM, México's National authority in industry-related standards and measurements), and a AOTF system setup by the present authors. This kind of data is used in automotive engineering to characterize color. As can be readily appreciated from the curves, data acquired with the AOTF system has appropriate correspondence with CENAM's data, while providing in excess of ten times more spectral information on a given auto-part. Figure as shown in (Rizzo Sierra et al., 2019).

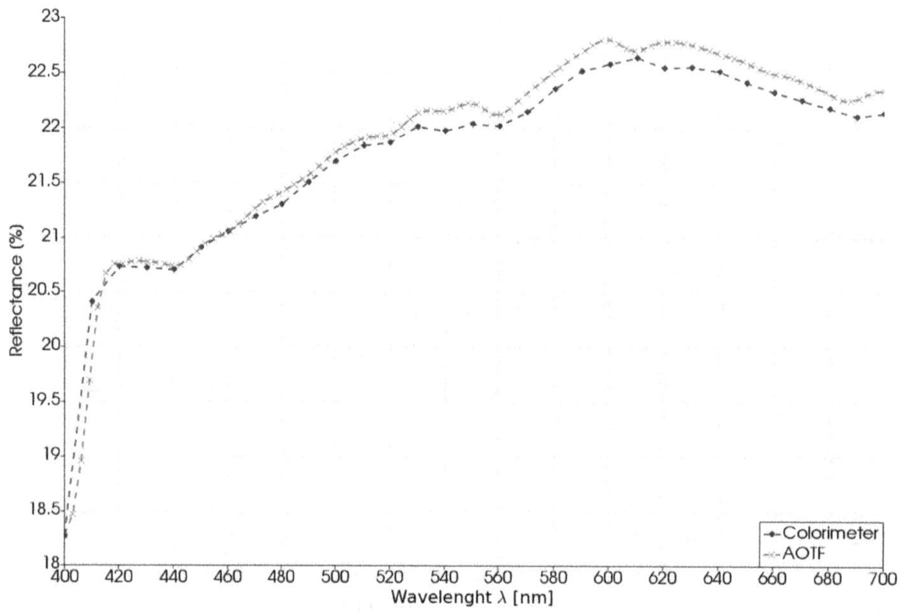

3. Improvement on time sampling frequency capabilities over existing spectrometry instruments. This is possible due to measurements established by potentially on-the-fly comparative irradiance data/imaging analysis/processing via artificial intelligence (AI) and machine learning (ML); instead of requiring data acquiring, processing, and post processing.
4. In addition, AOTF spectrometry allows implementing thermography functions on the studied atmospheric columns by choosing adequate spectral bands, which could be explored and implemented in subsequent projects. Then, it offers complementary information closely related to important subjects such as urban/rural ecology and climate change.

REFERENCES

Hair, J. W., Hostetler, C. A., Cook, A. L., Harper, D. B., Ferrare, R. A., Mack, T. L., Welch, W., Izquierdo, L. R., & Hovis, F. E. (2008). Airborne high spectral resolution lidar for profiling aerosol optical properties. *Applied Optics*, *47*(36), 6734–6752. doi:10.1364/AO.47.006734 PMID:19104525

Holben, B. N., Tanre, D., Smirnov, A., Eck, T. F., Slutsker, I., Abuhassan, N., Newcomb, W. W., Schafer, J. S., Chatenet, B., Lavenu, F., Kaufman, Y. J., Castle, J. V., Setzer, A., Markham, B., Clark, D., Frouin, R., Halthore, R., Karneli, A., O'Neill, N. T., ... Zibordi, G. (2001, June 16). An emerging ground-based aerosol climatology: Aerosol optical depth from AERONET. *Journal of Geophysical Research, D, Atmospheres*, *106*(D11), 12067–12097. doi:10.1029/2001JD900014

Isaza, C., Mosquera, J. M., Gómez-Méndez, G. A., Zavala-De Paz, J. P., Anaya-Rivera, E. K., Rizzo-Sierra, J. A., & Palillero-Sandoval, O. (2019). Development of an acousto-optic system for hyperspectral image segmentation. *Metrology and Measurement Systems*, *26*(3).

Just, A. C., Wright, R. O., Schwartz, J., Coull, B. A., Baccarelli, A. A., Tellez-Rojo, M. M., Moody, E., Wang, Y., Lyapustin, A., & Kloog, I. (2015). Using high-resolution satellite aerosol optical depth to estimate daily PM2. 5 geographical distribution in Mexico City. *Environmental Science & Technology*, *49*(14), 8576–8584. doi:10.1021/acs.est.5b00859 PMID:26061488

MODIS aerosol product information. (2019a). Retrieved from https://ladsweb.modaps.eosdis.nasa.gov/missions-and-measurements/products/MOD04_L2/

MODIS aerosol product information. (2019b). Retrieved from https://ladsweb.modaps.eosdis.nasa.gov/missions-and-measurements/productsMOD04_3K/

MODIS bands and spectral ranges. (2019). Retrieved from https://web.archive.org/web/20070715215437/http://edcdaac.usgs.gov/modis/table2.asp

Molina, L. T., Velasco, E., Retama, A., & Zavala, M. (2019). Experience from Integrated Air Quality Management in the Mexico City Metropolitan Area and Singapore. *Atmosphere*, *10*(9), 512. doi:10.3390/atmos10090512

Red Automática de Monitoreo Atmosférico de la ZMVT. (2019). *Técnicas de medición*. Retrieved from http://rama.edomex.gob.mx/tecnicas_medicion

Rizzo Sierra, J. A., Isaza, C., Anaya Rivera, E. K., Zavala De Paz, J. P., & Mosquera, J. (2019). Acousto-Optic Dispersion Applicability to Plastic Auto-Part Color Characterization. In Progress in Optomechatronic Technologies (pp. 51-64). Springer. doi:10.1007/978-981-32-9632-9_7

Van Donkelaar, A., Martin, R. V., Brauer, M., Kahn, R., Levy, R., Verduzco, C., & Villeneuve, P. J. (2010). Global estimates of ambient fine particulate matter concentrations from satellite-based aerosol optical depth: Development and application. *Environmental Health Perspectives*, *118*(6), 847–855. doi:10.1289/ehp.0901623 PMID:20519161

Volkova, K. A., Poberovsky, A. V., Timofeev, Y. M., Ionov, D. V., Holben, B. N., Smirnov, A., & Slutsker, I. (2018). Aerosol Optical Characteristics Retrieved from CIMEL Sun Photometer Measurements (AERONET) near St. Petersburg. *Atmospheric and Oceanic Optics*, *31*(6), 635–641. doi:10.1134/S1024856018060180

Chapter 3
Acoustic Design of Ordinary Spaces:
Offices, Schools, Healthcare Facilities, Restaurants, and Retail

Juan Negreira
https://orcid.org/0000-0002-7111-8554
Saint-Gobain Ecophon, Spain

ABSTRACT

When designing for wellbeing, noise is usually not properly accounted for (if at all) during the design phase of a building. However, noise is often rated as the number one cause of dissatisfaction in offices; it negatively affects patients and staff in hospitals, prevents quality learning and teaching in schools, and bests poor service as the most irksome complaint for restaurants users. The question that arises is then, "How can we design to avoid the negative effects of noise on the end-users to enable wellbeing in indoor spaces?"

INTRODUCTION

Noise is, according to data from the World Health Organization (WHO), the second largest environmental cause of health problems, just after the impact of air quality (particulate matter). As a matter of fact, more than one million six hundred thousand healthy life years (DALYs) are lost annually. Of these DALYs, 903,000 years are lost due to sleep disturbance and 45,000 years due to cognitive impairment in children. Excess noise is scientifically related to the appearance or worsening of certain medical conditions, both psychological and physiological.

The term "room acoustic design" often makes people think about performance spaces such as auditoria and theatres, as it is well-known that the quality of the activities performed inside them undoubtedly depend to a great extent on their acoustic design. Nevertheless, ordinary spaces (hereafter embracing this term offices, healthcare facilities, schools, restaurants, retail, industry...) are very seldom conceived with

DOI: 10.4018/978-1-7998-7279-5.ch003

acoustics as a design parameter (amid others), in spite of being one of the main indoor environmental quality (IEQ) factors. Acoustic specialists usually (when present) come into the project in the very last stages of it, or after the project is finished, when any counter action becomes more difficult and costly.

As a result, noise exposure while deploying activities in ordinary spaces with not-good-enough room acoustics has been widely proven to have negative effects on people in different environments. Noise has been shown to be the number one cause of dissatisfaction in offices (Jenssen, 2005); it affects negatively patients and staff in hospitals (Beldam, 2019 & Johansson et. al, 2012); it hinders quality learning and teaching in schools (Tiesler & Oberdöster, 2006), as well as noise bested poor service as the most irksome complaint for restaurants users (Negreira, 2019). Having the end-user, i.e. the people, in mind and in the centre of the design is of crucial importance when designing ordinary public rooms. Only in that manner the room will support the activities performed in it, enabling comfort and wellbeing.

How can then one design indoor environments in order to avoid the negative effects that noise exposure has on the end-users and thus improve acoustic comfort in them? The latter question will be addressed in this chapter, after presenting brief state-of-the-art regarding how sound affects people in different typologies of spaces as well as some basic acoustics concepts. Note that only room acoustics is dealt with in this chapter (matters of acoustic insulation -i.e. sound transmission between different spaces- are not delved into hereafter).

BACKGROUND

Picture yourself in a big cathedral. All the hard surfaces of the space make the sound bounce back and forth and you feel the energy of the sound without hearing exactly what is said just a few metres away. This is, in many cases, the exact same situation one has in ordinary spaces where people spend most of our time of their daily life. We often design for acoustics in performance spaces… don't people have ears outside of concert halls and auditoria?

Acoustically hard materials (where sound cannot penetrate to be absorbed and thus reflected back to the room) support sound levels to escalate when activities are performed. In these spaces, it is likely to encounter unpleasant environments (i.e. long reverberation, low intelligibility and high sound levels). This, in turn, can activate the so-called Lombard effect (involuntary tendency of speakers to increase their vocal effort in order to try to improve their audibility). Good room acoustics should be tailored for each situation depending on (i) the type of activity performed in the space, (ii) the people that perform the activities inside the room, and of course (iii) the room treatment. In the following, a brief state-of-the-art will be given.

Offices

Both traditional (cellular) and open-plan offices (becoming increasingly common) respond to the need for organisations to facilitate decision-making and knowledge transfer between workers, as well as to promote communication and collaboration between people, or even contribute to the corporate image of the firm. Fortunately, the wellbeing of the end-users is also a fundamental aspect that is increasingly gaining popularity when designing these spaces.

Noise (as part of the wellbeing), is usually left aside during the design phase, despite of it being the number one cause of complaints in offices, and is an underlying cause of stress and frustration in the workplace (Jenssen, 2005). About two-thirds of the people surveyed in (Oseland, 2018) consistently argue that noise has a negative effect on their job performance, and about 50% of these also argue that it affects their wellbeing and stress levels. In (Mark, 2015), the studies revealed that a typical office worker is interrupted every 3 minutes and 5 seconds and that, once that distraction ceases, it takes 23 minutes and 15 seconds to return to the same level of concentration as before. These interruptions are usually tackled (in order to compensate the time lost) by increasing the work rate, which implies greater stress, haste, frustration and time pressure. (Fried, 2002) demonstrated that noise exposure is correlated with sick leave; this correlation being greater the more complex the task performed by the worker is. In addition, these distractions have a significant impact in economic terms for the employer, especially if it is taken into account that the cost of human capital represents 82% of the company's costs in a period of 10 years (Brill, 2001).

Good room acoustics can help addressing these burdens of reduced productivity and wellbeing of workers. It has been shown that good acoustic conditioning in offices can: (i) reduce adrenaline levels by 30% (which implies a reduction in heart rate, stress, fatigue, etc.) (Evans, 2000); (ii) promote the resolution of complex tasks (Evans, 2000); (iii); increase 66% motivation for a task; (iv) increase the arithmetic yield by 20% (Banbury, 1998); (v) improve performance by 50% in tasks that require concentration (Weinstein, 1974) and (iv) reduce cognitive stress by 11% (Seddigh et al., 2015). With these data, the relevance of good room acoustics to improve the wellbeing of workers, and consequently productivity, seems essential.

There are many architectural challenges when it comes to creating a good acoustic design for an open office. On one hand, different people, each one of them with his/her personality and performing a different task, have to be accommodated in open spaces having many potential distractions. On the other hand, room acoustics is often overlooked because, among other factors, it is not always clear whether it forms part of the structure (is it the property manager who must provide the conditioned space?) or whether it is an element of interior design that the client has to consider when occupying the space that he/she rents.

All in all, and in order to optimise the workspaces in terms of productivity and wellbeing of the staff, it is important to carry out an "activity based acoustic design". In so doing, besides the room itself (size? furniture density? linings? ...). one should also take into account both the type of activity carried out in the space (will it be a noisy activity? will confidentiality be needed? ...), as well as the people who work in it (age? number? personality? ...).

Schools

During lessons, students and teachers are exposed to various types of noise (outside noise, noise arising from the activity itself inside the classroom, HVAC systems...). During the last four decades, extensive research has been performed aiming at showing that excessive noise exposure has a detrimental effect on the cognitive development of children as well as negative effects on teachers. Good room acoustic design, in turn, can influence to a great extent the latter negative effects, highlighting the need of considering acoustics when designing classrooms. Just in that manner, quality teaching and learning will be enabled.

(Tiesler&Oberdöster, 2006) observed a direct relationship between greater background noise and increased pulse in teachers. Heart rhythm is a recognised medical stressor that should be kept under control as much as possible, since 80% of the teachers have reported stress in the class at some point of their career. In this study, the heart rate was diminished 10 bpm with "help" of good acoustic design.

In addition to increased heart rate due to stress, 65% of teachers have or will at some point have voice problems during their career (Durup, 2015). In fact, according to the American Speech-Language-Hearing Association (ASHA), they are 32 times more likely to suffer from voice-related problems than other workers with similar professions. In UK primary schools, for example, up to 73,000 sick leave days per year are recorded due to vocal problems among teachers (data from the Royal National Institute for the Deaf -RNID).

The results in (Dockrell&Shield, 2008) showed that all the students were affected by the presence of noise, and this was reflected in that they got worse grades. However, it was observed that children with special educational needs were more affected by noise and therefore their results worsened to a greater extent than students with normal hearing. In connection with the latter, high noise levels have been pointed out as having a negative impact on student behavior (Tiesler, 2018).

Good room acoustics has proved, amid other: (i) to increase concentration and reduce tiredness in pupils (Schönwälder, 2008), (ii) to improve academic grades (Klatte, 2009), and (iii) to reduce stress and voice problems of teachers (Dockrell&Shield, 2008).

Moreover, other school spaces like canteens, sport halls, corridors… are often louder than for example playgrounds and even heavy traffic, and thus also negatively influencing end-users' wellbeing. Those should also be properly addressed from an acoustic point of view.

Healthcare Facilities

In the year 1958, Florence Nightingale expressed in her *Notes on Nursing* the following words: *"Unnecessary noise is the cruelest absence of care which can be inflicted upon either the sick or well"*, and today after more than 100 years of research it is still a fact that we are still struggling with noise wherever people live, work, sleep and recover.

WHO guidelines (Berglund et al., 2005) recommend that average sound levels should not exceed 35 dB in most rooms in which patients are being treated or observed. Moreover, WHO states that in ward rooms, the equivalent sound levels should be 30 dB and the noise peaks during the night should not exceed 40 dB. Although the WHO guidelines are hard to reach in reality (30 dB is what one would have in a private bedroom), the fact that WHO stresses low sound pressure levels in hospitals is very positive.

Hospitals and healthcare facilities are today really complex buildings – someone might say small cities- and one thing is for sure: it is never totally quiet in a hospital. It works around the clock. According to (Busch-Vishniac et al., 2005), noise levels in hospitals have increased in recent years, both during daytime and nighttime. This can be due to several factors: more patient density, there are more machines that carry out more complex tasks, demographic changes, and in general more sound sources. What it has not been solved in parallel with the development of medical techniques and procedures is to control the situation in regards to sound. As an example, (Johansson et al, 2012) recorded in their study peak levels of 82–101 dB (like having a circular saw next to one). Exposure to high noise levels in healthcare facilities can have, according to (Weise, 2010), many negative effects on patients' and staff's health: impair sleep, increase stress, delay post-illness rehabilitation, aggravate agitation, cause psychiatric symptoms, escalate restlessness, increase respiratory rates and increase heart rates.

Many of the spaces within a hospital are places where crucial decisions are made. On the accuracy of those decisions relies the health of patients. Therefore, healthcare facilities should be designed in way that facilitate clear communication, avoid having to force one's voice and thus reducing stress and minimising the risk of errors. They should also provide wellbeing for patients, keeping noise levels low to facilitate getting proper sleep, which is essential for a speedy recovery. In line with the latter, (Lange et al, 2015) investigated the suitability of the sound environment in a modern intensive care unit (ICU) in promoting sleep by analysing continuous audio recordings captured over the course of three weeks. They discovered that a patient was interrupted in her/his sleep up to 167 times in a 24-hour period because of a highly disruptive noise environment. (Hagerman et al., 2005) observed, over eight weeks, the effect of an acoustic intervention in a hospital in Huddinge, Sweden. They monitored 94 patients suffering from chest pain and they concluded that reducing the noise levels and the reverberation in the spaces (through use of an acoustic class A absorbing ceiling), led not only to a 56% reduced hospital readmissions but also to a significant fall (67%) in the need for extra intravenous beta-blockers in the group during the period with good acoustics. The latter was in line with (Minckley, 1968), who also detected that medication intake increased with noise levels.

Regarding the staff, noise in emergency departments is regarded by 60.5% of staff as being "very" or "somewhat" burdensome (Simon. et al., 2010). According to (Joint Comission, 2010), 70% of critical medical errors in emergency departments can be traced back to "communication shortcomings" such as multitasking and interruptions. The latter is a very important fact to bear in mind, since (Woloshynowych et al., 2007) claimed that 83% of communication in an emergency department is speech related, thus room acoustics being of paramount importance. In fact, good room acoustics can reduce stress and errors in operating rooms (Beldam, 2019).

The helpless of course often suffer the most. In neonatal intensive care units (NICU), quiet time is extremely important for neonatal kids, and exposure to high noise levels can, amid others: decrease oxygen saturation, raise blood pressure, increase heart and respiratory rates, worsen sleep, expose the baby to higher cortisol levels and increased caloric expenditure, induce weight-related side-effects, (Brown, 2009 & Slevin et. al, 2000 & Johnson, 1995 & Zahr, 1995). Multiple recurrent episodes of noise-induced stress reactions can even lead to apnea and bradycardia, increasing the risk of hypoxic episodes as well as worsening of sensory development, speech and language (Brown, 2009). Likewise, exposure to high noise levels can correlate with future attention deficit hyperactivity disorder (ADHD) and abnormal brain development (Mann et al.,1986).

Age-related hearing loss (presbyacusis) causes communication problems for approximately 37% of people between the ages of 61 and 70. This prevalence rises to 60% for people aged 71 to 80 (Baur et al. 2009). Impaired hearing not only adversely affects spatial orientation and increases the risk of falling, but also turns communication into a real effort and causes rapid fatigue/exhaustion. Frequent misunderstandings are known to lead to withdrawal, self-doubt, depression and dogmatism (Arneborg, 2004) as well as becoming socially and intellectually isolated. The severity of hearing loss correlates with reduced cognition and an increased incidence of depression in old age (Cacciatore et al. 1999 & Dalton, 2003). Good room acoustics helps to ensure optimal hearing conditions for the elderly, regardless if it is in a nursery home, or in a hospital during a doctor appointment.

All in all, the design healthcare facilities cannot ignore acoustics if it intends to consider the wellbeing of both staff and patients.

Restaurants and Retail

The "acoustic environment" of these types of spaces is orchestrated by the management of the place in order to fulfil the particular desired purposes. With noise (unwanted) and sound (desired) the behaviour of the customers can be modified to some extent.

Retail: In (You Stop the Music: How Sounds in Retail Stores Divide Shoppers), some of the participants confessed that the music played in a particular store cheered them so much that they were concerned about behaving in an inappropriate way (dancing or singing) inside the store. Those who had negative responses, on the contrary, were consumers who felt that the music in certain stores was "discriminatory", in the sense that it seemed to be directed at particular gender or age groups that excluded them. Volume also proved to be another major source of concern; the greater the volume, the greater the "imposition" that buyers felt. Some avoided "noisy" retail spaces while others reported having bought faster than they would have liked.

However, the aforementioned so-called marketing techniques does not imply that one has to use high levels of noise, since it can be counter-productive and even produce health-related effects. In the questionnaires reported in (Alnuman, 2020), they showed that headaches and difficulties in communicating with others are the most common noise-induced problems among workers of shopping centres, those occurring in 47.1% and 38.2% of respondents respectively.

Restaurants: bars and restaurants are places identified with socialisation, friendship, relaxation; and factories of opportunities and inspiration. Unfortunately, noise levels there are often of such extent that having a conversation with the people one goes with becomes nearly impossible without having to strain one's voice, which is very harmful and will most likely increase clients' complaints. As a matter of fact, it was shown that noise bested poor service as the most annoying source of complaint for restaurants users (Zagat, 2018).

In (Biswas, 2019), low-volume music and noise were shown to increase healthy food sales due to induced relaxation, while high noise levels tended to increase levels of excitement and agitation, which in turn resulted in unhealthy food choices. Other studies have shown that increased noise levels can increase beverage consumption, as the "arousal" produced encourages one to drink faster and ask for more (Guéguen 2004 & Guéguen 2008). These noise levels (and their type) can even alter taste and smell (Stafford, 2012 & Woods, 2011 & Fiegel, 2014). The latter are factors that can often go counter good acoustic design and comfort in certain types of establishments due to increased revenue by the owners. However, in (Negreira et al., 2019), it was shown that in addition to acoustic comfort and clientele satisfaction (reported by means of questionnaires and also reflected in an increase on online ratings), good room acoustics can also increase the revenue of a restaurant (11% in this particular case, with a ROI of 4 months).

BASIC ACOUSTICS

Soundwaves

Sound occurs when particles in the air are set into motion. When a sound source starts (e.g. a person talking, a dog barking, a loudspeaker playing music…) it creates differences of pressure in a medium (air, other fluids or solids, but not in vacuum), which in turn produces vibrations/oscillations in its particles. These particles create sound energy that travels in form of pressure waves until they reach our ears (at a speed of approximately 340 metres per seconds in the air). In the following, the main parameters needed in order to describe a sound are delved into. For the sake of simplicity, air will be considered as the sound propagation medium hereafter.

Sound Pressure Level (SPL) – dB and dBA

The sound level indicates how much energy the sound contains. The so-called amplitude of the wave is defined as the distance from a wave's crest to its trough. It is a measure of how much an air particle deviates from its equilibrium position when the pressure differences are created by the sound source. It is directly related to the amount of energy that the sound contains, which is in turn called the sound level – measured in decibels (dB).

The decibel scale is not linear, but logarithmic. This unit is used to express a change in value with respect to a reference. In acoustics (when calculating sound pressure level –SPL) this reference is considered to be $p_{ref}=20\ \mu Pa=2\cdot 10^{-5}$ Pa (corresponding to the minimum pressure difference our hearing system can theoretically detect around 1 kHz). The latter is done in order to palliate the fact that our auditory system is able to perceive a very wide range of pressure differences, i.e. it would not be practical to work with pressure units. Moreover, our hearing system reacts in a logarithmic way to sounds. The SPL (L_p) of a given sound during a certain time, producing a certain air pressure $\tilde{p}$ (which is the root-mean-square RMS of a given signal, i.e. some sort of average) can be calculated as:

$$L_p = 10 \cdot \log\left(\frac{\tilde{p}^2}{p_{ref}^2}\right) = 20 \cdot \log\left(\frac{\tilde{p}}{p_{ref}}\right).$$

SPL is frequency-dependent, although average values of many frequencies are often given. Without going into too much detail (it is outside the scope of this chapter), let's give an example: if a person speaking produces a sound pressure difference in the air of 0.02 Pa, then the SPL is:

$$L_p = 10 \cdot \log\left(\frac{0.02^2}{\left(2\cdot 10^{-5}\right)^2}\right) = 20 \cdot \log\left(\frac{0.02}{2\cdot 10^{-5}}\right) = 60\,\text{dB}.$$

The latter result is a way to express, in a "handy" way, that the person talking is creating in the air a SPL 1000 times higher than the minimum pressure difference a person without hearing loss could detect (i.e. $0.002/2\cdot 10^{-5}=1000$). Then, a dB-value is assigned to that. 60 dB is the typical conversation sound level at 1 metre distance. Instead, if the person would be screaming, creating a difference in air pressure 10000 times more than the minimum detectable (i.e. $0.2/2\cdot 10^{-5}=1000$), the SPL would now be instead, 80 dB.

Sometimes, instead of dB, SPLs are expressed in the units of dBA. Since human hearing is not equally sensitive to all frequencies (i.e. it feels different frequencies differently loud even if the theoretical "volume" in dB is the same), the sound signals are filtered so that the properties of human hearing are mimicked. Thus, low frequencies are weighted favourably (people are not that sensitive to them) while high-pitch frequencies are "punished" (see Table 1). For example, if a SPL of L_p=65 dB is measured at 500 Hz, it would correspond to a SPL, in dBA, of L_{pA}=(65-3.2)=61.8 dBA, which correlates better with how humans perceive sound. Again, average values are commonly encountered. In this way, it is not possible to transform from dBA to dB (and vicecersa) since it is not possible to "decompose" the average values into different SPL values for each frequency.

Table 1. dBA-filter

Frequency	125	250	500	1000	2000	4000	8000
dBA filter	-16.1	-8.6	-3.2	0	1.2	1	-1.1

As a summary, and aiming at giving the reader some understanding while keeping the topic "simple", some ideas/concepts about SPL are given hereunder:

- With individual exceptions depending on many factors (e.g. age, genetics), people can hear from 0 dB to the "pain threshold" of 120 dB (above which level permanent hearing damages can occur), see Fig. 17. A normal conversation is often held at a level of 60 dB (at 1 metre distance from the speaker). For typical SPL values, see Table 2.
- The SPL depends on the distance between the sound source and the listener/place of measurement. L_p should always be given, for a meaningful interpretation, accompanied by the distance.
    - In indoor spaces, a decrease of -3 dB is expected with doubling the distance. Where no reflections are present (outdoors, i.e. so-called free-field) the reduction with distance-doubling is -6 dB. E.g., if inside a classroom a measurement of 57 dB is reported 2 metres from the teacher, it can be stated that at 4 metres, the SPL will equal 54 dB (57-3).
- Levels of exposure above 80 dB during long periods of time can be harmful for the health.
- An increase in the sound level by 10 dB corresponds to the sensation of double the "volume".
- Due to the logarithmic properties, a doubling in the number of (equal) sound sources imply an increase in SPL of 3 dB. For example, if an engine produces 75 dB, two identical engines would generate (75+3) = 78 dB.
- Loudness and volume are psychoacoustic terms, meaning that they account for the subjective sound-sensation, which is not clearly measurable without ambiguity. Loudness correlates not only with physical strength (amplitude), but also with other parameters (frequency, spectral composition, duration of exposure…). The same sound will not create the same loudness perception by all individuals (people).
- Other sound-related quantities often expressed in dB:
    - Sound power: power emitted by the sound source. Sound power levels are connected to the sound source and are independent of distance (unlike SPL).
    - Sound intensity: its numerical value is coincident with the SPL values in dB (due to the reference quantity chosen). However, whereas SPL is a field quantity (i.e. defined by a value at a point –like temperature for instance), sound intensity is an energy quantity (besides de numerical value, it also needs a direction –e.g. like speed).

Wavelength and Frequency

The wavelength (denoted by the Greek letter Lambda λ) determines the timbre or the pitch of the sound (frequency); it is the distance (in metres) that it takes for a wave to complete a full cycle. The number of entire cycles per unit of time (second) determines the frequency of the wave and is measured in Hertz (Hz).

Table 2. Typical SPL values

Sound source (examples)	SPL (L_p) in dB
Aircraft (50 metres away)	130
Pain threshold	120
Circular saw (at 1 metre distance)	110
Club with loud music (at 1 metre distance)	100
Vacuum cleaner (at 1 metre distance)	70
Normal conversation (at 1 metre distance)	60
Library	40
Quiet bedroom at night	30
Hearing threshold	0

The audible spectrum is roughly between 20 and 20000 Hz, going from a dark (low frequency, e.g. traffic or HVAC noise) to a bright (high frequency, i.e. an alarm) timbre. The lower the frequency, the longer the wavelength (see Fig. 1). Due to the latter phenomenon, it is often harder to absorb/isolate lower frequencies. This is because the wave, when it impinges against a given surface (e.g. acoustic ceiling), does not need to go through that many cycles inside the material as a high frequency wave, thus loosing energy. Generalising, the thicker the tile of the acoustic ceiling, the better the absorption at low frequencies. This can also be compensated by the distance between the soffit and the suspended ceiling –the lower the installation, the better low frequency absorption.

Figure 1. Example/scheme of a low frequency wave (left) and a high frequency wave (right).

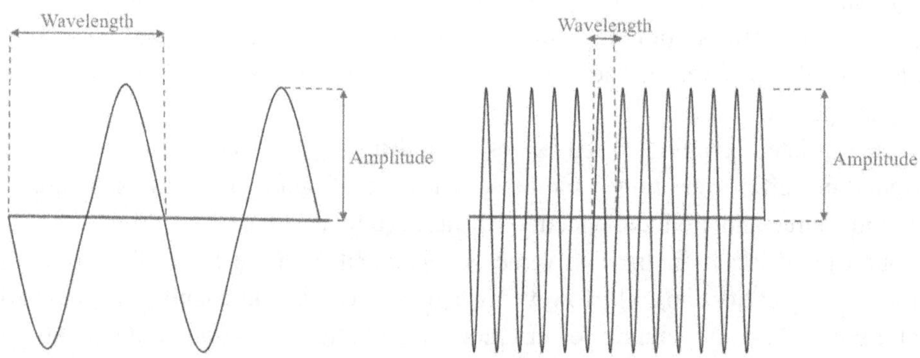

Let the time it takes for the high frequency wave of Fig. 1 to go through the 13 cycles shown be 0.013 seconds. Thus, the frequency of the wave would be:

$$f_{high} = \frac{\text{number of oscillations}}{\text{time}} = \frac{13}{0.013} = 1000\,\text{Hz}.$$

The low frequency wave, instead, would have (assuming the same time):

$$f_{low} = \frac{\text{number of oscillations}}{\text{time}} = \frac{2}{0.013} = 154\text{Hz}.$$

The two above calculations correspond to the simplest representation of a sound, i.e. the so-called tone (a sound composed of just one frequency). This is (simplifying) how pressing a key in a piano would sound like. However, in reality, sounds are composed of many more frequencies (depending of the type of sound), see Fig. 2. For example, a loudspeaker through which music is played sends out many instruments with many different frequencies simultaneously. These frequencies bounce around the room and the design will have to be addressed and adapted to this. In order to enable acoustic comfort, the designer has to analyse the sound sources, the absorption of the linings, the room shape, and the like.

Figure 2. Graphic representation of a tone (left) and a sound comprised of many frequencies (right).

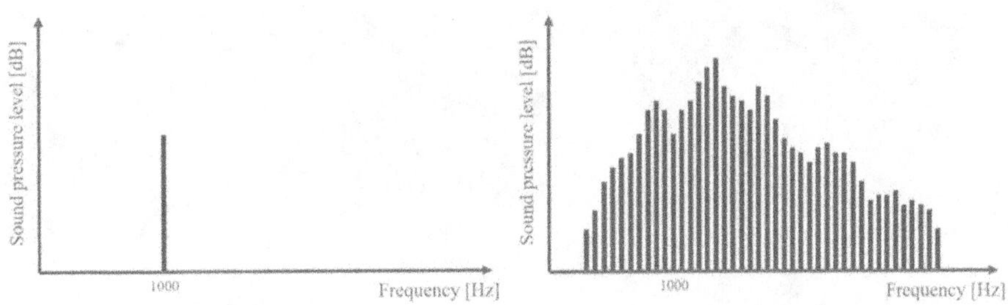

For the sake of simplicity, the spectrum (different frequencies) is often divided into frequency bands, where each band embraces and averages a certain frequency range. Within room acoustics, one typically works with the frequency bands of 125 Hz, 250 Hz, 500 Hz, 1000 Hz, 2000 Hz and 4000 Hz. These frequencies are those inside which the human voice falls.

The speed of sound c[m/s] in a medium (often air in the case of room acoustics) relates the wavelength of a sound λ[m] with its frequency f[Hz] according to the following equation:

$$\lambda = \frac{c}{f}.$$

Thus, a 1000 Hz wave would have a wavelength (in the air) of λ.340/1000=3.4 m.

Acoustic Absorption

When a sound wave hits one of the surfaces of a room (wall, ceiling or floor), part of the sound energy is reflected back to the room, another part penetrates into the surface (being absorbed and turned into heat – the amount depending on the material in question), and the rest is transmitted to other rooms (cf. Fig. 3).

Figure 3. Graphical definition of sound absorption: incident (3), absorbed (2), transmitted (1) and reflected (4) energy. Source of figure: Saint-Gobain Ecophon.

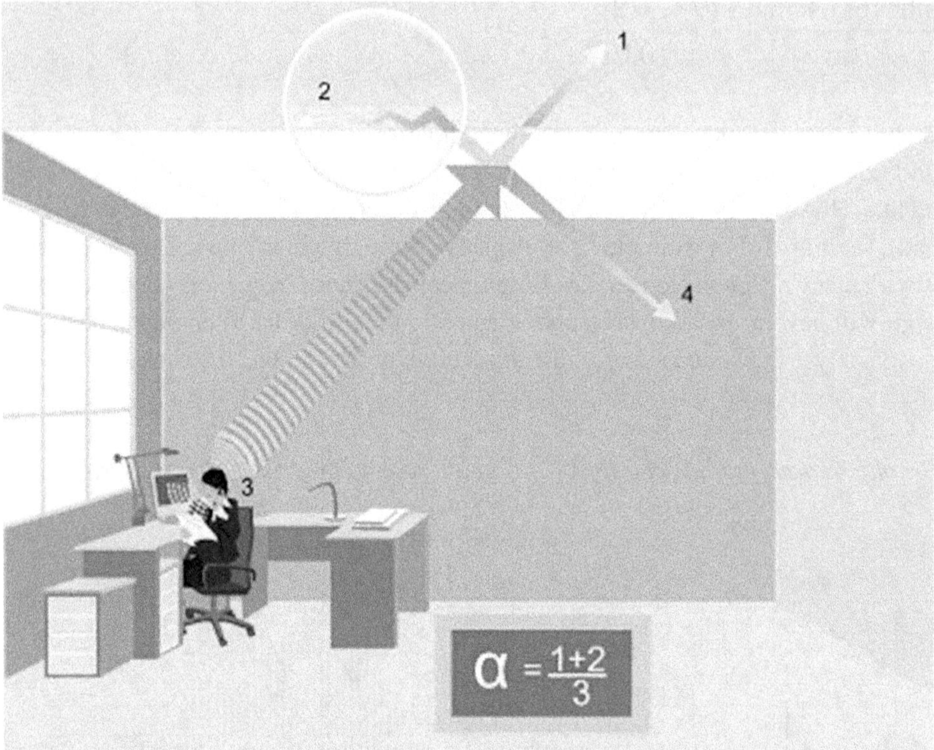

Acoustic absorption is defined as the ability of a material to convert the incident sound energy into heat; that is, the amount of energy that is not sent back into the room once it hits its surface. It is denoted by the Greek letter alpha (α) and it varies between 0 (a fully reflective material) and 1 (total absorption). It is a parameter of paramount importance when it comes to room acoustics of ordinary spaces, since it helps reducing reverberation, improving speech clarity and reducing sound propagation and sound strength.

The sound absorption coefficient of a material is measured following the test method outlined in the international standard EN ISO 354. The American "equivalent" standard is ASTM C 423. Although in general terms the two previous standards are similar, there are some differences between them. For the sake of simplicity, no further details regarding these will be given; just the general procedure will be explained.

Measurements are ideally made in a reverberation chamber (i.e. a room whose linings are very reflective), ensuring the existence of a diffuse field (that is, the sound has angles of incidence evenly distributed against the surface of the object to be measured). All the latter implies high reverberation and high sound levels, as well as low intelligibility inside that space. The measurement procedure is carried out by measuring the reverberation time in two different scenarios:

1) first with the empty room,
2) after introducing the material to be tested into the room (the area of the specimen of the absorbent material has to be sufficient for the measurements to yield relevant data).

The difference in reverberation time between the results of these two measurement results (having in mind that all the other parameters –linings, volume- are kept constant) allows one to determine the absorption coefficient α of the material in question (see Fig. 4).

Figure 4. Left: Scheme of the layout used for absorption coefficient measurements according to ISO 354. A reverberant chamber of volume V with diffusers (in order to assure a diffuse field inside the space) is shown together with the material of area S whose absorption (α) is to be measured. Right: laboratory technician preparing a measurement campaign according to ISO 354. Source: Saint-Gobain Ecophon.

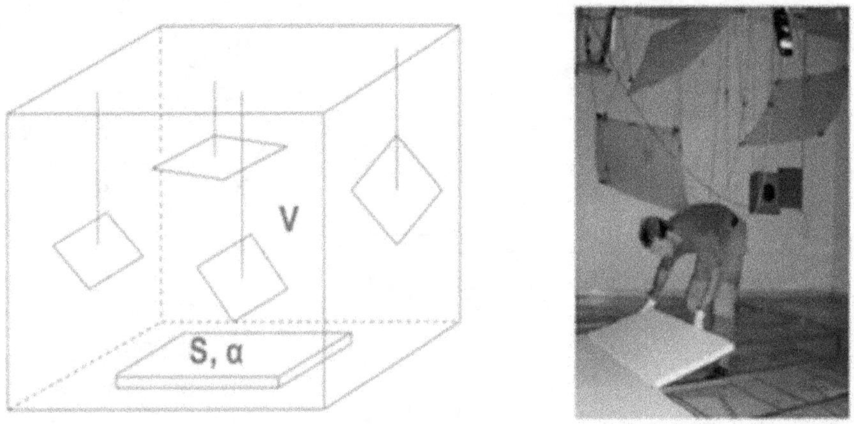

Single Value Absorption Indexes

The absorption, and therefore the reverberation time, depend on the frequency; that is, a material can absorb differently at different frequencies due to the variation in wavelengths (see Fig. 1). Thus, the result of this test is a curve that gives us the practical absorption coefficient α_p for each octave of frequency (see Fig. 5). α_p is an indicator of how well (installed in a particular manner) absorbs sound, and is expressed as a percentage. The values therefore range (theoretically) between 0 (fully reflective material) and 1 (fully absorbent material). For example, an α_p of 0.75 means that 75% of the sound energy that hits the material is absorbed and not returned (reflected) back to the room. Note that sometimes, instead of the practical absorption coefficient α_p (in octaves), values of α_s in third octave bands (i.e. more resolution) are given (for the sake of simplicity, only α_p will be shown).

Having a frequency-dependent absorption can sometimes make communication between professionals difficult, especially for those not having a basic understanding of acoustics, neither it is practical. The ISO 11654 standard proposes a method to obtain a single value weighted absorption coefficient α_w that, in some way, summarises the overall performance of an acoustic solution in terms of acoustic absorption. In addition, the standard also sets a classification in which acoustic absorption classes of materials are established based on α_w (Table 3). Along with the absorption class of the material, the plenum/ods (overall depth of the system – distance from the floor to the soffit) must also be specified in order to fairly compare different test results.

In a graphical way (Fig. 6), the influence of the weighted absorption coefficient could be illustrated as follows. Let an area of 10 m^2 be a particular soffit, which is lined with an acoustic ceiling. If the ceiling

Figure 5. Example of results of a sound absorption coefficient measurement (per octave band frequency) according to ISO 354. The room acoustic solution tested is the acoustic ceiling Saint-Gobain Ecophon Master A (glasswool, 40 mm tiles), with an ods (overall depth of the system –distance from ceiling to soffit) of 200 mm. The results are performed by the laboratory CSTB on behalf of Ecophon.

RESULTS

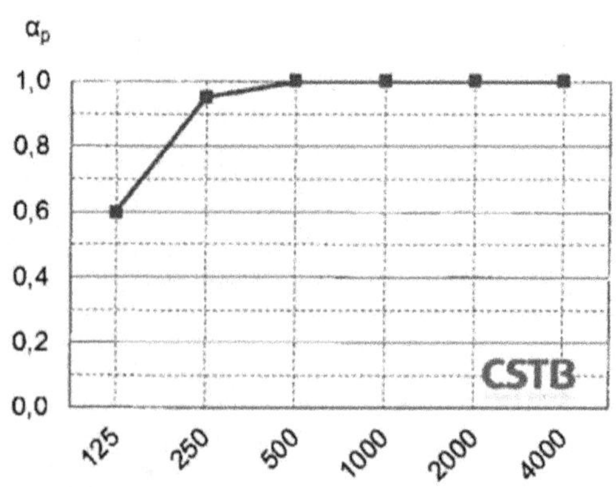

f	α_p
125	0,60
250	0,95
500	1,00
1000	1,00
2000	1,00
4000	1,00
Hz	

α_w= 1,00
classement / class: A

It is strongly recommended to use this single number rating in combination with the complete sound absorption coefficient curve.

is Class C (e.g. $\alpha_w = 0.6$), it could be stated that only 60% of the material is “actively” of “effectively” absorbing noise, while the remaining 30% would be reflecting. However, if the α_w is instead 0.97 (that is, Class A absorber), almost all the material installed in the ceiling (except 3%) would be absorbing noise. The latter means that one would optimise, to some extent, the use of the material and money spent on the ceiling the higher the absorption class is.

Sometimes, instead of α_w, the “American version” NRC (Noise Reduction Coefficient, measured according to the standard ASTM C 423) is stated in the specification sheets of an acoustic solution. In the same way as α_w, NRC is an average indicator that indicates a percentage of energy absorbed by a material. Although they are similar, neither of the descriptors can be directly deduced from the other,

Table 3. Table B1 of ISO 11654 – sound absorption classes

Sound absorption class	α_w
A	0.90; 0.95; 1.00
B	0.80; 0.85
C	0.60; 0.65; 0.70, 0.75
D	0.30; 0.35; 0.40; 0.45; 0.50; 0.55
E	0.25; 0.20; 0.15
Not classified	0.10; 0.05; 0.00

Figure 6. Graphic representation of the "meaning" of α_w. The higher the α_w, the more effective absorption area included (thus improving room acoustics).

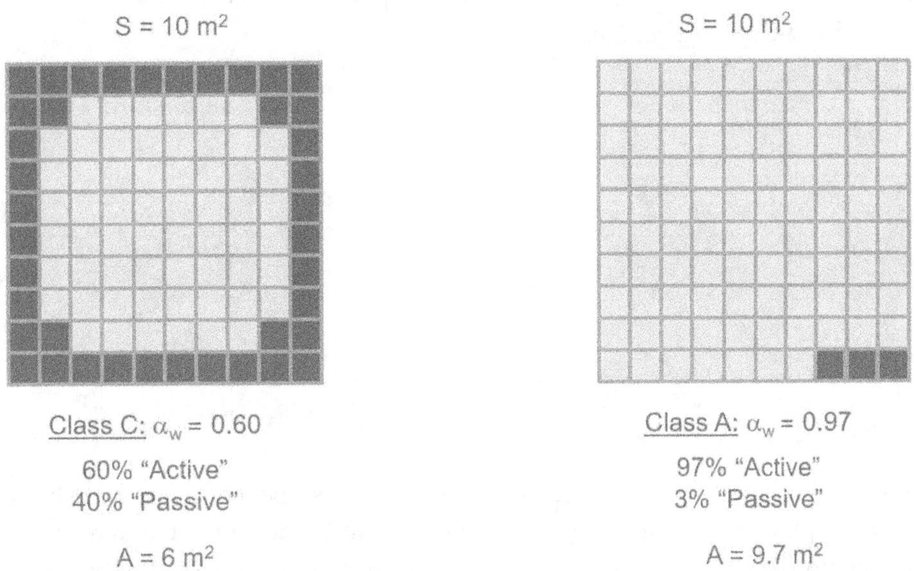

since there is no mathematical relationship between them. This is due to the way these indicators are obtained. While α_w uses a method of comparing the practical absorption coefficient α_p with a reference curve (giving different weights to different frequencies between 125 Hz and 4000 Hz), NRC makes a simple arithmetic mean (giving the same weight to all frequencies) of the α_p values (of 250 Hz, 500 Hz, 1000 Hz and 2000 Hz) obtained in the test. Furthermore, NRC ignores frequencies below 250 Hz and above 2 kHz. However, in most cases, the reality is that both indexes are used interchangeably when doing basic calculations (depending on the norms used and/or the data available).

NRC is sometimes substituted for the SAA (Sound Absorption Average) value, which is also defined in the standard ASTM C423. The difference between NRC and SAA is that the SAA value is the average of the practical absorption coefficients α_p of the thirds of an octave (12 in total) ranging from 200 to 2500 Hz (that is, it includes more values in the mean, but it still does not give different weights to low and high frequencies). However, its use is not as common as NRC.

Another index often employed is α_m (for example, in the Spanish Building Regulations – CTE DB HR). This index is simply obtained as an arithmetic mean of the absorption coefficient at 500, 1000 and 2000 Hz. It is often also used interchangeably with NRC and α_w for calculations. In Appendix 2, a short list with typical absorption values for different materials can be found.

Free Hanging Units (FHUs)

In the case of baffles and rafts, measuring the practical absorption coefficient α_p can be difficult. If the absorbent is small or does not have a well-defined surface that is exposed to sound, it is not relevant or possible to calculate the absorption coefficient (Fig. 7). In these cases, the standards in force advice to use the absorption per object A_{obj} instead. Being able to have an absorption area per object is a very useful and important property of the Sabine equation (which will be seen later on), which means that

Figure 7. Absorption measurements according to ISO 354. Left: procedure for a full ceiling (easy to determine the area exposed to sound). Right: FHU (e.g. acoustic raft) where the surface exposed to sound is harder to determine and thus the absorption is given by means of absorption area per object. Source of figure: Saint-Gobain Ecophon.

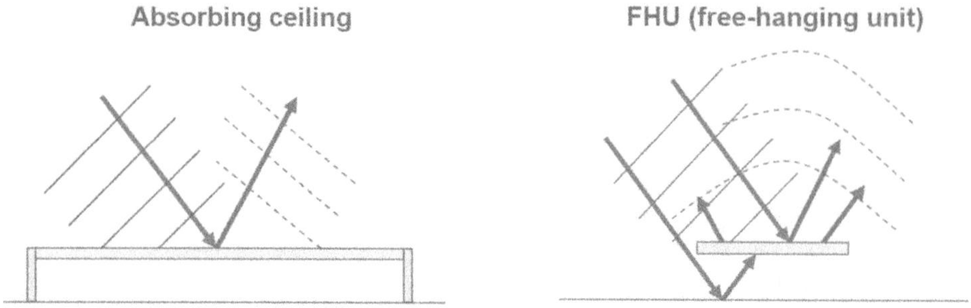

even for "non-flat" objects such as furniture, people, etc., the absorbent efficiency can be quantified by the equivalent absorption area expressed in m^2 per object. The procedure to measure is also defined in the ISO 354 standard. The best way to compare an absorbent ceiling with a raft or baffle is to calculate the reverberation time for each room and situation.

Figure 8. Typical laboratory layout (with diffusers hanging) of a measurement of absorption in FHUs according to ISO 354 (left) and a picture of an office hall with FHUs Ecophon Solo Square. Source of figure and picture: Saint-Gobain Ecophon.

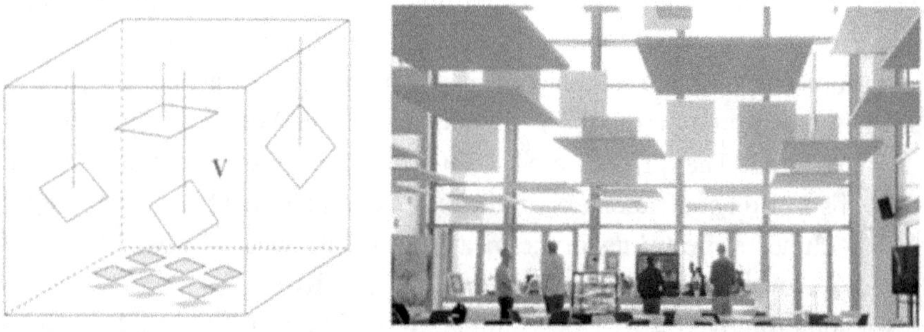

In Figure 8, the measurement procedure to obtain the equivalent absorption area for rafts or baffles as individual objects is shown. As in the case of absorbent ceilings, a difference in absorption area is obtained by measuring the difference in reverberation time with the reverberation chamber full and empty. Normally more than one FHU is needed to perform the measurements so that the changes in reverberation time during measurements are noticeable. Subsequently, this difference in absorption area is divided by the number of FHUs that were considered during the test, thus obtaining the absorption area in m^2 per one object (Fig. 9).

Figure 9. Example of results of the sound absorption measurements according to ISO 354. The room acoustic solution tested is the FHU (raft) Saint-Gobain Ecophon Solo 2400x1200 mm (glasswool, 40 mm tiles), with an ods (overall depth of the system –distance from ceiling to soffit) of 400 mm. The results are performed by the laboratory CSTB on behalf of Ecophon.

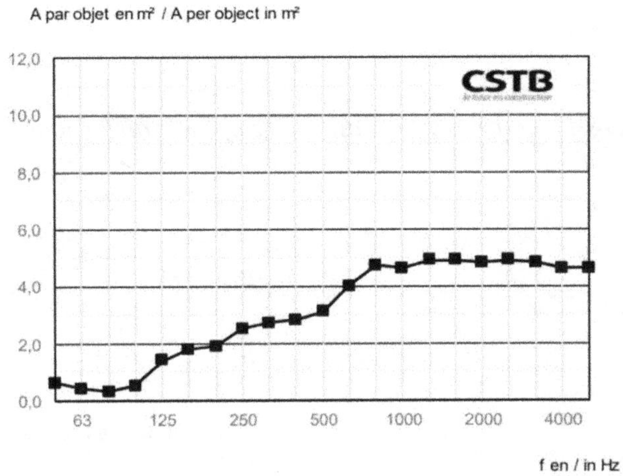

f	A_{obj}	
	1/3 Octave band	Octave band
50	0,6	
63	0,4	0,4
80	0,3	
100	0,5	
125	1,4	1,2
160	1,8	
200	1,9	
250	2,5	2,4
315	2,7	
400	2,8	
500	3,1	3,3
630	4,0	
800	4,7	
1000	4,6	4,7
1250	4,9	
1600	4,9	
2000	4,8	4,9
2500	4,9	
3150	4,8	
4000	4,6	4,7
5000	4,6	
Hz	m²	

Types of Absorbers

In general terms and in a simplified way, the following types absorbers can be distinguished:

- Porous absorbers: they are composed of an open-cell solid skeleton (e.g. mineral wool) surrounded by air, where sound can travel through from one end to the other. When sound impinges onto a porous absorber, it penetrates in it due to the small dimensions of the pores. Losses, i.e. absorption, occur due to thermal conduction and viscous friction. They are very effective absorbers, especially in mid- and high-frequencies; in low frequencies, the thickness of the material and/or the overall depth of the system has to be increased to gain absorption to compensate for the longer wavelengths. Their absorption depends on the thickness, mounting conditions, porosity, density and air flow resistivity. These are the most versatile and widely used absorbers for ordinary spaces.
- Membrane absorbers: they consist of a non-porous and flexible panel placed at a certain distance from the partition or floor. By utilising the resonant properties of the membrane they are able to absorb sound over a narrow frequency range when sound energy is dissipated by means of the plate vibration.
- Resonators: aka Helmholtz resonators. Comprised of a volume of air (behaving as a spring) contained in a cavity with at least one opening connected to the room through a neck (whose air behaves as a mass). These two elements (spring-mass) give rise to a resonant system, which will present an absorption peak at that particular resonance frequency. Their principle is the same as a

glass bottle when blowing air into it (i.e. the "effectively-absorbed" frequency is the one can hear when blowing air into the bottle). Slat absorbers also share the same absorption mechanism.

- Multiple resonators/perforated plates: It consists of a thin flat plate with small holes punched in it. Their absorption principle is similar to the resonators described above. However, often an acoustic porous lining is installed on top of the plate so that it widens the bandwidth of absorption. The absorption depends on the diameter and percentage of perforations, the mounting conditions as well as the quality of the acoustic lining.

Figure 10. Different types of absorbers together with a schematic curve of their absorption coefficient. Source of figures: Saint-Gobain Ecophon.

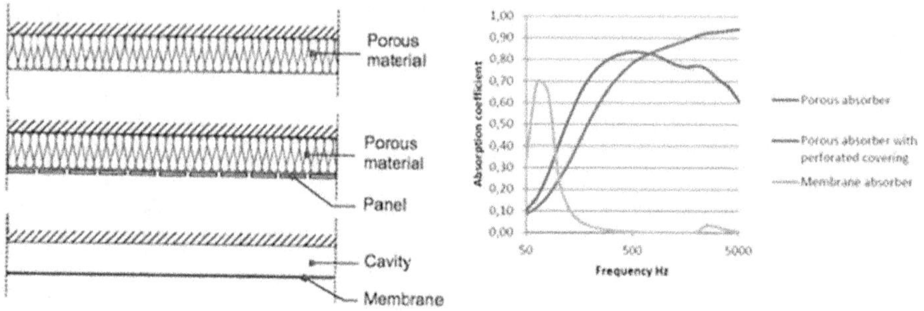

Acoustic Parameters

International standards facilitate that things work as intended, through regulations, recommendations or definition of test or calculation methods. They provide worldwide recognised specifications for products, services and systems alike. The standards also ensure that companies operate safely, efficiently and provide a high quality product or service to their customers. Fortunately, the "acoustic awareness" about the impact that noise has on our daily lives and our health, regardless of the environment considered (work, school, hospital...), is growing. Due to the latter, the development of acoustic norms is proliferating little by little, although more research is still needed in order to optimise and adapt to each type of space the room acoustic descriptors. In the following section, several room acoustic parameters will be described (some of them specified in national and international standards).

Reverberation Time

The reverberation time is defined in the standard ISO 3382 series as the time it takes (in seconds) for a sound to decrease its noise level by 60 dB after the source emission has stopped. Reverberation time is most commonly measured, for practical reasons, through a decay of 20 or 30 dB (denoted T_{20} and T_{30} respectively), 5 dB after the excitation noise ceases, and then extrapolated to the full 60 dB range (denoted T_{60}). The general nomenclature can also be T or RT (reverberation time).

Figure 11. Graphical representation of the reverberation time (T, in seconds). The RT may be different for different frequencies due to the absorption of the materials being often frequency dependent.

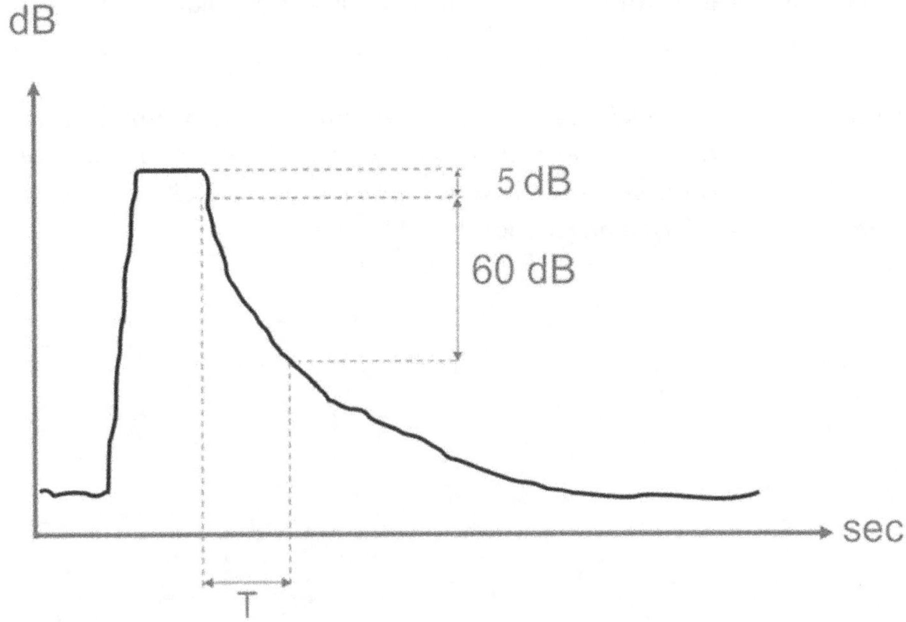

The reverberation time informs us about how long the sounds remain in a room before they disappear. The reverberation time is directly proportional to the volume (that is, the more volume a space has, the greater the reverberation is) and inversely proportional to the absorption (the more absorption that is entered into the space, the more the reverberation is reduced). The RT is calculated according to an equation often referred to as Sabine's law:

$$T_{60} = 0.16 \cdot \frac{V}{A}.$$

where V [m^3] is the volume of the enclosure considered and A [m^{2}Sabine] or simply given in [m^2] is the equivalent absorption area; that is, the sum of the "absorption efficiencies" of all linings in the space. It indicates how much sound is really being absorbed, and it can be expressed as:

$$A = \sum_{i=1}^{n} \alpha_{w,i} \cdot S_i.$$

being $\alpha_{w,i}$ the weighted absorption coefficient of each one of the materials present in the room, and S_i their corresponding physical surface (length times width in case of a rectangular area for example - see Figure 6).

The absorption of each material is dependent on the frequency, and thus so will be the reverberation time (see Fig. 12). However, the requirements in standards are often expressed in average values of different frequencies. For more information on acoustic absorption, see the corresponding section in this chapter.

Figure 12. Graphic representation of RT (in seconds on the horizontal axis) in thirds octave bands. Note that low frequencies tend to have more reverberation (that is, they take longer to disappear) than high / high frequencies. The image corresponds to measurements made with a B&K 2270 sound level metre and post-processed with the B&K Qualifier software.

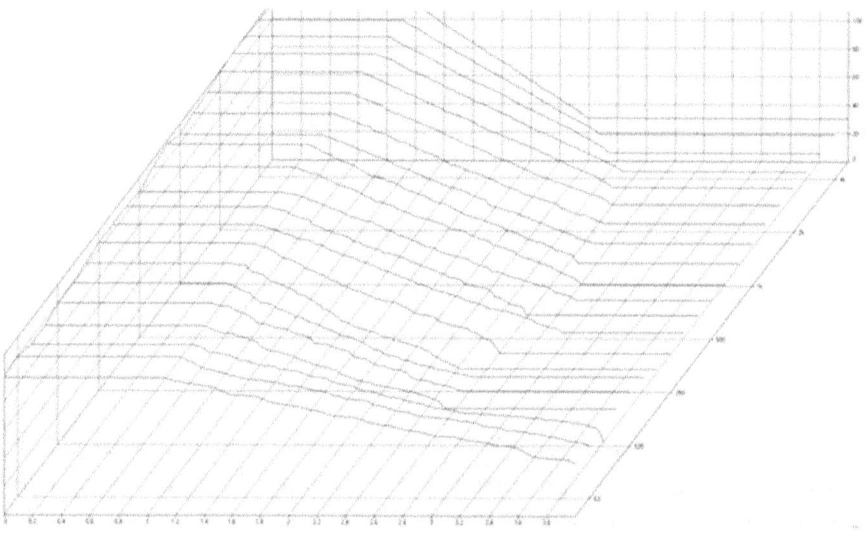

Sabine's law starts from the hypothesis of the existence of a diffuse field (that is, that the sound has angles of incidence evenly distributed against a surface of the enclosure). This is difficult to achieve in reality due to the (usually) non-homogenous distribution of the absorption in ordinary rooms (often, if present, the absorption is installed on the ceiling).

In order to illustrate how different actions in a room can modify the reverberation time of a space, the following example (together with Fig.13) is given:

- *"Sabine"*: shows the line predicted by the use of Sabine's law (a diffuse field which implies a uniform estimated decay).
- *"No boxes":* room with a Class A acoustic absorbent ceiling. It can be seen as:
    - Firstly, the sound pressure decreases (in the upper left corner) with a certain slope/incline.
    - After a while (by decreasing -10 dB in this case), the angle of the decay curve changes slightly, becoming "slower" than in the first part. This is due to the fact that initially the sound corresponding to the vertical reflections that impact directly on the ceiling is absorbed (where the absorption is concentrated). Once these reflections are absorbed, there are still

many reflections parallel to the ceiling and floor (called grazing field) that bounce between parallel walls, since their absorption is very low.

- *"Boxes on the wall":* if objects to one of the walls are added, they do not only absorb sound, but they do make the acoustic field more diffuse (by spreading the sound). In this way, it is clearly depicted how the curve gets closer to the "Sabine" case.

Therefore, it can be seen that with several room acoustic solutions combined, the RT can be modified. Starting from an absorption in the ceiling to lower noise levels, one can then further reduce the RT (and improve other parameters), for example, by introducing irregularities so that the sound field becomes more diffuse (through furniture, absorption in the walls...). Due to the fact that in reality the field is rarely diffuse, when calculating RT of ordinary rooms using Sabine's law, one could be underestimating the real RT (measured and perceived by end-users). Sabine's law can, nevertheless, give a fairly good orientation of the RT in a space; and many standards recommend its use.

Figure 13. Reverberation time measurements with different room acoustic treatments. Source of graphics: Saint-Gobain Ecophon.

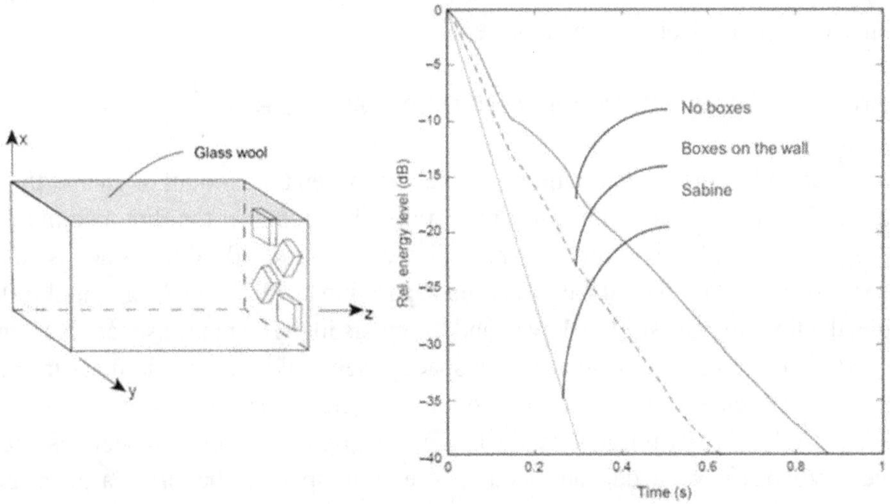

Some things that are worth keeping in mind regarding reverberation time are:

- Often T_{20} is used in practice. This means that the slope of the decay curve is evaluated in the rage -5 dB to -25 dB (instead of -5 to 60 dB according to the definition).
- EDT (early decay time), defined as the RT measured during the first 10 dB decay is sometimes used as an indicator; since it does not disregard the early reflections of the sound (i.e. the first 5 dB decay). Due to that, it is considered to be more related to the subjective performance of sound, since the early reflections affect the comfort of the end users.
- At steady-state circumstances, i.e. when a constant sound power is fed into the room, the sound field is fairly diffuse in the sense that waves are travelling in all directions and the use of practical

absorption factors is suitable. However, during the decay process, i.e. after the sound source is turned off, the sound field will become non-diffuse and normally the measured reverberation times are longer than estimated by Sabine formula (cf. Fig. 13).

- In rooms with acoustic ceilings, the RT is not only dependent on the amount of absorption in the room and the room volume as stated by Sabine's law. In these rooms, the reverberation time is influenced by:
    - The volume and shape of the room.
    - The absorption of the acoustic ceiling. Especially the absorption for waves that hit the ceiling surface at large (steep) angles of incidence (grazing waves).
    - The amount of sound scattering and absorbing furniture and equipment in the room. Especially scattering objects along the walls are important for the sound diffusion.
    - The absorption for walls and floor.
    - At high frequencies, there will even be a small contribution due to the air absorption.
- The Just Noticeable Difference (JND), i.e. the RT minimum difference that people are able to detect is, according to the norm ISO 3382-1, 5%.

Reverberation time is often the only parameter regulated in room acoustic regulations (for the sake of simplicity, National Standards will not be described in this chapter). In Appendix 1, an example of RT calculation according to Sabine's law is presented.

Speech Clarity and Other Intelligibility-Related Parameters

Speech clarity is defined as the relationship, in decibels, between the amount of energy that reaches the listener in the first 50 milliseconds (i.e. early reflections that enhance the direct sound) with respect to the energy arriving after those 50 milliseconds. The threshold of 50 milliseconds is considered (for ordinary spaces and speech) as the critical time limit separating useful from detrimental reflections. For younger people, the limit may be slightly lower, and for music in performance spaces is 80 milliseconds.

C_{50} is derived from the impulse response of a space when making acoustic measurements. It is an objective measure of the clarity or intelligibility of speech; the fewer late reflections and the larger the density of direct sound and early reflections, the better. The higher its value, in decibels, the more intelligible the speech will be (its value depending on the use of the space). The formula can be expressed as:

$$C_{50}\left[\mathrm{dB}\right]=10\cdot\log\left(\frac{\mathrm{energy}\left(0-50\,\mathrm{ms}\right)}{\mathrm{energy}\left(50\,\mathrm{ms}-\infty\right)}\right).$$

The speech clarity is influenced by:

- The location and the amount of absorption (e.g. an absorbing wall panel on the rear wall in large/long rooms reduces late reflections).
- Reflecting surfaces, preferably close to the speaker or sound source, will increase the speech clarity as it enhances the direct sound towards the listeners.

- The shape of the room: it is preferable to have a room shape that supports a short distance between the speaker and the listeners.
- The signal to noise ratio (i.e. the speech level in relation to the background noise): the higher it is (due to noise being prominent over the non-desired sound) the better
- Sound-scattering objects on the walls or wall absorbers: these will help eliminating disturbing echoes that can occur between walls ("flutter echo").

Sometimes, the clarity of speech is expressed in percentage, with a parameter called definition (D_{50}[%]), which is also related through a mathematical formula with the clarity of speech, according to:

$$D_{50}\left[\%\right]=\frac{\text{energy}\left(0-50\text{ms}\right)}{\text{energy}\left(50\text{ms}-\infty\right)}.$$

$$C_{50}\left[\text{dB}\right]=10\cdot\log\left(\frac{D_{50}}{1-D_{50}}\right).$$

A speech clarity value of 0 dB means that the same number of early reflections (0-50 ms) as late (50 ms – final) exist, while a negative value means that there are more late than early reflections (poor intelligibility). Acceptable values depend on the use and volume of the room being studied. To give some guidance, from 2-3 dB the clarity would already be quite good. Values of 6 dB would imply very good clarity. A C_{50}=3 dB value, for example, would mean that there is 1000 times more early energy in the first 50 milliseconds than there is from the 50 milliseconds to the end. A value of C_{50} = 8 dB corresponds (according to the formula) to a definition of D_{50} = 0.86 (86% of the energy is in the 0-50 milliseconds time window).

Another intelligibility-related parameter is the speech transmission index (aka. STI). In the same way as definition (D_{50}), STI is an expression of how large a percentage of the speech is understandable. STI=1 corresponds to 100%, STI=0.75 corresponds to 75%, etc. Speech transmission is standardised in the norm IEC 60268-16. In contrast to speech clarity, which is a parameter extracted from the impulse response of the room, STI considers the listener and the source position.

The parameters C_{50} and STI have already been introduced in several national standards (e.g. Italy, Norway and Hungary) for ordinary spaces, although it is nowadays still not common to encounter it. The Just Noticeable Difference (JND), i.e. the minimum C_{50} increment that people are able to detect is, according to the norm ISO 3382-1, 1 dB.

Sound Strength

Auditory strength is the level at which people experience sound. Measured in decibels, it quantifies how much of the sound reflected in a room contributes to the general sound level of the space; that is, it is an indicator of the natural amplification of the space due to its shape, volume and linings. The lower its value, the better (for places where a "calm" environment is desired, such as schools, offices or hospitals - in the case of an auditorium it would be different). In this way, the room will not amplify the sound and therefore the overall noise level will not increase.

The idea behind the measurement of sound strength is to measure the sound level produced by a calibrated source emitting noise in the room under study and compare it to the sound level that the same setup would produce inside an anechoic chamber (i.e. where reflections are non-existent). The sound level difference between both cases is due to the room reflections' effect on the sound level.

It is important consider the sound strength in a room where specifically noisy activities are carried out, since a high G value could imply that the noise level in the room could easily escalate. In addition to this, sound strength is important to pay attention to in small rooms with low reverberation time. A room may have a short RT and still contribute significantly to the noise level. The G value is therefore particularly useful for small spaces where the regulatory requirements may not be sufficient. Although the sound strength value depends on the usage of the room, a value lower than 20 dB is recommended for ordinary spaces. A room with low sound strength affects the behaviour of users, tending to speak lower, something similar to what happens when one enters a library, in which the general noise level is low and there is no need to raise the voice. The Just Noticeable Difference (JND), i.e. the minimum G increment that people are able to detect is, according to the norm ISO 3382-1, 1 dB.

Strength is mainly influenced by:

- The sound absorption of the room.
- Distance between sound source and receiver.

All in all, it can be concluded that in order to have a global acoustic description of a space, more acoustic parameters apart from the often used (alone) reverberation time, are needed. Each one of them focus on a different part of the impulse response of a room, as it is depicted on Fig. 14.

Figure 14 .Typical impulse response of a room (in blue). In a schematic way, the part of the response each of the room acoustic parameters focuses on is shown (reverberation time in green, speech clarity in yellow and sound strength in red)

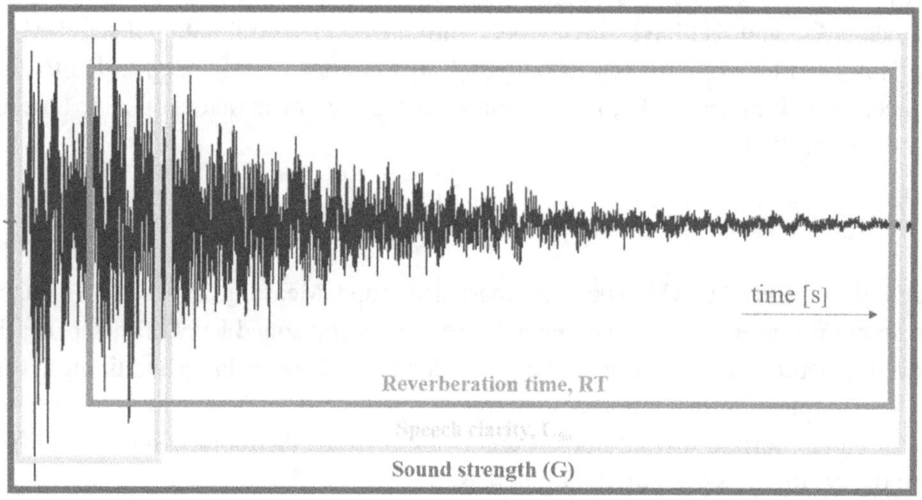

Sound Propagation

In big open spaces, such as open-plan offices and corridors, the reverberation time and the other above mentioned parameters may not be enough to describe the acoustic quality of a space, since other parameters related to the sound decay and background noise are needed. The international standard ISO 3382-3 specifies methods for measuring the acoustic properties of open plan offices so as to describe how noise behaves in these open spaces and to allow good privacy between workstations.

In spaces of this nature, sound propagates more easily and effectively. The shorter the sound propagation distance, the less the number of distracted people will be, located close (or not so close) to the sound source. Several factors can affect the room acoustics of these spaces, e.g. the absorption present in the office (both in ceilings and walls), the height of vertical partitions (and their quality), background noise, how protected each workstation is, the distance between them and of course the morphology of the room (dimensions, shape). Furthermore, the interaction between several of these factors mentioned above is fundamental.

The measurement procedure proposed by the standard makes use of a sound source simulating a person speaking and the measurements are carried out with the space completely finished (without people, but with normal daily background noises such as ventilation, traffic... and furniture) so that the acoustic evaluation is as realistic as possible. The idea is to perform measurements on a straight line that crosses workstations, starting close to the source and going away from it. At each point along that imaginary line different acoustic parameters are measured, in order to (through some post-processing) determine:

- Reduction of sound pressure level of speech (dBA) with doubling the distance: $D_{2,S}$
- Sound pressure (in dBA) at 4 metres distance from the source: $L_{p,A,S,4m}$
- Distraction distance r_D (in metres). It is defined as the distance at which the STI is less than 0.5.
- Average value of background noise in (dBA): $L_{p,A}$

Although the standard states that "Open plan offices with good acoustic conditions are rare", it gives some example of target values: $D_{2,S} \geq 7$ dB, $L_{p,A,S,4m} \leq 48$ dB. The materials, geometry and design of the room affect the sound propagation over distance. The most effective way of reducing sound propagation over distance is, however, screening with acoustic materials.

Another norm soon-to-be-published dealing with open plan offices is the ISO 22955. It is intended for stakeholders working in the planning, design, construction or layout of open-plan offices with the aim of providing end users a good level of acoustic comfort. It shall be used as a basis for discussion and dialogue between the stakeholders involved in creating office spaces. It deals not only with the acoustics of open-plan spaces but also with the cognitive effects of noise.

Privacy is of paramount importance in open-plan offices, since confidential conversations and tasks that require concentration need a great deal of privacy. A way of classifying suspended ceilings based on their ability to contribute to acoustic privacy (together with a screen) in office landscapes is the articulation class (AC). Defined in the standard ASTM E-1110, it describes the ceiling's ability to dampen noise between different areas, and can be used as a tool for classifying and comparing acoustic ceiling systems. The higher the AC is, the better the speech privacy is in open-plan environments. It is recommended to use a suspended ceiling with an articulation class of minimum 180 to achieve an acceptable level of communication privacy. The AC value takes into account, indirectly, the angle dependent absorption of a ceiling system (which is the case in most real scenarios, where sound sources are more directional). The AC value is a way of improving the specification of a ceiling system together with a high absorption class.

Another important parameter for privacy is the acoustic attenuation (evaluated by the standard ISO 10848-2). It evaluates (in the laboratory) the airborne flanking acoustic insulation (through the plenum) of a suspended ceiling, expressed through the index D_{nfw}. The higher it is, the better the system prevents sound to travel from one room to the adjacent one through the plenum. This is very important, for example, in spaces where partition walls do not reach all the way up to the soffit and privacy is needed between rooms. In those cases, a ceiling solution with a high value of D_{nfw} (larger than 35 dB) should be chosen.

THE SENSE OF HEARING

Hearing is the only sense that never rests or sleeps; it is always awake. Our auditory system has developed during thousands of years outdoors, where it had to adapt to survive the many threats cavemen faced daily long time ago. However, nowadays people spend an amount of time that can reach up to 90% of our lives in indoor spaces, where the sound field is completely different to the outdoor one our hearing was developed for. While outdoors in nature there is often no plain hard surfaces where the sound energy can reflect (it often spreads freely sideways and towards the sky), indoors (e.g. in a classroom, an office, a ward) one is often surrounded by acoustically hard surfaces (e.g. gypsum, masonry, concrete) where the sound can bounce. This allows sound levels to escalate, and thus creating the uncomfortable environments and potential health effects previously seen.

In broad strokes, it can be said, in a simplified manner, that good room acoustic design is that which is able to create and mimic inside a room (the more the better) the sound field existent outdoors. That is the environment that our hearing was developed for and where people feel more comfortable in. In this manner, when using acoustic ceilings and wall panels in the architectural design of indoor spaces, the idea behind it is to try to mimic the "natural sky of the forest", where sound is not reflected back into the room, and the breath of it through wall panels.

But… how does one recognise sounds and locate them with so much precision? It is thanks to auditory system. In broad strokes, it can be said that it is comprised of (i) ear, which converts sound energy into neural signals and (ii) brain, which receives and process the information contained in the sound.

As previously seen, sound energy travels in form of pressure waves in the air until they reach our ears. Inside the ear (composed of outer ear, middle ear and inner ear – cf. Fig.15) very complex natural processes are performed. After the sound is carried through the auditory canal, the tympanic membrane (eardrum) together with the bones of the middle ear convert the sound pressure waves into fluid waves inside the cochlea (filled with salt water) by jerking a bone (3 different ones in reality). Subsequently, the last bone hits the cochlea and converts the mechanical vibrations into waves due to the fluid inside the cochlea. Around the cochlea are lined the so-called basilar membranes, equipped with hair cells which move harmonically with the vibrations of the cochlear fluid and the basilar membrane. That movement triggers a signal that travels from the hair cell into the auditory nerve, and then onward to the brain. That impulse is then interpreted as a specific sound (its depending on the hair cell that moves and excites the nerve). Hearing impairments are often cause by damage in this hair cells (see Fig. 16). Another task for the brain to perform is the source location, i.e. where the sound is coming from. To that end, it compares the sounds that come into the two ears and by time and intensity differences it is capable of doing so.

Figure 15. A diagram of the anatomy of the human ear. Green is outer ear. Red is middle ear. Purple is inner ear. Source of figure: L. Chittka; A. Brockmann; Perception Space – The Final Frontier.

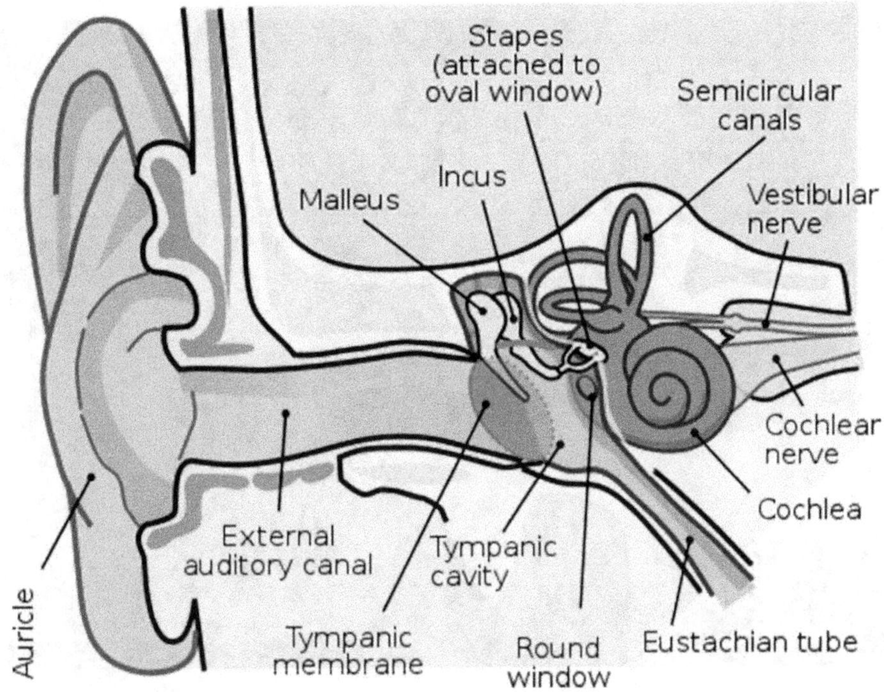

Humans are able to hear (generalising) frequencies between 20 Hz and 20 kHz. The hearing threshold is (in its lower limit) frequency dependent; it increases with decreasing frequency. That is, in order to be able to hear a low frequency sound, a higher sound level is needed, compared with a high pitch tone. The upper threshold is limited by irreversible damages in our hearing, and it falls around 120 dB, regardless of the frequency.

The so-called "speech banana" (see Fig. 17) is the area where the conversation falls: it ranges between 250 Hz and 8000 Hz and sound levels between 35 dB (whisper level) and 80 dB (when screaming) approximately. As it can be seen in Fig. 17, vowels have a lower frequency than consonants. Presbyacusis (age-related hearing loss) makes the audible region to shrink, hence worsening the ability to hear high frequencies (see Fig. 17).

Sound and Message

When designing indoor spaces, the success and acoustic comfort of the majority of the activities performed inside them are very much dependent on the quality of the message that the end users convey and/or receive. What happens to the message when is conveyed in a place with bad room acoustics? Generally speaking, inadequate room acoustics can make communication difficult and blur the message due to the

Figure 16. Healthy hair cells in the cochlea: Damage can be caused by noise, e.g. gluing the cells together or making them loose stiffness. In cases of complete degeneration, hair cells may even brake off. Source of picture: Dr. David Furness - Wikipedia.

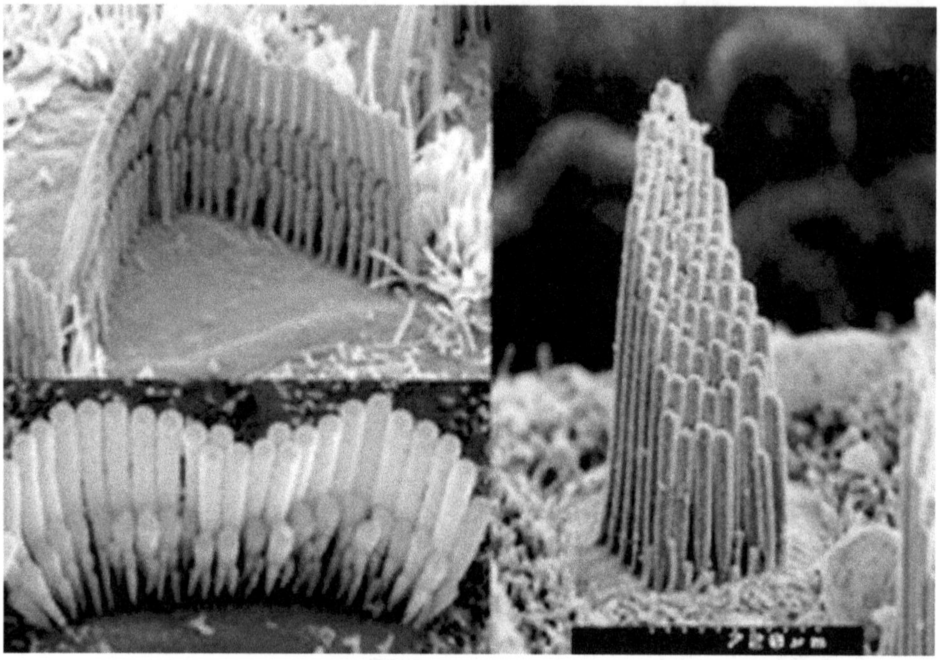

accumulation of noise in the room and its way of interacting with the energy present in speech sounds. When speaking, the balance energy/information can be simplified as follows:

- Vowels contain little information but a lot of energy; when pronounced, nothing prevents the sound from coming out.

Figure 17. Hearing region of a person without hearing loss (left) and with hearing loss (right). The speech banana, where the letters are contained, is also shown. Source of figures: Saint-Gobain Ecophon.

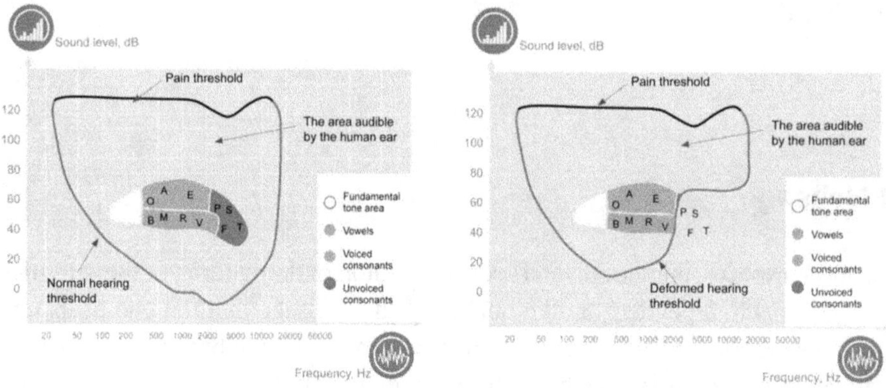

- Consonants, in contrast, are characterised by their low energy (i.e. volume) and a lot of information, due to the obstruction of the air flow that we produce when pronouncing.

If a long reverberation time (due to a room not being properly designed) is added to speech, the vowels will mask and "eat up" the consonants as they have much more energy. The resulting message will be, in visual terms, "fuzzy/blurry". Furthermore, as a consequence of not listening or understanding the message that someone is trying to convey to us, people tend to involuntarily raise the voice; the noise level increases, but without increasing clarity. This is called the Lombard effect. Good room acoustics will enable acoustic comfort and thus wellbeing for the end-users and the success of the activities to be performed.

Figure 18. Graphic representation of how an increase in the volume of the voice (height of the yellow cup) in a place with a lot of reverberation could cause the vowels (that contain the volume of the speech but little information) to mask and "eat up" the consonants (that contain the information and little energy) due to the widening of the yellow cup. The "pronounced" word above is "acústica" (Spanish for acoustics).

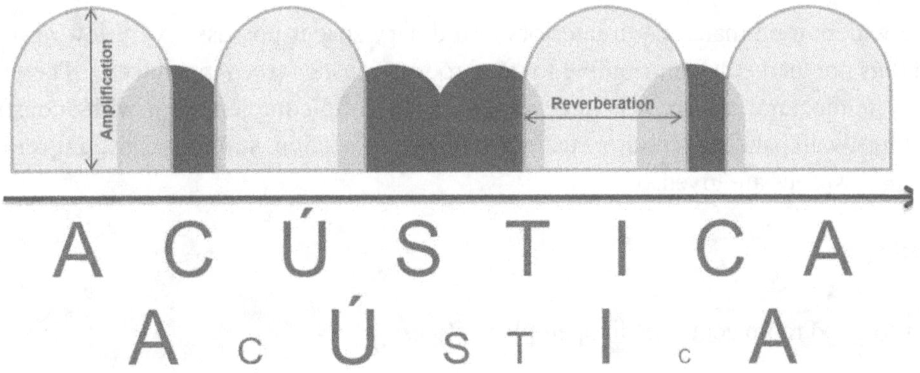

PSYCHOACOUSTICS

Noise is defined as unwanted sound. In that definition, there is intrinsically a subjective component, due to which sound (and noise) waves have a large variety of physical, physiological and psychological effects on people. Psychoacoustics is the part of acoustics that studies the psychological and physiological responses in people associated with sound exposure, i.e. how people perceive sounds.

Efforts for controlling noise in buildings is often focused on physical solutions, such as acoustic ceilings and vertical barriers. However, the requirements for the spaces of the 21st century - especially in connection with open office environments– encourage a more complex approach that includes not only physical but also psychological and physiological solutions. The challenge is to create workspaces that accommodate different personalities doing different tasks in an end-user centered design approach.

There is evidence that the most productive teams have a rich mix of personality types. Nevertheless, most workplaces are more suitable for the extrovert types due to the prevalence of open office landscapes. The survey presented in (Oseland&Hodsman, 2018) revealed that personality type does affect noise perception, in particular extroversion and neuroticism. Psychological profiling, could, in the same way as it is often used for recruitment purposes, also be used for putting people together who prefer and function better in certain acoustic environments. An even better opportunity is to create suitable spaces for different types of personality and to allow employees to choose where they want to work.

The perception of noise is influenced by the relation to the noise source. In general, people tend to be less disturbed by sound sources that they understand and feel comfortable with. It is crucial to the wellbeing of the employees that they have a sense of being able to control their sound environment. People in need of noise reduction often also tend to avoid confrontations. An official noise corporate policy could be beneficial in many cases.

(Oseland&Hodsman, 2018), in their comprehensive review about acoustics in the workplace, reviewed more than 100 research reports from the 1950s aiming at providing (for acousticians, architects, interior designers and property developers) knowledge about healthy, happy and productive work environments for everyone. The reader is referred to that latter reference, as psychoacoustics is a very broad topic outside the scope of this chapter.

DESIGN TIPS

Most of the widely-used materials in interiors in ordinary spaces possess a very low absorption coefficient and thus not markedly contributing to good room acoustics (see Appendix 2). Therefore, besides an adequate architectural design, it is of crucial importance to complement it with acoustic treatment such as ceilings, wall panels, furniture, etc. In the following section, several acoustic tips to design four typical ordinary spaces are given.

Open Offices

Three steps to good room acoustics in open plan offices:

- Step 1: Make sure to use a sound absorbing ceiling (ideally an absorption Class A with articulation class larger than 180).
- Step 2: Use sound absorbing and insulating screens to minimise disturbance between workspaces.
- Step 3: Use free hanging units over workspaces to further support the sound environment.

Figure 19. Steps to good room acoustics in open plan offices. Source of figure: Saint-Gobain Ecophon

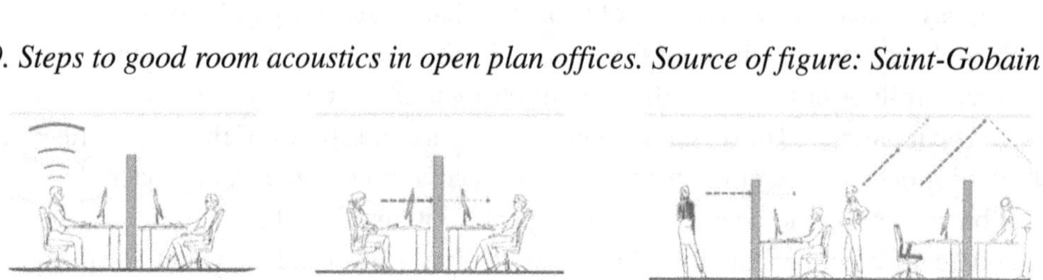

Seven steps to ensure success of open plan offices:

1. Inform about the benefits and risks when sitting in an open plan.
2. Have clear codes of conduct.
3. Invest in sound absorbing ceilings and screens to minimise disturbance. Requirements to the building programme can be added to assure the room acoustic comfort:
   a. Sound propagation requirements for open spaces (e.g. for good room acoustics, according to ISO 3382.3: $D_{2,S}$ ≥7 dB, $L_{p,A,S,4m}$ ≤ 48 dB and r_D ≤ 5 m)
   b. Reverberation time and speech clarity requirements for smaller rooms (e.g. T≤0.5 s & C_{50}≥3 dB for superior comfort).
4. Have sufficient number of silent rooms with adequate sound insulation between them.
   a. Sound insulation is not dealt with in this chapter, but values of airborne sound insulation between rooms larger than 35-40 dB are strongly recommended.
5. Provide portable technical solutions.
6. Make available a wide variety of spaces (for resting, for formal and informal meetings, etc.).
7. If a sound masking systems is to be installed, make sure that space it is properly treated from a room acoustic perspective. Otherwise there is a risk of noise levels increasing when introducing more sound into the space (due to lack of absorption).

Classrooms

Traditional Classrooms: three steps to good room acoustics in classrooms:

- Step 1: Acoustic insulation: external sources, installation noise, and noise penetration from adjacent spaces must be taken care of adequately though use of proper construction solutions.
- Step 2: Lower noise levels from activities inside the classroom.
- Step 3: Lower the reverberation time, and enable good speech intelligibility.

The latter requirements can be assured by properly designing a traditional classroom. How?

1. Reduce reverberation time and sound levels by using a wall-to-wall Class A absorbent ceiling.
   a. Reverberation levels below 0.5 seconds are strongly recommended.
2. Use elements that absorb low frequencies (e.g., glass wool blankets over the ceiling).
   a. It has been shown that the existence of low frequencies (HVAC noise, outside traffic...) makes attention and concentration difficult.
3. Improve speech clarity by acting on walls (wall panels, diffusers ...). The presence of absorption on the walls reduces reflections parallel to the ceiling and floor, thus improving speech intelligibility.
   a. Speech clarity levels above 3 dB are strongly recommended.
   b. Wall absorption will be placed on two adjacent vertical surfaces and at the height of the speech, although the one opposite the teacher is the most important.
   c. The area of wall panels to be installed should be at least 20% of the floor area.
   d. Making the design non-regular by, e.g. tilting walls, using shelves, coat racks, etc. will minimise reflections between parallel surfaces and thus improve acoustic comfort.

4. In order to guarantee the comfort of the teacher, a small reflective area on the ceiling above the speaker is recommended. It will not only reinforce the direct sound towards the audience, but also allow the teacher to hear his/her own voice more clearly (thus protecting the voice).

Figure 20. Scheme of acoustic design of a traditional classroom. Source of figure Saint-Gobain Ecophon.

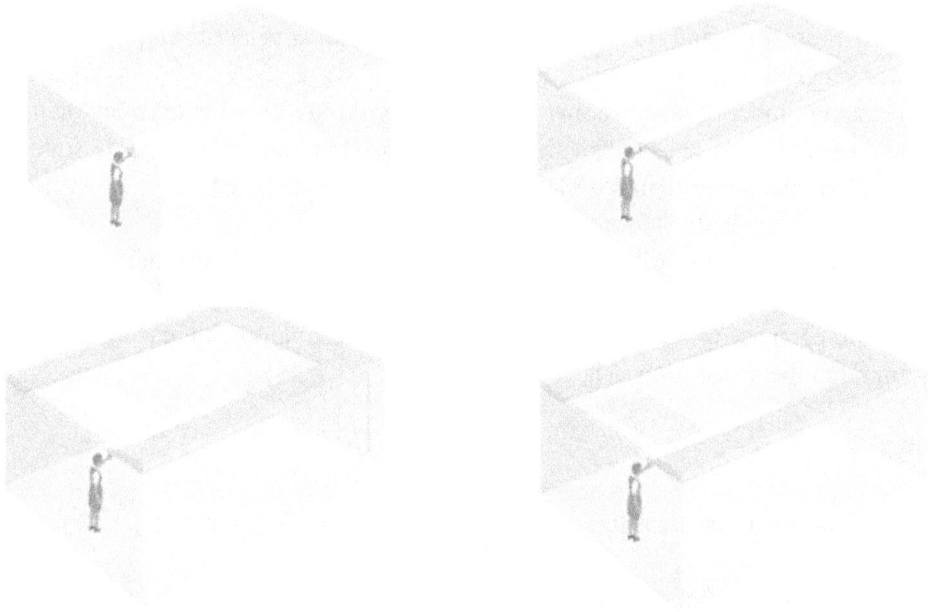

Open Classrooms: these spaces are becoming increasingly more common. Although there are many proven potential pedagogical benefits, open schools entail an important acoustical challenge. The success of spaces of this sort and the associated pedagogical philosophy depends firstly on the behaviour of both staff and students, as well as the compromise of the school management. Everyone should be aware of the open school concept, believe in it, and behave accordingly. Some points to keep in mind when it comes to the acoustic issue are:

- An "activity-based acoustic design" should be adopted. Zoning according to activities and separating noisy from requiring concentration is vital for the "acoustic success" of such spaces.
- The key is to absorb sound locally and prevent sound propagation, taking into account indirect paths (reflections, etc.) through the use of materials, furniture... that produces adequate absorption, reflection, diffusion.
    - It is important to always think about the general rule "line of sight/line of sound" in order to reduce propagation ("what you can see, you can hear"). Avoiding reflections that produce unwanted propagation is essential. To that end, suitable furniture (coat racks and mobile shelves...) can be used as space separators.

Indirect acoustic measures (regardless of whether one designs traditional or open classrooms) are advisable. Examples of such actions can be to use soft elements below the legs of the chairs (e.g. wheels, rubber pads) that will prevent background noise levels to increase when dragging them (students will tend to speak louder when background noise levels are high). Moreover, carpets, installed in circulation areas, can help both to prevent the noise level from increasing, and to absorb (marginally) high frequencies at the source when walking with hard soles on them.

Healthcare

In general, to control the noise levels inside hospital wards, it is of crucial importance:

- Step 1: Reduce reverberation time and sound levels in the spaces.
- Step 2: Support the speech intelligibility, so that communication is optimised, avoiding communication (potentially fatal) errors and stress of patients and staff.
- Step 3: Limit sound propagation in long corridors and open spaces (e.g. nurse stations) that can "pollute" other areas, distracting and being detrimental to patients' privacy and recovery.
- Step 4: Allow privacy aspects so nobody feels uncomfortable due to their conversation being heard in the outside of the ward.

The acoustic measures to be adopted to achieve the latter are:

1. Install absorbing ceilings (ideally Class A and an articulation class larger than 180).
    a. If special hygiene and disinfection requirements are needed, there are solutions in the market that address both acoustics, aesthetics and hygiene simultaneously.
    b. Reverberation levels below 0.5 are strongly recommended
2. In places where there is crucial communication between staff (e.g. operating rooms) or between staff and patients (e.g. examination rooms), install absorption on the walls in order to improve speech clarity.
    a. Speech clarity levels above 3 dB are recommended.
3. Good insulation between rooms is also of crucial importance due to privacy-issues.

Restaurants

In general, to control the noise levels inside restaurants, it is of crucial importance to take three steps:

- Step 1: Reduce reverberation time and sound strength so that sound levels in the space do not escalate.
- Step 2: Support the speech clarity, so that conversations inside groups can be held without straining the voice.
- Step 3: Allow privacy aspects so nobody feels uncomfortable due to their conversation being heard in the table next to them.

In order to assure the latter requirements, the following general acoustic design tips are given:

1. Invest in absorbing ceilings (class A preferably) or FHUs in order to reduce noise levels. Provide walls with some sort of absorption (absorbing panels, thick curtains) or irregularities (non-parallel surfaces, tilted walls, shelves…) in order to improve intelligibility.
   a. Although the reverberation time depends on the volume of the space, values lower than 0.7 seconds are recommended. If the dining area is an open plan, sound propagation requirements may also be added to the building programme.
2. Zoning: try to separate potentially noisy areas (kitchen, HVAC room, vending machines if present…) from the dining area.
3. Limit background noise through different measures: limit the density of tables so that less sources are present in the space, use "soft" materials in circulation areas, control (if present) the volume of the music being played, use soft pads under chairs' and tables' legs, etc.

ACKNOWLEDGMENT

The author would like to help Saint-Gobain Ecophon for the images, pictures and knowledge provided as well as many of his colleagues for their invaluable help during the writing process of this chapter.

REFERENCES

Alnuman, N., & Altaweel, Z. (2020). Investigation of the Acoustical Environment in A Shopping Mall and Its Correlation to the Acoustic Comfort of the Workers. *Applied Sciences (Basel, Switzerland), 10*(3), 1170. doi:10.3390/app10031170

Arneborg, E. (n.d.). Altersschwerhörigkeit – Symptome, Ursachen, Folgen, Diagnostik, Therapie [Age-related hearing loss – symptoms, causes, consequences, diagnosis, therapy]. In *ASTM C423: Sound absorption and sound absorption coefficients by the reverberation room method*. American Society for Testing and Materials.

ASTM E1110:2019: Standard Classification for Determination of Articulation Class. American Society for Testing and Materials. Pennsylvania, USA.

Banbury, B., & Berry, D. C. (1998). The disruption office-related tasks by speech and office noise. *British Journal of Psychology, 89*(3), 499–517. doi:10.1111/j.2044-8295.1998.tb02699.x

Baur. (2009). *Einfluss exogener Faktoren auf Altersschwerhörigkeit, HNO*. Springer Medizin Verlag.

Beldam, M.-B. (2019). Impact of acoustics on staff performance in operation rooms. Proceedings of Internoise.

Berglund, B., Lindvall, T., & Schwela, D. H. (1999). *Guidelines for community noise*. Technical Report World Health Organization.

Biswas, D., Lund, K., & Szocs, C. (2019). Sounds like a healthy retail atmospheric strategy: Effects of ambient music and background noise on food sales. *Journal of the Academy of Marketing Science, 47*(1), 37–55. doi:10.100711747-018-0583-8

Brill, M., & Weidemann, S. (2001). *BOSTI: Disproving Widespread Myths about workplace design.* Kimball International.

Brown, G. (2009). NICU Noise and the Preterm Infant. *Neonatal Network, 28*(3), 165–173. doi:10.1891/0730-0832.28.3.165 PMID:19451078

Busch-Vishniac, I. J., West, J. E., Barnhill, C., Hunter, T., Orellana, D., & Chivukula, R. (2005). Noise Levels in John Hopkins Hospital. *The Journal of the Acoustical Society of America, 118*(6), 3629–3645. doi:10.1121/1.2118327 PMID:16419808

Cacciatore, F., Napoli, C., Abete, P., Marciano, E., Triassi, M., & Rengo, F. (1999). Quality of Life Derterminants and Hearing Function in an Elderly Population: Osservatorio Geriatrico Campano Study Group. *Gerontology, 45*(6), 323–328. doi:10.1159/000022113 PMID:10559650

Código Técnico de la Edificación – Documento Básico de Protección Contra el Ruido (2009) – CTE DB HR [Spanish Building Regulations].

Dalton, D. S., Cruickshanks, K. J., Klein, B. E., Klein, R., Wiley, T. L., & Nondahl, D. M. (2003). The Impact of Hearing Loss on Quality of Life in Older Adults. *The Gerontologist, 43*(5), 661–668. doi:10.1093/geront/43.5.661 PMID:14570962

Dockrell, B., & Shield, J. (2008). *The effects of classroom and environmental noise on children's academic performance.* JASA.

Durup, N., Shield, B., Dance, S., Sullivan, R., & Gómez-Agustina, L. (2015). How classroom acoustics affect the vocal load of teachers. *Energy Procedia, 78*, 3084–3089. doi:10.1016/j.egypro.2015.11.761

EN 16487:2015: Acoustics - Test code for suspended ceilings - Sound absorption. European Standardization Organization.

Evans, G. W., & Johnson, D. (2000). Stress and open office noise. *The Journal of Applied Psychology, 85*(5), 779–783. doi:10.1037/0021-9010.85.5.779 PMID:11055149

Fiegel, A., Meullenet, J. F., Harrington, R. J., Humble, R., & Seo, H. S. (2014). Background music genre can modulate flavor pleasantness and overall impression of food stimuli. *Appetite, 76*, 144–152. doi:10.1016/j.appet.2014.01.079 PMID:24530691

Fried, & … . (2002). The joint effects of noise, job complexity and gender on employee sickness absence, Journal of Occup and Organiz. *Psychology*, 75.

Guéguen, N., Hélène, L. G., & Jacob, C. (2004). Sound level of background music and alcohol consumption: An empirical evaluation. *Perceptual and Motor Skills, 99*(1), 34–38. doi:10.2466/pms.99.1.34-38 PMID:15446627

Guéguen, N., Jacob, N. C., Le Guellec, H., Morineau, T., & Lourel, M. (2008). Sound Level of Environmental Music and Drinking Behaviour: A Field Experiment with Beer Drinkers. *Clinical and Experimental Research, 32*(10), 1795–1798. doi:10.1111/j.1530-0277.2008.00764.x PMID:18647281

Hagerman, I., Rasmanis, G., Blomkvist, V., Ulrich, R., Eriksen, C. A., & Theorell, T. (2005). Influence of intensive coronary care acoustics on the quality of care and physiological state of patients. *International Journal of Cardiology, 98*(2), 267–270. doi:10.1016/j.ijcard.2003.11.006 PMID:15686777

IEC 60268-16: Sound system equipment - Part 16: Objective rating of speech intelligibility by speech transmission index. International Electrotechnical Commission. Geneva, Switzerland.

ISO 10848-2:2017: Acoustics – Laboratory and field measurement of flanking transmission for airborne, impact and building service equipment sound between adjoining rooms – Part 2: Application to Type B elements when the junction has a small influence. Organization for Standardization, Geneva, Switzerland.

ISO 11654:1997. Acoustics – Sound absorbers for use in buildings–Rating of sound absorption, International Organization for Standardization, Geneva, Switzerland.

ISO 3382-1:2009. Acoustics – Measurement of room acoustic parameters – Part 1: Performance spaces, Organization for Standardization, Geneva, Switzerland.

ISO 3382-2:2008. Acoustics - Measurement of room acoustic parameters - Part 2: Reverberation time in ordinary rooms, Organization for Standardization, Geneva, Switzerland.

ISO 3382-3:2012. Acoustics – Measurement of room acoustic parameters – Part 3: Measurement of room acoustic parameters — Part 3: Open plan offices, Organization for Standardization, Geneva, Switzerland.

ISO 354:2013. Acoustics – Measurement of sound absorption in a reverberation room, International Organization for Standardization, Geneva, Switzerland.

ISO/FDIS 22955: Acoustic quality of open plan-offices. Organization for Standardization, Geneva, Switzerland.

Jensen, K.L., Arens, E., & Zagreus, L. (2005). Acoustical quality in office workstations, as assessed by occupant's surveys. *Proceedings of Indoor Air.*

Johansson, L., Bergbom, I., Person-Waye, K., Ryherd, E., & Lindahl, B. (2012). The sound environment in an ICU patient room – A content analysis of sound levels and patient experiences. *Intensive & Critical Care Nursing, 28*(5), 269–279. doi:10.1016/j.iccn.2012.03.004 PMID:22537478

Johnson, A. N. (2001). Neonatal response to control of noise inside the incubator. *Pediatric Nursing, 27*(6), 600–605. PMID:12024534

Joint Commission. (2010). *Sentinel Event Data.* Root Causes by Event Type.

Klatte, M. & Lachmann, T. (2009). *A lot of noise about learning: acoustic conditions in classrooms and what they mean for teaching.* Academic Press.

Lange, M. F. (2015). The sound of the intensive care unit - 3 weeks of continuous sound recording. *Proceedings of DASAIMs yearly meeting 2015.*

Mann, N. P., Haddow, R., Stokes, L., Goodley, S., & Rutter, N. (1986). Effect of Night and Day on Preterm Infants in a Newborn Nursery. *British Medical Journal, 293*(6557), 1265–1267. doi:10.1136/bmj.293.6557.1265 PMID:3096460

Mark, Gudith, & Klocke. (n.d.). *The Cost of Interrupted Work: More Speed and Stress*. University of California, Irvine.

Minckley, B. B. (1968). A study of noise and its relationship to patient discomfort in the recovery room. *Nursing Research, 17*(3), 247–250. doi:10.1097/00006199-196805000-00018 PMID:5184904

Negreira, J., Svensson, C., Oseland, N., & Canto, R. (2019) Good acoustics as an extra source of income in restaurants – A case study. Proceedings of Internoise.

Nightingale, F. (1859), *Notes on Nursing*. Academic Press.

Oseland, N., & Hodsman, P. (2018). A psychoacoustical approach to resolving office noise distraction. *Journal of Corporate Real Estate, 20*(4), 260–280. doi:10.1108/JCRE-08-2017-0021

Schönwälder, H.-G., Ströver, F., & Tiesler, G. (2008). *Health promoting influences on performance ability in school education*. Academic Press.

Seddigh, A., Berntson, E., Jönsson, F., Danielson, C. B., & Westerlund, H. (2015). The effect of noise absorption variation in open-plan offices: A field study with a cross-over design. *Journal of Environmental Psychology, 44*, 34–44. doi:10.1016/j.jenvp.2015.08.004

Simon, M., Tackenberg, P., Hasselhorn, H.-M., Kümmerling, A., & Büscher, A. (2005). *Auswertung der ersten Befragung der NEXT-Studie in Deutschland*. Wuppertal University.

Slevin, M., Farrington, N., Duffy, G., Daly, L., & Murphy, J. F. (2000). Altering the NICU and measuring infants' responses. *Acta Paediatrica (Oslo, Norway), 89*(5), 577–581. doi:10.1111/j.1651-2227.2000.tb00342.x PMID:10852196

Stafford, L. D., Fernandes, M., & Agobiani, E. (2012). Effects of noise and distraction on alcohol perception. *Food Quality and Preference, 24*(1), 218–224. doi:10.1016/j.foodqual.2011.10.012

Tiesler, G. (2018). Communication behaviour and workload of students and teachers in highly absorbent classrooms. Proceedings of Euronoise 2018.

Tiesler, G., & Oberdöster, M. (2006). *Acoustic ergonomics of school*. Publication Series from the Federal Institute for Occupational Safety and Health - Research Report - Fb 1071.

Weinstein, N. D. (1974). Effect of noise on intellectual performance. *The Journal of Applied Psychology, 59*(5), 548–554. doi:10.1037/h0037338

Weise, C. H. (2010). *Investigation of patient perception of hospital noise and sound level measurements: before, during and after renovations of a hospital wing*. Architectural engineering – Dissertations and Student Research (Master Thesis Report).

Woloshynowych, M., Davis, R., Brown, R., & Vincent, C. (2007). Communication patterns in a UK emergency department. *Annals of Emergency Medicine, 50*(4), 407–413. doi:10.1016/j.annemergmed.2007.08.001 PMID:17881316

Woods, A. T., Poliakoff, E., Lloyd, D. M., Kuenzel, J., Hodson, R., Gonda, H., Batchelor, J., Dijksterhuis, G. B., & Thomas, A. (2011). Effect of background noise on food perception. *Food Quality and Preference*, *22*(1), 43–47. doi:10.1016/j.foodqual.2010.07.003

You Stop the Music: How Sounds in Retail Stores Divide Shoppers. (n.d.). Available here: https://bit.ly/2PTo22F

Zahr, L. K., & de Traversay, J. (1995). Premature infant responses to noise reduction by earmuffs: Effects on behavioral and physiologic measures. *Journal of Perinatology*, *15*(6), 448–555. PMID:8648453

APPENDIX 1

Example of Calculation of Reverberation Time

A rectangular room has the dimensions given in the figure below. The ceiling is covered with two different materials, namely *AbMat.1* and *AbMat.2*, while the back wall consists of two different materials, namely *AbMat.3* and *AbMat.4*. The absorption coefficients (for a diffuse field) for all materials are presented in the table below. The surfaces which are not covered with any of said materials can be considered as fully reflective. Answer the following:

- What is the reverberation time of the room above according to Sabine's formula?
- If the previously estimated reverberation time is to be reduced (in order to meet a particular standard) by 35%, and one only has access to a new material (*AbMat.5*) whose absorption coefficient is $\alpha_w = 0.65$ to place it on the long walls. Which area should be covered so that the previous requirement is met?
- If the previous reverberation time is to be achieved by using free hanging units instead of the *AbMat.5*, how many rafts should be installed if their absorption area per object is 1.2 m^2?

Figure 21.

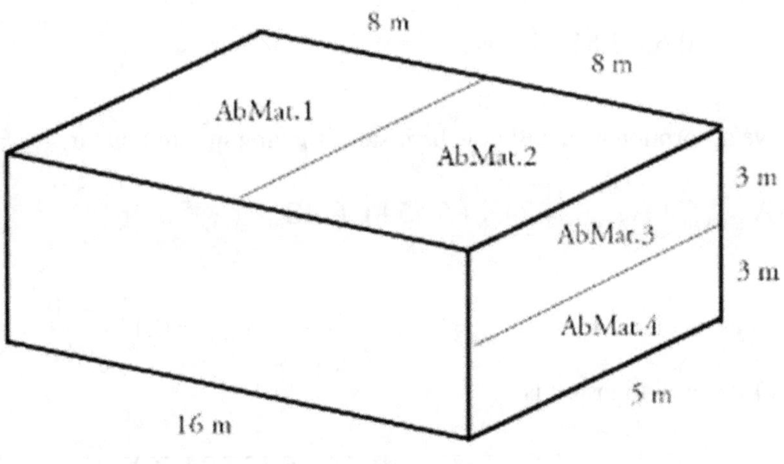

Table 3.

Material	Absorption coefficient α_w
AbMat.1	0.24
AbMat.2	0.37
AbMat.3	0.15
AbMat.4	0.22

Sabine's law: $T_{60} = 0.16 \cdot \frac{V}{A}$. with $A = \sum_{i=1}^{n} \pm_{w,i} \cdot S_i$.

The effective absorption area (A[m^2]) can be first calculated as:

$A_{LongWalls} = A_{Floor} = A_{FrontWall} = 0$.(totally reflective surfaces, i.e. α_w=0)

$$A_{ceiling} = \propto_{AbMat1} \cdot \frac{S_{Ceiling}}{2} + \propto_{AbMat2} \cdot \frac{S_{Ceiling}}{2} = (8 \cdot 5 \cdot 0.24) + (8 \cdot 5 \cdot 0.37) = 24.4m^2.$$

$$A_{RearWall} = \propto_{AbMat3} \cdot \frac{S_{Wall}}{2} + \propto_{AbMat4} \cdot \frac{S_{Wall}}{2} = (3 \cdot 5 \cdot 0.15) + (3 \cdot 5 \cdot 0.22) = 5.55m^2.$$

Thus, the total effective absorption area is: $A = \sum_{i=1}^{n} \pm_{w,i} \cdot S_i = 24.4 + 5.55 = 29.95m^2$.

The volume of the room is: $V = 16 \cdot 5 \cdot 6 = 480m^3$.

Hence, the reverberation time can be calculated simply as: $T_{60} = 0.16 \cdot \frac{V}{A} = 0.16 \cdot \frac{480}{29.95} = 2.56s$.

If a reduction of 35% of the reverberation time is to be achieved, then:

$$T_{60,New} = 0.65 \cdot T_{60,Old} = 0.65 \cdot 2.56 = 1.66s.$$

The new effective absorption area will now be instead (having in mind that α_{AbMat5}=0.65):

$$A_{New} = A_{Ceiling} + A_{RearWall} + A_{AbMat5} = 24.4 + 5.55 + 0.65 \cdot S_{AbMat5}.$$

Where A_{New} can be calculated as: $T_{60,New} = 0.16 \cdot \frac{V}{A_{New}} \Rightarrow A_{New} = 0.16 \cdot \frac{480}{1.66} = 46.26m^2$.

Thus, the area of material to install is:

$$24.4 + 5.55 + 0.65 \cdot S_{AbMat5} = 46.26 \Rightarrow S_{AbMat5} = \frac{(46.26 - 5.55 - 24.40)}{0.65} = 25.1m^2.$$

If now FHUs (with A_{obj}=1.2 m^2) are to be used instead of AbMat.5 in order to achieve a reverberation time of 1.66 seconds, and knowing that the absorption area to be introduced (calculated above) is A_{new}=46.26 m^2, then:

$$A_{New} = A_{Ceiling} + A_{RearWall} + A_{FHUs} \Rightarrow 46.26 = 24.4 + 5.55 + N^o{}_{FHU} \cdot 1.2.$$

$$N^{o}_{FHU} = \frac{(46.26 - 5.55 - 24.40)}{1.2} = 13.59 \approx 14\text{FHUs}.$$

APPENDIX 2

In Table 4, some absorption coefficients of typical materials are listed.

Table 4. Typical weighted absorption coefficients.

Constructive solution / material	α_w / α_m
Bare concrete	0,04
Painted concrete	0,07
Bare masonry	0,04
Painted masonry	0,02
Plasterboard	0,01
Stone	0,02
Wood	0,08
Parquet	0,05
Cork	0,06
Fabric	0,17
Carpet ≤ 10 mm	0,17
Carpet ≥ 10 mm	0,30
PVC	0,05
Linoleum	0,03
Ceramic tiles	0,02
Glass	0,04
Metal	0,02
Acoustic ceilings	See Table 3

Data Source: list of constructive solutions of the Spanish Building Code Regulations (CTE DB-HR)

NOTE 1: Note that most of the widely-used materials in interiors in ordinary spaces possess a very low absorption coefficient and thus not markedly contributing to good room acoustics. Therefore, it is of crucial importance to complement an interior design with acoustic ceilings, acoustic wall panels, architectural adapted design, furniture, etc.

NOTE 2: other references which treat acoustic materials as constructive elements can be found in:

- Cox T.J. & D'Antonio P. (2009). Acoustic Absorbers and Diffusers: Theory, Design and Application, Tailor&Francis.
- Kuttruff H. (1973). Room acoustics. Tailor&Francis.

NOTE 3: The best way of knowing an absorption coefficient is checking the manufacturers' data sheets. Remember always to compare solutions tested under the same conditions/standard.

Chapter 4
Bamboo Utilization as a Sustainable Building Material:
Bamboo in Buildings

Paul C. Okonkwo
Dhofar University, Salalah, Oman

Israr Ul Hassan
Dhofar University, Salalah, Oman

Wesam H. Beitelmal
https://orcid.org/0000-0001-6386-0639
Dhofar University, Salalah, Oman

ABSTRACT

The extraction of building materials from their resources through harvesting, preservation, and utilization has become a significant segment of human contribution to the global ecosystem since the industrial revolution. Bamboo is the world's fastest-growing woody plant, and bamboo grows multiple times quicker than most species. Housing is one of the focused demands for bamboo, and as a result of the current scarcity of home units, the demand for bamboo is increasing. Bamboo building construction is portrayed by a basic edge approach like that applied in traditional building design and construction. Applying bamboo as an environmentally friendly material is seen as a movement towards creating a sustainable environment and reducing greenhouse emissions. The need to employ government policy in addressing the production and application of bamboo is reported, and the challenges of bamboo in the global market are highlighted in this chapter.

DOI: 10.4018/978-1-7998-7279-5.ch004

INTRODUCTION

Building materials, innovations, and practices have advanced throughout the ages. The investigation and progress in building improvement began with the usage of regular materials like stone, soil, leaves, natural lumber, etc. A couple of issues related to the strength of the regular materials like soil, leaves, wood, etc., lead to the investigation and development of sustainable structural materials (Reddy, 2004). While blocks and bricks burning were the earliest technologies used for thermal energy to produce durable building materials, metal, lime, and lime-based items; on the other hand, they represent one of the significant manufactured energy-consuming materials used for building construction (Venkatarama Reddy, 2009). It was demonstrated that between 2% and 38% of energy is consumed by conventional building materials (Bribián, Capilla, & Usón, 2011), including steel, solid, aluminum, and glass, which are high energy content materials, paving the way for the search for an alternative renewable and sustainable building material. Subsequently, the innovation of natural inorganic binders like pozzolanic materials has given rise to lime-pozzolana (LP) cement, resulting in the discovery of building material known as Portland cement. Portland cement and steel brought progressive changes in the building industry since the early part of the 20th century, followed by plastics and plastic products that later entered the building industry (Cao et al., 2017).

Buildings have an instantaneous impact on the surroundings, ranging from the use of raw substances in the course of construction, renovation, and maintenance to the emission of harmful materials at some stage in the building's lifestyle cycle (Hu, Cabeza, & Yan, 2020; Nejat, Jomehzadeh, Taheri, Gohari, & Majid, 2015; Syla, 2019). To address global warming, environmental economics, and sustainable improvement have emerged as imperative concerns to the global world. Many environmental discussions have focused on the concept of ecologically sustainable development (ESD) which is designed based on the building development viewpoint to address the green use of resources to satisfy the requirements and desires of present and future generations. The building and the environment are undistinguishably connected. Since buildings sway on the environment during their life cycle, the selection of materials utilized in the building will affect the general building performance just as the environment. It became inevitable that the building has found itself at the center of issues regarding environmental effect due to materials used in their construction. The impact of building on the environment is linked not only with the indoor air pollution but also on the global climate and ozone depletion. It then requires that incorporating sustainable building materials into the design of the building will have a significant impact on increasing the life span of buildings as well as reducing the carbon emission during the building life cycle. Chen et al. (Chen, Okudan, & Riley, 2010) reported that appropriate sustainable material selection will help in attaining the objective of sustainable development in the building industry. Because of the pattern of development from zero energy material to more current materials for the building development, it became evident that more energy is spent on building development. Besides, a portion of the advanced building materials is moved over significant distances before they are utilized in building development. Attributable to the worldwide requirement for carbon emission reduction and hence the pressure to comply with carbon neutral targets, is required that materials that are recyclable, natural, sustainable, and environmentally friendly should be used for the construction of buildings.

The selection of sustainable building materials requires analyzing and developing the building materials for their interaction with the environment and sustainability. Setting up standards and rules that qualify building materials to line up with the standards and goals of practical improvement in development is required. Sustainable materials are materials that are regular and offer explicit advantages to the clients such as low support, energy proficiency, the improvement of tenant wellbeing, comfort, and expanded efficiency while being less harmful to nature and the environment (Latha, Darshana, & Venugopal, 2015). Although several attempts have been made to set up complete methods for evaluating a thorough scope of sustainability considerations in building materials, most of the studies have focused on the environmental protection and impact of buildings with limited attention paid to the social and economic factors that are related to sustainability (Mahdavi, Clouston, & Arwade, 2011; Vogtländer, Van der Lugt, & Brezet, 2010). Several building codes and standards have been launched, aimed at encouraging product manufacturers to embark on advancing their supply-chain sustainability efforts with verse level of sustainability objectives at the building design stage where material appraisal and choice normally occur.

To ensure that appropriate sustainable building materials are selected, appropriate codes, standards, and guidelines have to be put in place (Gatóo, Sharma, Bock, Mulligan, & Ramage, 2014; Rojas, Lew, & Naeim, 2010). As the search for natural, renewable, and sustainable building material continues, Bamboo has presented itself as the potential candidate being globally available and rapidly renewable due to its comparatively low-energy-intensive and structural properties (P. Sharma, Dhanwantri, & Mehta, 2014). Bamboo is renewable, sustainable, low-cost, and environment friendly material and has amazing strength quality which in effect addresses the scarcity and strength challenges faced by the wood-based industry. However, the absence of proper construction regulations and norms is a boundary to designers and modelers in utilizing bamboo material which affects the overall building material selection. Proper standards are required for design and testing of full culm bamboo to give the establishment from which developers, architects and engineers who plan and develop buildings.

Though Bamboo has been utilized for quite a long time as a material for development, furniture, artworks, and food, among others, its demand as a sustainable material in the building industry is quite increasing (Mahdavi et al., 2011). Recently, the utilization of bamboo has been changed and basic structures developed from full culm bamboo have shown a route forward for complex bamboo building structures (Raj & Agarwal, 2014; P. Sharma et al., 2014). The increased enthusiasm for, and the advancement of, bamboo in current building material development have been driven by expanding the requirements for economical materials to fulfill the rising needs according to fast urbanization. The study will explore the uses and application of Bamboo as a sustainable material for the building industry. This study reflects the key tendencies in the sector of sustainable building materials with a focus on the uses and application of bamboo in the building industry. This study centers around certain issues relating to the sustainability, carbon emission and impact of using bamboo to the environment as well as outlining future prospects and challenges.

ORIGIN AND STRUCTURE OF BAMBOO

Bamboo is classified as a grass member from a bigger grass family and can be effectively found in tropical and some mild territories of the world (Clark, Londoño, & Ruiz-Sanchez, 2015). Bamboo material has cultural and ecological significances in many countries where the material provides economic and social benefits. Certain conditions such as temperature, rainfall, soil type, etc affect the distribution of different bamboo species (Jack, 1931; Liese, 1988; Yudodibroto, 1985). Fig. 1 shows the Phyllostachys bambusoides, cultivar White Crookstem specie of bamboo growth in Georgia, USA.

Figure 1. Phyllostachys bambusoides, cultivar white crookstem (Scurlock, Dayton, & Hames, 2000)

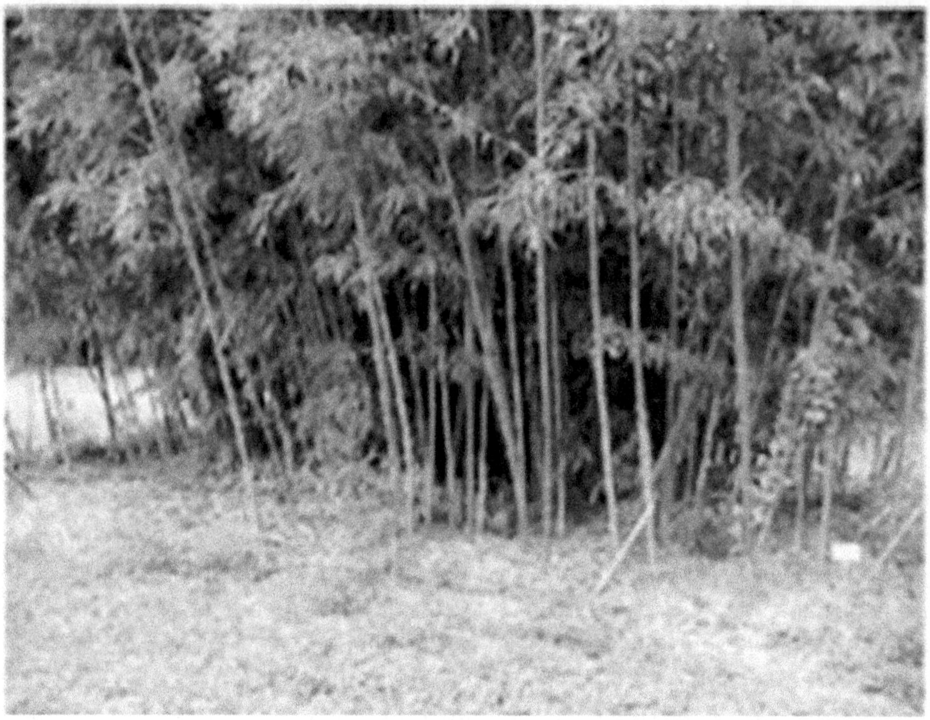

The resilience, fast growth rate and possibility of multiple harvesting within a few years offer a better advantage over other forestry species. Bamboo plants are mainly composed of roots, rhizomes, stems, branches, leaves, and shoots as shown in Fig. 2.

Bamboo has a structure comprising of a tube-shaped pole with a jointed stem known as a culm as shown in Figure 2. The thickness of a bamboo reduces alongside the height of the culm, while the density of the strands increments from the bamboo culm's inner wall to the external wall. While bamboo stems are round, jointed, and hollow, the culm involves internodes which are secluded by nodes. The length and thickness of the internodes are differed; depend upon the species and nature. The basic life structures of the internodes are described by shape, size, and vascular gatherings of the bamboo culm. In the outer culm, the vascular groups are smaller and the internal are larger. The culms are the most fundamental piece of bamboo and changes in size, width, and color. The culm includes the strands of cellulose fibers and the lignin system. Spaces between connecting strands of fibers are stacked up with lignin and the quantity of strands increments toward the outer surface of the culm. As one of the speediest growing plants, bamboo can achieve full stature going from 15-30m in a period of one to four years (Liu, Fox, & Xu, 2000). Bamboo is essentially a giant grass that originates from sub-families of bambusoideae and Poaceae or Gramineae (Guo, Chen, Li, & Yang, 2001). Each species can be perceived by its root system in which there are three known root systems including, sympodial, monopodial, and amphodial (Scheba, Blanchard, and Mayeki, 2017). The sub-family bambusoideae includes both woody and herbaceous bamboos. Bamboo normally develops in groups and its developmental character can be separated into two sorts:

Figure 2. Bamboo tissue (Bian, Zhong, Zhang, Yang, & Gai, 2020).

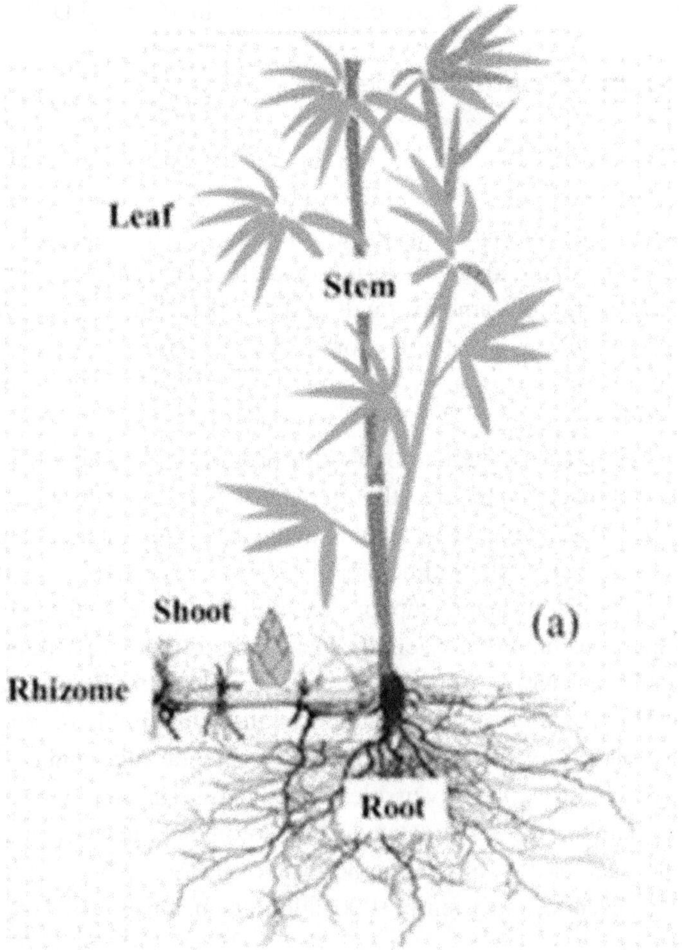

a. Monopodial and
b. Sympodial Bamboo

Monopodial bamboo roots grow by spreading on a level plane in a shallow depth of the soil. Progressively, new shoots are developed at a relatively long distance from the parent's plant. While Monopodial bamboo is predominantly found in temperate climates, sympodial bamboo is found in the tropical climate and the roots grow very close to the parents' plant forming a cluster of numerous stems or sticks. There are several bamboo species found on the planet and every species can be recognized and distinguished by their root system.

The bamboo forest has a high harvest cycle and can be harvested in a short period, in addition to having a high rate of carbon absorption in comparison with timber. The strength of bamboo likewise relies upon the age and species, which decides their appropriateness to be utilized in construction when they attain the maturity age of around 1-4 years. At maturity, bamboos possess an optimum strength and are suitable to be utilized for heavy-duty applications (Awalluddin et al., 2017). It has likewise been discovered that bamboos' compressive strength increases along with their stature, notwithstanding the increasing compressive strength from the inner to the outer part of their culm (Correal D & Arbeláez C, 2010).

Bamboo Harvesting and Production Methods

Bamboo culms grow up as shoots from the rhizome structure and attain at a greatest tallness under a year. Dependent upon the species and its usage, the culm for the most part needs a long time to accomplish its harvestable quality, regularly up to 4 years. Due to variation in species, some of the bamboo stands can mature early. When harvesting bamboo, clear-cutting or cutting is regularly performed. Clear-cutting is accepted to diminish the energy of bamboo stands and recuperation of the stand takes a lot of time (Banik, 2015). Selective harvesting is a certainly more economical method for harvesting and management of bamboo plantation. Another strategy for bamboo harvesting includes bamboo culms being normally cut with a machete.

During the ground laying process, the bamboo culm or part of the culm is buried in the ground. Regular watering is required to enable its growth. On the other hand, when the rhizome system is cut for replacement, the material has to be well-watered to avoid losing its water content (Akinlabi, Anane-Fenin, & Akwada, 2017). Akinlabi et al. (Akinlabi et al., 2017), suggested that harvested culms should be immersed in reservoirs filed with water to support leaching of starches and sugar from the culms. For hollow bamboos, utilizing this technique can deliver a neat and tidy cut with zero possibility for water to accumulate in the cavity of the rest of the stump. Be that as it may, the methodology could result in the rhizome structure crumbling the bamboo stand. Bamboo stands can nimbly produce consistent income for local producers and ecological growth guaranteed through enduring bamboo incorporation in the country's business strategy. Countries have given rules and guidelines in gathering bamboo (Banik, 2015). For instance, the country bamboo harvesting standard in Colombia underwrites that developed culms are to be cut to a furthest reach of 25% of the bamboo stand each year. With an ideal stand density of around 4000 culms for each hectare, consistently 1000 culms can be sensibly harvested on every hectare.

BAMBOO MATERIAL PRESERVATION

Bamboo is considered as one of the building materials that are strong with the elasticity of more than 28,000 N for each square inch, contrasted with steel which is 23,000 N for every square inch (Anagal, 2010). However, the utilization of bamboo as building material must go through a preservative measure. Structurally, bamboos are not made up in a way that enables preservative treatment on them. Though the bamboo's external stems, with its high silica content and waterproof-shell, considerably oppose insects attack, the protection prevents additive from entering the culm. Furthermore, the bamboo is secured with an impermeable, waxy layer, allowing the preservative to enter the bamboo stem through the conducting vessels which are not more than 10% of the cross-section during preservation treatment (Fei, Liu, Jiang, Cai, & Yu, 2013). The bamboo preservation techniques fall into two classifications:

a. Traditional preservation
b. Chemical preservation

Traditional Preservation

In numerous countries, traditional preservation techniques such as curing, smoking, drenching, and lime-washing are utilized in bamboo preservation. In as much as the impact of these techniques is not yet known, the strategies are famous as they can be applied with low cost and with low expertise levels (Kumar, Shukla, Dev, & Dobriyal, 1994). For the curing process, the harvested bamboo culms are left in the open, with branches, and leave flawless. Transpiration measure, which proceeds even in the wake of felling, causes the starch substance to fall. The smoking treatment of the culms over fire is highly preservative against parasites and insects. The dousing process includes submerging the culms in stale or running water for half a month to filter out the sugar contents in the bamboo. Following the dousing process, the wet bamboo is air-dried under shade before washing with lime water to secure the bamboo against parasitic attack.

Chemical Preservation

When considering using bamboo in modern industry or large-scale projects for housing or other buildings, chemical preservations are unavoidable. However, it is smarter to stay away from additives with synthetic compounds like arsenic as they can be dangerous to the environment as well as those handling them (Kaur, Satya, Pant, & Naik, 2016). Utilizing effective and safe chemicals for the preservation of bamboo can be achieved by using boron-based element chemicals, such as copper-chrome-boron (CCB) (Saikia, Dutta, Kalita, Bora, & Goswami, 2015). To enhance its resistance against fungal and termite attacks, bamboo is commonly preserved using borax boric acid solution through several processes, for example, submersion, gravitational or vertical douse dispersion, and infusion utilizing a blower machine. Preserving bamboo with borax boric acid can increase the life expectancy of bamboo as well (Saikia et al., 2015). One of the major advantages of utilizing this chemical is that there is no waste as the chemical by-product from the bamboo preservation process is utilized as fertilizer. Akinlabi et al. (Akinlabi et al., 2017) reported that the use of salt as one of the preservatives currently minimise the risk of hazardous chemicals being released into the environment by other preservatives, as well as consequent health problems. Notwithstanding, the utilization of the chemical in the preservation cycle of bamboo has emerged different discussions about the effect of the wastewater on the environment and requires government policies to address the challenges (Okokpujie, Akinlabi, & Fayomi, 2020).

Properties of Bamboo

As building materials, bamboo has a strong fiber and the compressive strength of bamboo is significantly higher than concrete, while the elasticity is close to the steel (Li, 2004). Bamboo fiber likewise has higher shear than wood (Li, 2004). Bamboo offers a tremendous commercial and domestic products opportunities as a result of its amazing mechanical, physical, and chemical properties (Li, 2004). Bamboo is a trademark common cellulosic composite in which cellulose strands are introduced in the lignin and hemicellulose cross section. The geometry of bamboo's longitudinal profile has a useful assessed structure, which can withstand unprecedented breeze loads (Awalluddin et al., 2017). Bamboo has distinctive mechanical properties in the three measurements: axial, radial, and tangential. The compression properties of the bamboo corresponding to the longitudinal direction are fundamentally higher than the perpendicular direction. Bamboo composites are regularly utilized for basic items as opposed to the raw bamboos. This is as a result of conceivable variation of properties along with the longitudinal and radial directions as well as the physical dimension of the items required. In any case, bamboo is a natural material and it is exposed to extraordinary variability and unpredictability because of different conditions, for example, long periods of development, soil and ecological conditions, and the location of the bamboo culm inside the bamboo (Shah, Sultan, Jawaid, Cardona, & Talib, 2016; Xiao, Yang, & Shan, 2013). Thus, it is seen that the mechanical properties of bamboo vary massively across the sections of the bamboo (Tan et al., 2011). Bamboos are accessible as various species and the mechanical and physio-compound properties vary from one species to another species. Although there are several unique types of bamboo, the mechanical and chemical properties of the bamboo are not fixed for all the species. The mechanical property relies upon sort of species, length, horizontal layer, and age of the bamboo. The maturing of a bamboo culm also influences its properties. The external layer has a more defined function in supporting bamboo than the internal layer based on its formation and location in the stem structure. To modernly utilize bamboo strips productively, it is prudent to use external surface material to deliver high-quality bamboo composites. The mechanical and physical-compound properties of the bamboo just as bamboo composites are additionally affected by the climatic and biological variables, development strategies, and harvesting procedures. Hence the inception of the bamboo must be thought of whenever finding particular applications. The hollow cross-segment and solid diaphragms at normal stretches add to the quality of the bamboo pole.

BAMBOO AS A BUILDING MATERIAL AND APPLICATIONS

Bamboo is an adaptable material because of its high strength to weight proportion, simple functionality, and availability. Bamboos also are generally appropriate as a sustainable material for building structures because of its great mechanical and physical properties. For load conveying structural composite items, mechanical properties, for instance, rigidity, compressive strength, shear, flexural strength, and bending elasticity modulus are fundamentals. Bamboo is chemically treated due to their low natural durability and can be used in different appliances, for example, rooftop structure, rafters, for flooring, doors, and windows, walling, ceiling, manhole covers, and so on. Bamboo production does not involve a lot of energy utilization and in this manner adoption of bamboo for housing assists with safeguarding the environment. Bamboo is a renewable plant with an exceptionally short turn period and the bamboo housing is being effectively utilized globally due to its material properties (B. Sharma, Gatoo, Bock, Mulligan, & Ramage, 2015). Bamboo is being broadly utilized in different applications such as, supporting posts, frames, allotments, roofs, dividers, ceilings, entryways, windows, and tying. Bamboo has been utilized as a construction material because of its simple accessibility, simplicity of functionality, and its strength. Janssen et al. (JANSSEN, 2000) compared the bending properties of bamboo with other building materials as shown in Table 1.

For flooring tiles and facade, compressive strength, hardness, abrasive resistance, and slip resistance are essential, while for structural assemblies, nail withdrawal strength is basic. Bamboo is also used as rough material for mash, paper, and board undertakings. Bamboos are additionally basic in numerous conventional applications, for example, for fencing, water pipes, umbrella handles, and enhancing crafted works. The utilization of bamboo, which can truly push the little and medium scale endeavors, are very important for optimal use of bamboo.

Table 1. Comparison of bending properties of bamboo to other common building materials (JANSSEN, 2000)

Building Materials	Specific Gravity	Modulus of Elasticity (GPa)	Modulus of Rupture (Mpa)	Modulus of Rupture to Specific Gravity Ratio (MPa)
Giant timber bamboo	0.52	10.7	102.7	197.5
Loblolly pinc	0.51	12.3	88	172.5
Douglass-Fir	0.45	13.6	88	195.6
Cast iron	6.97	190	200	28.7
Aluminum alloy	2.72	69	200	73.4
Structural steel	7.85	200	400	50.9
Carbon fiber	1.76	150.3	5,650.00	3,205.10

The restored enthusiasm in the past five decades about bamboo has prompted change in the structures in which bamboo is utilized and the perspective of the house made with bamboo has also changed. In traditional construction, bamboo can be used as whole culms, split lengthwise, pressed flat, or woven into mats. The bamboo is regularly joined by lashing with plants, part bamboo or rattan, making a generally frail joint between bamboo shafts. Generally, bamboo culms are utilized as essential building materials for building houses or it outlines by plastering the bamboo with cement or clay which have increased the development of bamboo housing (De Flander & Rovers, 2009). In present-day times, engineered bamboo is utilized to make pre-assembled bamboo houses with the assistance of bamboo-based boards, veneers, and laminated boards. This innovation advancement can be successfully embraced for the development of low-cost (single-storied) building contingent on the plan of the house and nature of the interior finish, and upon the neighborhood conditions. A lot of advancement has occurred to improve the innovation and strategies that can be utilized to make bamboo appropriate for construction. There has been an improvement in the preservation and security technology of bamboo just as in jointing strategies with the goal that the utilization of bamboo can be increased as a building construction material. These advances are helping in increasing the sturdiness of bamboo as a construction material. Researches on structural engineering and improvement of bamboo composites have opened new landscapes for lightweight, strong and tasteful development for an assortment of uses with appropriate bamboo treatment. The basic building system can be characterized into a semi-structured active and non-structure dynamic system. While the structure dynamic system is an organized system that just can withstand the axial forces, tension, or compression, the non-structure dynamic system is an organized system that can only withstand tension, compression, and bending moment (B. Sharma et al., 2015). In building construction, organic shapes are designed on the roof, and the roof structure can be made and created from spatial or surface structure. Categorically, bamboo can be used as a building material in the following applications:

Application of Bamboo in Trusses and Roof Skeletons

Due to the required strength, bamboo rafters are used to build frames and trusses for fixing the roof in building structural design. The building roofs skeleton comprises of bamboo bracket or rafters over which strong bamboo purlins are laid and lashed to the beam using galvanized iron wire. A mesh of divided bamboo is made and is lashed to the purlins to cover the roof, creating a roof skeleton.

Bamboo Walling/Roof

The bamboo material is light in weight, and it is useful for earthquake inclined territories since the possibility of falling of the bamboo wall or roofs are less because of adaptability. Regardless of whether it falls, it tends to be re-raised effectively with less human and property misfortune and the least expense. Bamboo dividers can be developed in various manners as shown below:

- Whole stem strips of bamboo are nailed to one or both sides of the bamboo frame.
- Split bamboo mats are secured to the bamboo posts or mats be woven. Often, mud is applied to the two sides of such mats.
- Bamboo strips are nailed to bamboo casing or posts for inside walling.
- Cement or lime plastering is applied to the mud covering for better appearance and cleanliness.
- For partitioning of walls, only a single layer of bamboo strips is used.

Bamboo as Flooring and Furniture Materials

Bamboo is used as an effective flooring material because of its high wear and tear resistance properties and the entire building floor can be covered utilizing bamboo sheets, mats, and so forth. Bamboo flooring is a quality product that can be utilized broadly and has a huge, worldwide consumer market. It has certain advantages over wooden floors because of its perfection, brightness, strength, high resistance, protection characteristics, and adaptability. Bamboo flooring has a soft natural luster and keeps up the normal gleam and tastefulness of bamboo fiber. This flooring is alluring to the demanding markets in Europe, Japan, and North America (Takahashi & del Bambú–PERUBAMBU, 2006). Traditional bamboo furniture and design are often sent in conservative level packs, to be assembled on the spot for particular furniture design. The new design of bamboo furniture is significantly better in addressing the issues of traditional bamboo furniture, for example, high work and transportation costs, low productivity, instability, quality fluctuating, and susceptibility to bugs and fungi. Simultaneously, the designed bamboo holds the specific physical, mechanical, chemical, environmental, and stylish features of bamboo. The bamboo furniture offers superb toughness and lightweight attributes at a much cheaper cost globally.

APPLICATION OF BAMBOO IN BUILDING CONSTRUCTION

Some of the popular buildings made with bamboo are generally constructed using a basic frame structure. One of the applications of bamboo in building construction is the green school building constructed utilizing bamboo as fundamental structure materials in Indonesia. This structure is considered as the originator of bamboo recovery in Indonesia (Nurdiah, 2016a).

Although bamboo is a traditional structural material in Indonesia, its low cost has made bamboo a potential candidate for common building material in Indonesia. The construction of the Green School building shown in Fig.3 has resulted in a different phase of investigation in the building structure, construction process, and development methods (Nurdiah, 2016a). The school complex comprises several

Figure 3. Green School (a) Main hall "Mepantigan"; (b) Main building "The heart of Green School"; (c) The bridge (Nurdiah, 2016a).

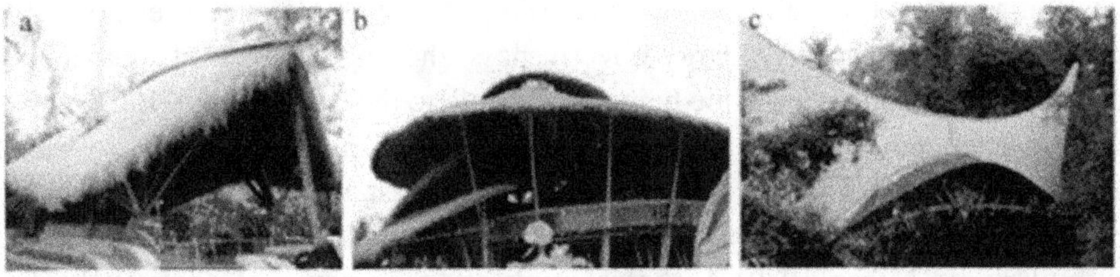

masses in which each mass has a capacity of accommodating different functional apartments such as, classroom, multifunction hall, research facility, multifunction corridor, office, understudy and instructor's residence, and so forth. Fig. 3 shows that the rooftops are the most recognizable and noticeable of the mass, where each mass has distinctive rooftop shapes. While the arch-shaped building is located as the entrance (Fig.3a), the main building situated in the middle, is a two and three storey-building. The masses have organic shapes as well as a bridge that has hyper-structure as shown in Fig. 3c. Apart from the construction and development of the Green School, different other buildings utilizing bamboo as a building material have been designed and constructed globally as shown in Fig. 4.

Figure 4. A reformed bamboo building (Zhou, Huang, Li, & Su, 2012).

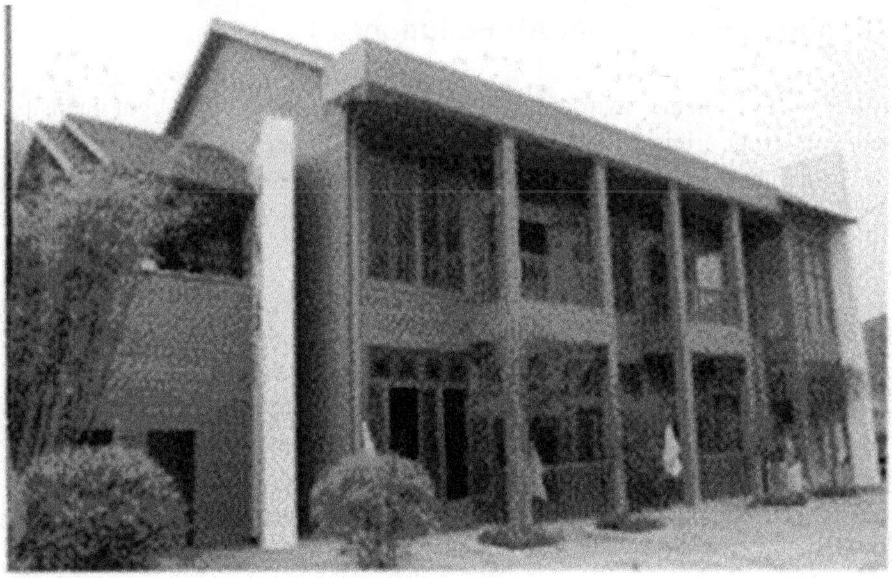

Alongside the increasing popularity of bamboo it has been used in designing and constructing commercial buildings (De Flander & Rovers, 2009; Nurdiah, 2016a).

SUSTAINABILITY OF BAMBOO

Sustainable building materials are alluded to as materials that are regular and offer explicit advantages to the clients regarding low support, energy effectiveness, the improvement of inhabitant wellbeing, comfort, the increase of productivity while being less unsafe to the environment. Bamboo as a sustainable material rises up out of the way that bamboo, when harvested in a reasonable way, can have a more beneficial outcome on the environment as building materials. Sustainable harvesting of bamboo can be refined by cutting explicitly 20% of developed stems since they will be replaced each year by a relative ascent of youthful shoots (Minae, 1989). Technical implications on potentially harvestable bamboo, impact on soil erosion and the intended use of bamboo stems may be considered when harvesting bamboo for sustainability. Since bamboo can be harvested every 1–4 years, it was recommended that the yearly harvesting of bamboo keeps the clump or the bamboo forest healthy (Tripathi, 2008). When bamboo is harvested, the root system is safe and is prepared to create more shoots that develop into a full-grown bamboo tree (Manandhar, Kim, & Kim, 2019). Bamboos have an exceptionally quick growth rate and have been seen as appropriate for afforestation (Zakikhani, Zahari, Sultan, & Majid, 2017). In any case, one investigation noticed that any place bamboo is planted for reforestation and soil protection, it can be inter-planted with various other crops (Ministry of Forestry and Mines 2011) because a great deal of leaves fall onto the surface giving new supplements to the entire vegetation system (Minae, 1989). Bamboo can be planted in regions that have been recently desolated by deforestation or in flood fields (Basumatary, Middha, Usha, Brahma, & Goyal, 2015). Albeit a few bamboos can adjust to changing environments, most require generally warm and muggy conditions.

Impact of Bamboo on the Indoor Air Pollution

Bamboo plays a critical role in the environment. It not only helps in reducing light intensity and protects against ultraviolet rays, but primarily reduces in-door air pollution (Nurdiah, 2016b). Planting bamboo indoor can provide a safer option to clean the air at home instead of using air purifiers. Atanda (Atanda, 2015) reported that 35% of carbon dioxide can be reduced by bamboo and significant amount of oxygen delivered, making bamboo a good candidate to reduce in-door air pollution.

Cost of Bamboo Material

Bamboo is frequently embraced as a less expensive building material. However, the assumption may be valid in situations where bamboo is accessible locally, but the transportation and logistical expenses could altogether increase the bamboo material cost. Due to the high demand for bamboo in flooring, bikes, and so on in developed nations, like Europe and America, even with the increasing cost of bamboo, bamboo is still cheaper than other woods. This advantage as well as the genuine propensity towards sustainability open the door for bamboo to enter into the housing industry (Kaur, Pant, Satya, & Naik, 2016). Bamboo can be prepared into present-day items, like engineering bamboo that may effectively rival with other wood items in cost and performance (Lobovikov, Schoene, & Yping, 2012), yet at present bamboo has been a specialty market for the wealthier populace. An exploratory investigation on utilizing bamboo to make covers with the tensegrity arch indicated that bamboo can be utilized for the construction of the basic building, which is easy to assemble and lightweight which brings about the economy of material and labor cost (Moreira & Ghavami, 2001). The concept of sustainable products and improvement of bamboo bio-composites can be viewed as an astute harmony between the requests of society's increasing interest for bamboo products, the conservation of forest health, and diversity of material resources and revenue generation (Endalamaw, Lindner, & Pretzsch, 2013). The significant issue is that the commercialization of most profoundly esteemed bamboo products has been recognized to cause significant effects on the sustainability of construction materials (Endalamaw et al., 2013). With the increasing revenue generation from bamboo, fast and uncontrolled bamboo harvesting has prompted serious exhaustion of bamboo and deforestation. Likewise, the option of transportation from the country of assembling to the country of utilization adds enormously to the embodied energy and cost, disrupting the sustainability advantage of bamboo.

Government Policy on Bamboo

The issue behind the helpless improvement of bamboo used in the construction industry is ascribed to poor policy formation. Realizing bamboo as an end product used in the construction industry needs to cut across these three phases of the policy which include, regulatory, distributive, and redistributive phases. (Davidson, Castro-Delgado, Arias, & Mann, 2006; Okokpujie et al., 2020) This policy should include a great deal of cognizant exertion from the government, stakeholders, and policymakers of the country. It should likewise help in the bamboo's sustainability implementation policy and the product used in the construction industry. The fundamental objective of the open regulatory policy of bamboo application in the construction industry is to keep everything under control and forestall practices that will risk humankind and protect the working environment. Bamboo from a few examinations has demonstrated to be an excellent material for building construction (Van der Lugt, Van den Dobbelsteen, & Janssen, 2006). Notwithstanding, actualizing bamboo for the construction industry needs precise guidelines and policy (Ogunwusi, 2013). For example, there is a need to heat treat bamboo before being utilized in basic critical structural systems. Governments can accomplish this objective by limiting residents, groups, or industrial associations participating in inappropriate treatment and utilization of bamboo in structural applications that will influence the social and political order.

Another objective for the development of bamboo regulatory policy should be to ensure the financial activities of the country are protected. In any case, precluding manufacturing companies from doing ill-advised harvesting of bamboo plants, which will be negative to the development of the economy of the nation, is exceptionally required in implementing the government policy. Distributive open policy on the utilization of bamboo in the construction industry is extremely noteworthy as the residents should gain from being part of the bamboo revenue generation and monitoring process. The distributive policy should provide guidelines for bamboo utilization and applications, for example, bamboo utilized for building houses, scaffolds, and development of streets. This absence of awareness within the decision-makers and its application is preventing the bamboo-based construction industry from taking shape. The aspect of the policy that addresses the bamboo implementation in the construction industry will urge residents to go into huge scope bamboo cultivating and bamboo change into various end products. This approach will expand the revenue generation of the local and state government, thereby causing tremendous growth in economic development. Hence, individual, private, and public corporations will realize the prospect to invest in bamboo cultivation and processing, knowing that bamboo can be a significant source of revenue.

Durability and Challenges of Bamboo

The essential concern of a bamboo utilization in the building construction or different applications is the strength of the material. The service life of bamboo is regularly considered as being unreasonably short for any valuable venture since bamboo has less normal durability than most woods, inferable from a lack of explicit chemical that happens in numerous sorts of wood yet missing in bamboo. Assessment on the qualifications among various types of bamboo for a specific application would think about the selection of species with better standard strength. Regardless of the level of natural durability of such a chosen bamboo species that will meet the expected service life prerequisite for a particular item of application, the selection of bamboo ought to rely upon the bamboo harvesting and treatment cycles. The challenge that bothers the low natural durability is the hollowness of the bamboo culm, particularly when stood out from the start to finish gigantic cross-segment of wood. On account of bamboo, a loss of 2 mm as a result of fungi or insects attack may mean the loss of one-fourth of its thickness. In most tropical countries, the high relative dampness of the air adds to the strength issues of bamboo. A high dampness content in the bamboo makes total drying troublesome and hence provides an opportunity for parasitic attack thereby presenting vulnerabilities in its application in housing, furniture, etc.

Bamboo culm offers some unmistakable opportunities for the mass building while effectively adding to the eco–reclamation, carbon emission, and employments of the distraught rural communities. Consequently, the investigation of the physicochemical properties of different bamboo species is significant for its effective use. Although climate conditions, storage conditions, and harvesting methods influence the life expectancy of bamboo culm, varying from 1–3 years without treatment, organism, termite, borer beetles are the principal destroyer of bamboo in storage. Microorganisms and underground termites break down the culm under storage, with at least one of these parasites attacking the culms in the progression order. It requires that effective treatment and storage of bamboo are essential to protect bamboo industry, generate revenue and increase its applications.

CONCLUSION

Bamboo which is a fast-growing sustainable material can be regarded as one of the most traditional and established building materials utilized by humankind. Through the challenges of natural forests to fulfill wood demands, bamboo has become one of the fundamental material alternative resources. One of the most significant motivations to work with bamboo is its ease that will effortlessly protect millions who could not typically manage the cost of a rooftop over their heads and its tremendous elasticity makes it an exceptionally useful building material in territories with high risk of earthquakes. At present, there is a huge gap in the flexibly and application of bamboo material in building constructions and it is an excellent open door for bamboo materials to possess the market, since they have endless benefits contrasted with other building materials. Be that as it may, a wide advancement of the use of bamboo should be done to make bamboo material better acknowledged by individuals and cooperate bodies around the globe. Utilization of bamboo material in the construction industry will contribute a great deal to the feasible advancement and sustainability of the building construction industry and protection of the environment applying appropriate regulations on their uses in the construction.

REFERENCES

Akinlabi, E. T., Anane-Fenin, K., & Akwada, D. R. (2017). *Bamboo*. The Multipurpose Plant. doi:10.1007/978-3-319-56808-9

Anagal, V. (2010). *Sustainable urban solid waste management-a case study of Pune*. Academic Press.

Atanda, J. (2015). Environmental impacts of bamboo as a substitute constructional material in Nigeria. *Case Studies in Construction Materials*, *3*, 33–39. doi:10.1016/j.cscm.2015.06.002

Awalluddin, D., Ariffin, M. A. M., Osman, M. H., Hussin, M. W., Ismail, M. A., Lee, H.-S., & Lim, N. H. A. S. (2017). *Mechanical properties of different bamboo species*. Paper presented at the MATEC Web of Conferences.

Banik, R. L. (2015). Harvesting Techniques. In *Bamboo* (pp. 193–226). Springer. doi:10.1007/978-3-319-14133-6_7

Basumatary, A., Middha, S. K., Usha, T., Brahma, B. K., & Goyal, A. K. (2015). Bamboo, as potential sources of food security, economic prosperity and ecological security in North-East India: An overview. *Research in Plant Biology*, *5*(2).

Bian, F., Zhong, Z., Zhang, X., Yang, C., & Gai, X. (2020). Bamboo–An untapped plant resource for the phytoremediation of heavy metal contaminated soils. *Chemosphere*, *246*, 125750. doi:10.1016/j.chemosphere.2019.125750 PMID:31891850

Bribián, I. Z., Capilla, A. V., & Usón, A. A. (2011). Life cycle assessment of building materials: Comparative analysis of energy and environmental impacts and evaluation of the eco-efficiency improvement potential. *Building and Environment*, *46*(5), 1133–1140. doi:10.1016/j.buildenv.2010.12.002

Cao, V. D., Pilehvar, S., Salas-Bringas, C., Szczotok, A. M., Rodriguez, J. F., Carmona, M., Al-Manasir, N., & Kjøniksen, A.-L. (2017). Microencapsulated phase change materials for enhancing the thermal performance of Portland cement concrete and geopolymer concrete for passive building applications. *Energy Conversion and Management*, *133*, 56–66. doi:10.1016/j.enconman.2016.11.061

Chen, Y., Okudan, G. E., & Riley, D. R. (2010). Sustainable performance criteria for construction method selection in concrete buildings. *Automation in Construction*, *19*(2), 235–244. doi:10.1016/j.autcon.2009.10.004

Clark, L., Londoño, X., & Ruiz-Sanchez, E. (2015). Bamboo taxonomy and habitat. In *Bamboo* (pp. 1–30). Springer. doi:10.1007/978-3-319-14133-6_1

Correal, D. J. F., & Arbeláez, C. J. (2010). Influence of age and height position on Colombian Guadua angustifolia bamboo mechanical properties. *Maderas. Ciencia y Tecnología*, *12*(2), 105–113. doi:10.4067/S0718-221X2010000200005

Davidson, D., Castro-Delgado, S., Arias, J., & Mann, J. (2006). Unveiling a Ghost of Amazonian Rain Forests: Camponotus mirabilis, Engineer of Guadua Bamboo 1. *Biotropica*, *38*(5), 653–660. doi:10.1111/j.1744-7429.2006.00194.x

De Flander, K., & Rovers, R. (2009). One laminated bamboo-frame house per hectare per year. *Construction & Building Materials*, *23*(1), 210–218. doi:10.1016/j.conbuildmat.2008.01.004

Endalamaw, T. B., Lindner, A., & Pretzsch, J. (2013). Indicators and determinants of small-scale bamboo commercialization in Ethiopia. *Forests*, *4*(3), 710–729. doi:10.3390/f4030710

Fei, B., Liu, Z., Jiang, Z., Cai, Z., & Yu, Y. (2013). Mechanical properties of Moso bamboo treated with chemical agents. *Wood and Fiber Science*, *45*(1), 34–41.

Gatóo, A., Sharma, B., Bock, M., Mulligan, H., & Ramage, M. H. (2014). Sustainable structures: bamboo standards and building codes. *Proceedings of the Institution of Civil Engineers-Engineering Sustainability*. 10.1680/ensu.14.00009

Guo, Z.-H., Chen, Y.-Y., Li, D.-Z., & Yang, J.-B. (2001). Genetic variation and evolution of the alpine bamboos (Poaceae: Bambusoideae) using DNA sequence data. *Journal of Plant Research*, *114*(3), 315–322. doi:10.1007/PL00013993

Hu, S., Cabeza, L. F., & Yan, D. (2020). Review and estimation of global halocarbon emissions in the buildings sector. *Energy and Building*, *225*, 110311. doi:10.1016/j.enbuild.2020.110311

Jack, J. (1931). Use of Bamboo in Subsoil Drainage. *Journal - Royal Sanitary Institute*, *52*(1).

Janssen, J. (2000). *Designing and building with bamboo. International Network for Bamboo and Rattan*. INBAR.

Kaur, P. J., Pant, K., Satya, S., & Naik, S. (2016). Bamboo: The material of future. *International Journal Series in Multidisciplinary Research*, *2*(2), 27–34.

Kaur, P. J., Satya, S., Pant, K. K., & Naik, S. N. (2016). Eco-friendly preservation of bamboo species: Traditional to modern techniques. *BioResources*, *11*(4), 10604–10624.

Kumar, S., Shukla, K., Dev, I., & Dobriyal, P. (1994). *Bamboo preservation techniques: a review*. Academic Press.

Latha, P., Darshana, Y., & Venugopal, V. (2015). Role of building material in thermal comfort in tropical climates–A review. *Journal of Building Engineering*, *3*, 104–113. doi:10.1016/j.jobe.2015.06.003

Liese, W. (1988). *Bamboo as an alternative material in the context of diminishing resources*. Paper presented at the International Bamboo Workshop, Cochin, India.

Liu, W., Fox, J. E., & Xu, Z. (2000). Leaf litter decomposition of canopy trees, bamboo and moss in a montane moist evergreen broad-leaved forest on Ailao Mountain, Yunnan, south-west China. *Ecological Research*, *15*(4), 435–447. doi:10.1046/j.1440-1703.2000.00366.x

Lobovikov, M., Schoene, D., & Yping, L. (2012). Bamboo in climate change and rural livelihoods. *Mitigation and Adaptation Strategies for Global Change*, *17*(3), 261–276. doi:10.100711027-011-9324-8

Mahdavi, M., Clouston, P., & Arwade, S. (2011). Development of laminated bamboo lumber: Review of processing, performance, and economical considerations. *Journal of Materials in Civil Engineering*, *23*(7), 1036–1042. doi:10.1061/(ASCE)MT.1943-5533.0000253

Manandhar, R., Kim, J.-H., & Kim, J.-T. (2019). Environmental, social and economic sustainability of bamboo and bamboo-based construction materials in buildings. *Journal of Asian Architecture and Building Engineering, 18*(2), 49–59. doi:10.1080/13467581.2019.1595629

Minae, S. (1989). *Socio-economic issues in bamboo production and utilization in Kenya: present and future potentials*. Academic Press.

Moreira, L., & Ghavami, K. (2001). The influence of initial imperfections on the buckling of bamboo columns. *Proceedings of the International Workshop on the role of Bamboo in Disaster avoidance.*

Nejat, P., Jomehzadeh, F., Taheri, M. M., Gohari, M., & Majid, M. Z. A. (2015). A global review of energy consumption, CO2 emissions and policy in the residential sector (with an overview of the top ten CO2 emitting countries). *Renewable & Sustainable Energy Reviews, 43*, 843–862. doi:10.1016/j.rser.2014.11.066

Nurdiah, E. A. (2016a). *The potential of bamboo as building material in organic shaped buildings*. Petra Christian University.

Nurdiah, E. A. (2016b). The potential of bamboo as building material in organic shaped buildings. *Procedia: Social and Behavioral Sciences, 216*, 30–38. doi:10.1016/j.sbspro.2015.12.004

Ogunwusi, A. (2013). The impact of forest policy and land tenure system on bamboo development in Nigeria. *Public Policy and Administration Research, 3*(5), 13–20.

Okokpujie, I., Akinlabi, E., & Fayomi, O. (2020). Assessing the policy issues relating to the use of bamboo in the construction industry in Nigeria. *Heliyon, 6*(5), e04042. doi:10.1016/j.heliyon.2020.e04042 PMID:32478193

Raj, A. D., & Agarwal, A. B. (2014). Bamboo as a Building Material. *J. Civ. Eng. and Env. Tech, 1*(3), 56–61.

Reddy, B. V. (2004). Sustainable building technologies. *Current Science*, 899–907.

Rojas, F., Lew, M., & Naeim, F. (2010). An overview of building codes and standards in Chile at the time of the 27 February 2010 Offshore Maule, Chile earthquake. *Structural Design of Tall and Special Buildings, 19*(8), 853–865. doi:10.1002/tal.676

Saikia, P., Dutta, D., Kalita, D., Bora, J. J., & Goswami, T. (2015). Improvement of mechano-chemical properties of bamboo by bio-chemical treatment. *Construction & Building Materials, 101*, 1031–1036. doi:10.1016/j.conbuildmat.2015.10.106

Scurlock, J. M., Dayton, D. C., & Hames, B. (2000). Bamboo: An overlooked biomass resource? *Biomass and Bioenergy, 19*(4), 229–244. doi:10.1016/S0961-9534(00)00038-6

Shah, A. U. M., Sultan, M. T. H., Jawaid, M., Cardona, F., & Talib, A. R. A. (2016). A review on the tensile properties of bamboo fiber reinforced polymer composites. *BioResources, 11*(4), 10654–10676.

Sharma, B., Gatoo, A., Bock, M., Mulligan, H., & Ramage, M. (2015). Engineered bamboo: State of the art. *Proceedings of the Institution of Civil Engineers-Construction Materials, 168*(2), 57–67. doi:10.1680/coma.14.00020

Sharma, P., Dhanwantri, K., & Mehta, S. (2014). Bamboo as a building material. *International Journal of Civil Engineering Research, 5*(3), 249–254.

Syla, A. (2019). *Global Warming and role of Construction Materials in consume energy*. Academic Press.

Takahashi, J., & del Bambú–Perubambu, A. P. (2006). Bamboo in Latin America: Past, Present and the Future. *Bamboo for the Environment, Development and Trade*, 4.

Tan, T., Rahbar, N., Allameh, S., Kwofie, S., Dissmore, D., Ghavami, K., & Soboyejo, W. (2011). Mechanical properties of functionally graded hierarchical bamboo structures. *Acta Biomaterialia, 7*(10), 3796–3803. doi:10.1016/j.actbio.2011.06.008 PMID:21704742

Tripathi, Y. (2008). Bamboo entrepreneurship-Opportunities for rural employment. *Indian Forester, 134*(9), 1199–1210.

Van der Lugt, P., Van den Dobbelsteen, A., & Janssen, J. (2006). An environmental, economic and practical assessment of bamboo as a building material for supporting structures. *Construction & Building Materials, 20*(9), 648–656. doi:10.1016/j.conbuildmat.2005.02.023

Venkatarama Reddy, B. (2009). Sustainable materials for low carbon buildings. *The International Journal of Low Carbon Technologies, 4*(3), 175–181. doi:10.1093/ijlct/ctp025

Vogtländer, J., Van der Lugt, P., & Brezet, H. (2010). The sustainability of bamboo products for local and Western European applications. LCAs and land-use. *Journal of Cleaner Production, 18*(13), 1260–1269. doi:10.1016/j.jclepro.2010.04.015

Xiao, Y., Yang, R., & Shan, B. (2013). Production, environmental impact and mechanical properties of glubam. *Construction & Building Materials, 44*, 765–773. doi:10.1016/j.conbuildmat.2013.03.087

Yudodibroto, H. (1985). Bamboo research in Indonesia. *Proceeding from the International Bamboo Workshop.*

Zakikhani, P., Zahari, R., Sultan, M. T. H. H., & Majid, D. L. A. A. (2017). Morphological, mechanical, and physical properties of four bamboo species. *BioResources, 12*(2), 2479–2495. doi:10.15376/biores.12.2.2479-2495

Zhou, A., Huang, D., Li, H., & Su, Y. (2012). Hybrid approach to determine the mechanical parameters of fibers and matrixes of bamboo. *Construction & Building Materials, 35*, 191–196. doi:10.1016/j.conbuildmat.2012.03.011

Chapter 5
Beyond the Water Environmental Management in the Operational Building Phase for Its Application to the Peruvian Context

Estela Karem Samamé Zegarra
https://orcid.org/0000-0003-2317-5076
UNASAM, Peru

ABSTRACT

The world population is expected to be 9.3 billion by 2050, with a high increase in the urban population. It is worth considering that 71.7% of the surface of the earth covered by water, but only 3% of this water can be used as drinking water. In cities, buildings are recognized as one of the largest users of freshwater resources in construction and operation. The water use impact is different in some countries because some use conventional water treatments while other ones rely on advanced desalination. Climate change and population growth are clearly putting pressure on the world's water supply, so the first environmental assessment plan for buildings was launched in 1990 by the BRE in the United Kingdom where the water category is included in its environmental assessment.

INTRODUCTION

The relationship that cities and buildings built with water have can be described from different dimensions over time in many documents, books, conferences, etc. Water as a source of water has been a symbol and fundamental resource for all living beings for decades, providing psychological, health and hygiene benefits, satisfying the fundamental needs of people in cities for their subsistence; helping thermal comfort when the resource is used to treat hot air in hot desert areas and used as a resource for the construction of new buildings, remodeling, etc. As project strategies too, for example Frank Lloyd

DOI: 10.4018/978-1-7998-7279-5.ch005

Wright with his Kaufmann residence work better known as the Cascade House that integrates water into the project, the Barcelona pavilion by Mies Van Der Rohe, Chandigarh Le Corbusier and the work of Luis Barragán, in Mexico, where he mentions "Architecture, besides being spatial, is also musical. This music is interpreted by the water (…) The walls create silence, the water makes music and surrounds us. "

In a South American context, the Inca empire has also built marvelous technologies in Peru (Hidráulica Inca, nd), such as those seen today in Tipón, a work of engineering with spectacular terraces and elegant stone walls, in addition to Its decorative canals and waterfalls, water still flows through its canals and ponds to this day, visitors say. It is possible to continue mentioning a series of other works of architecture and hydraulic engineering that used water to incorporate it as part of a poetic ensemble of beauty and recovery or reuse, such as the emblematic structures of the Nazca aqueducts; Pre-Inca construction that recovers water from underground aquifers, an extensive network of underground channels and reservoirs made of stone built about 1600 years ago.

The role of architecture and construction in cities in relation to water resources has been to meet human needs, however, the responsibility to manage it in today's climate crisis should be increased and quantified since periods of droughts and other consequences are most acute in the hot and arid regions of the world such as Peru. (Miranda, 2018) (Ministerio de Ambiente, 2015) (Pérez, 2017) (Revista peruana Geo-Atmosférica RPGA, 2010) to them is added not only water availability but also quality for human use within homes or other buildings .

For this reason, this book chapter will present the contributions of certifications or studies that go beyond the evaluation of the environmental management of water in the operational use of buildings to improve some regulations or certifications for buildings within a Peruvian context. The sustainable or environmental certifications for residential buildings that are certifying buildings in Peru and that evaluate the water category will also be presented in parallel.

THE IMPORTANCE OF WATER CONSERVATION IN PERU

In a Peruvian context, experts on the subject of Sustainability and Construction mention that the water resource is a priority to conserve (Biondi, 2012), likewise in an interview with Dr. Martín Wieser in April 2018 with the question: If there was a certification specifically for social housing in Peru, which of the three Impact categories (energy, water, materials) would you consider most important for a weighting? It said that "Apart from that, I think that in the specific case of Lima and the Peruvian coast, the issue of Water / Drainage should have, if not the highest consideration, yes much more than what is assigned to it in the LEED or EDGE certifications."

Peru is a privileged country due to its water supply because it has an average annual volume of 2 046 287 MMC of water, ranking among the 20 richest countries in the world with 72,510 cubic meters / inhabitant / year (Fernández), however poor distribution of the population in its three regions Costa, Sierra and Selva with reference to the water availability of its hydrographic units, added to the poor management of the water of the inhabitants, generates inequalities of opportunity to drinking water and serious problems of water stress, adding to this, the contamination of this resource. The majority of the Peruvian population (about 70%) lives on the coast and it is precisely this region that receives approximately 1.8% of the country's available water (PUPC, 2018) (OXFAM, nd). To give an example, One of the cities on the coast is the capital, Lima, which is home to 9,674,755 inhabitants by 2020, representing 29.7% of the total population of Peru (32,625,948 inhabitants) (INEI, 2020) and its Rimac river only has a flow annual average of 42 m3 / s. Lisa Bunclark, specialist doctor in sustainable water management, thinks the following: "If we look at the entire country, we do not have water stress at the national level. If we look at the volume of water and the number of people, it is not a problem. The problem is that the water is not in all the areas we need ". (Bunclark, 2020) According to Oxfam, between 7 and 8 million Peruvians do not have access to drinking water.

People who do not have access to household services are forced to rationalize the use of water: limit personal hygiene, house cleaning and consumption according to Vargas and Carrión. According to INEI, between February 2017 and January 2018, 10.6% of the population that does not have access to water through the public network consumes water from tanker trucks (1.3%), wells (1.2%), and rivers and ditches. (3.2%).

The areas of Peru most at risk of running out of water according to a report published by the World Resources Institute (WRI) are the coastal areas of the regions: La Libertad, Lambayeque, Piura, Tumbes, Ica, Arequipa, Moquegua and Tacna, which are the most affected, and are approaching "day zero". The report indicates that governments still have time to mitigate the effects of this crisis. "By taking action now and investing in better management.

For Lima, Mirbel Epiquien, researcher of the Territory, Socio-Ecology and Ecosystem Services (TSESE) group of INTE-PUCP and head of Environmental Management and Ecosystem Services of Sedapal, mentions that climate change can "accelerate processes of prolonged drought and scarcity " in the capital. "The problem has already been felt for 20 years, and as a consequence other basins, such as the Mantaro, are used to feed Lima."

Professor Liliana Miranda in Peru (Miranda, 2018), through an interview, mentions that the water resource is important because it is used to produce electricity through hydroelectric plants. Climate change has the consequences of drought and this has already been felt through the El Niño phenomenon (Senamhi, nd) After this statement, it is worth mentioning that hydroelectric production, as seen in figure 3, is 42.7% of consumption In total, it is considered the second source of energy production in the country after natural gas and other fuels (53%). A percentage corresponds to solar and wind energy (3.2%).

Another current reality up to now facing the housing sector in Peru is informality in construction. Of the 10 million existing homes, 7 million are informal, this means that 70% of homes live in informality, without regulations in a framework of self-construction, according to the Ministry of Housing, Construction and Sanitation and Capeco.

And added to this is contamination; A study carried out by students from the University of San Ignacio de Loyola in Peru concluded that it is necessary to establish healthy water policies, which include, for example, the collection of information on the quality of wastewater in the main cities of Peru, especially those that exceed one million inhabitants or that include high levels of environmental contamination and the implementation of a domestic water control system, among others. (Larios- Meoño, González Taranco, & Morales Olivares, 2015)

On the other hand, at the global level, there are currently several scientific studies that analyze the conservation of important resources within the construction sector such as water. The UK was the first country to launch voluntary BREEAM environmental certification in 1990.

From the appearance of BREEAM, other sustainable certifications have been born for new construction buildings, renovations, cities, etc., with the aim of mitigating the impact from the construction sector, environmental certifications such as LEED, HQE, DNGB, among others, where they evaluate the water resource with their own methodologies.

In Peru, for example, by 2021, there are already 3 types of certifications that some buildings are using, which are: Bono Verde, LEED and EDGE certification. The last two are international certifications, however, EDGE has been designed to be used in developing countries and the national Bono Verde certification is only responsible for evaluating the sustainability of social residential buildings. All these environmental certifications evaluate water efficiency from the environmental point of view, however, some researchers mention that the water resource is not approached holistically. The few studies that focus on water management present evaluation and qualification indicators related to the environmental management of water in the operation stage of buildings, with less impact on an analysis throughout the life cycle from the extraction of the materials. The water incorporated in the materials is not considered in any of the environmental classification or certification of buildings. However, although LCA has been used to assess the impact of energy use, a comprehensive assessment of the impact of water use has not been performed using LCA. according to Robert H. Crawford & Stephen Pullen (2011)

On the other hand, other building evaluation and certification systems consider water from a human perspective, focusing on its quality for consumption or intake. For example, the concept of international WELL certification covers the aspects of water quality, distribution and control, includes characteristics that address the availability and principles of drinking water contaminants such as heavy metals, organic contaminants, agricultural and additives, control Legionella infection as well as features aimed at managing water to prevent damage to building materials, such as insulating materials that are sensitive to moisture and other environmental conditions.

Environmental certifications that evaluate the efficiency of water in residential buildings in Peru.

In this section we will see the three environmental certifications that are being used in Peru to evaluate the water category in residential buildings. These certifications approach it from the hydric efficiency.

The general description of them is addressed, such as the entity or body that promotes them, levels of achievement that can be achieved, type of buildings that it evaluates or number of certified buildings; and more specifically, in the water category, the evaluated criteria of the three certifications will be reviewed, which are: Mi vivienda verde or Bono Verde (Fondo Mivivienda, 2020), EDGE Certification (IFC, 2018) and LEED (Leed for Homes, 2011)

MI VIVIENDA VERDE CERTIFICATION (BONO VERDE- V7)

It is a sustainable housing certification program promoted by the Peruvian state and that is part of the Fondo Mivivienda of the FONAPE corporation (National Fund for the Financing of State Business Activity), it is a voluntary certification, whose first procedure manual is published in 2016.

This program encourages the buyer of certified homes or apartments through financial aid and preferential rates. Buildings can be certified in the design stage, that is, in the preliminary or project stage (new construction), being able to achieve three levels of achievement: Grade I +, Grade II +, and Grade III +.

With a record of 331 certified projects by 2020, the Mi Vivienda Verde methodology is given through the technical evaluation of documents such as plans, reports, specifications and / or technical product sheets, national or international quality certificates, letters of commitment., licenses and eligibility criteria. Only homes in the range from $ 16,662 to $ 118,744 can qualify for the evaluation, since it is a social program, as stated by Arch. Lucas Sarmiento, Supervisor of Real Estate Projects of Fondo Mivivienda, in March 2020.

Mi Vivienda Verde v7 requires compliance with 6 categories, being the following: Water, Energy, Bioclimatic, Materials, Waste and Urban Sustainability. (Fondo Mivivienda, 2020)

In water, the certification to obtain the Bono verde - Version 7, considers 9 indicators within the sub-criteria: Rational water consumption and Water reuse, of which the first 7 are mandatory for all the first two levels (grade 1+, grade 2+) that correspond to the use of low consumption hydrosanitary equipment (installation of taps, shower heads, water reserve tanks, technical irrigation in gardens) and the installation of independent meters. However, to reach the higher grade corresponding to 3+, it is mandatory to add the fulfillment of 2 indicators to the 7 indicators mentioned above. These correspond to the Reuse of water: The installation of a gray or black water treatment plant for the irrigation of gardens and another system for use in toilets.

Regarding the instruments or tools used for the evaluation in the design stage, Bono Verde uses a check list that details the technical specifications and the evidentiary documents for approval - compliance with the indicators and does not use or demand the use of a simulation calculator of water consumption of the project, later in use of the building it is necessary to send a consumption report through invoices that evidences the low water consumption, however in the construction stage there is no control of the implementation of the indicators.

EDGE

EDGE "Excellence in Design for Greater Efficiencies" is a program for developing countries of the International Finance Corporation (IFC), a member of the World Bank Group, financed by the Government of the United Kingdom, launched in July 2014 and by 2020 used in more of 140 countries of the world including Peru.

This voluntary certification can be used to certify buildings at any stage of their useful life cycle, which includes the conceptual idea, design, a new construction, existing buildings and renovations of Residences, Hotels, Hospitals, Shops, Offices and of Education evaluating buildings through the use of a free online software application (Edge, nd), which predicts the savings of three resources: Water, Energy and Materials, comparing the building to be certified with a standard local model case for also estimate the cost of capital and period of return on investment, all this is possible since it contains a database of climate, costs, consumption patterns and algorithms of cities to predict performance results.

With the evaluation of buildings, 3 levels of certification can be achieved: EDGE Certification, EDGE Advance and EDGE Zero Carbon, being the EDGE Certification the easiest to achieve since it requires the building to sustain a minimum saving of 20% in energy operational, 20% savings in water consumption and 20% savings in embedded energy of construction materials as a minimum. The three levels of achievement can be obtained in 2 main stages: preliminary certification (design stage) and final certification (post-construction stage) (IFC, 2018).

Regarding the EDGE certification with the new Beta 3.0 version (Edge, 2021), it will evaluate 8 more indicators in the Water category, compared to version 2.1. Therefore, you would now have 14 indicators. The indicators added in this version are: Low consumption bidet evaluation, use of low consumption dishwashers, kitchen rinse spray valves, energy efficient washing machines, pool covers, efficient garden irrigation system, water recovery condensed and smart meters.

On the other hand, in the previous version 2.1, the mandatory indicators to declare for the evaluation of the percentage (%) of water savings are 5: The consumption in L / m of the shower heads, bathroom and kitchen taps and the consumption of the L / flush of the toilets of one or two flushes evaluating these with the use of a calculator incorporated in the online software tool where the flows, types and number of devices are entered to obtain an average flow weighted in liters per minute or liters per download, likewise, design drawings, technical sheets of the manufacturers and additional calculations are requested to obtain the evaluation in the preliminary certification stage, then delivery vouchers and photographs of the implementation for the on-site audit for the final certification,which are performed by a certified EDGE auditor.

It is worth mentioning that EDGE allows to be selective with the WATER indicators that appear in the online software for its evaluation, its qualification methodology is not through summative scores but by percentage of savings above a baseline, therefore it is allowed select the indicators that are required until reaching a minimum of 20% savings to achieve certification.

LEED FOR HOMES

The LEED certification system (1998) is under the guidelines of the North American regulation ASHRAE 90.1-2007 and contemplates within its evaluation the Regional Priority category, awarding 4 points for addressing exclusive environmental problems in the region. The system is also used in 135 other countries (USGBC, 2012a)

The LEED toolkit consists of versions for new construction and major renovations, existing building operations and maintenance, commercial interiors, core and exterior development, retail, schools, homes, neighborhood development, and healthcare (USGBC, 2012c)

Regarding the version for homes, it was created in 2008 LEED for Homes (Leed for Homes, 2011), where its comprehensive evaluation, that is, in the design stage and later a verification visit is required mid-construction, as well as at the end of construction. LEED for Homes is available for building design and construction projects for single-family homes and multi-family projects of up to eight stories. It should be mentioned that in Peru there is currently no building certified with this version, but there are departments under the Corel and Shell modality as stated by the architect Leslie Berdiales, an accredited Leed specialist in Peru during an interview in March 2021.

The criteria evaluated in this version are nine: Integrative Process, Location and Transportation, Sustainable Sites, Water efficiency, Energy and Atmosphere, Materials and Resources, Indoor Environmental Quality, Innovation and Regional Priority and the levels that can be reached is by the sum of points where ≥ 40 points are obtained at Certificate Level, ≥ 50 points at Silver Level, ≥ 60 points at Gold Level, and ≥ 80 points at Platinum Level (US Green Building Council, 2017).

Leed for homes (V4) within the evaluation of the criterion called Water Efficiency, evaluates four indicators, being the use of the water consumption meter the mandatory prerequisite compared to the other three that correspond to: The reduction of the total demand for water, the management of water use inside the building and outdoors, which are evaluated online evidencing their compliance with supporting documents.

This certification gives a total score of 12 points for the evaluation of Water Efficiency of 110 points considered for the evaluation of the other environmental criteria, the 12 points can be compared in a check list and are given in this way:

1 point to 12 points are achieved according to the reduction of% of integral water, for example, if 20% of the total use of water is reduced (this includes the reduction of the use of water inside and out-

side) above the traditional practices of use, 3 points out of 12 points would be awarded. The tools used to calculate the average flow rate and percentage savings in LEED for water use inside and outside the building are the Water Reduction calculator and the EPA WaterSense Water Budget calculator.

On the other hand, if you want to apply to an evaluation of the indicators that correspond to the management of indoor water use (taps, sanitary ware and selection of washing machines), the points awarded are from 1 point to 6 points which are measurable If they meet the technical conditions, for example, for efficient faucets with WaterSense certificate, 2 points are awarded if 3.7 liters per minute are not exceeded at a pressure no greater than 414kPa.

Likewise, for the management of water use in gardens, from 1 point to 4 points are awarded per% reduction of grass and increase of native plants, providing complete information by other means of the native plants of some states of North America as a guide.

International Certifications that Evaluate the Quality of Water in Residential Buildings

There are other international certifications that evaluate the water category from another perspective, from quality, here we describe two certifications, one American and the next French, the WELL certification and the HQE certification that have not currently entered Peru, however, WELL if you have certified professionals in the country and it is promoted by entities such as the Peru Green Building Council.

WELL

The WELL environmental evaluation and certification system is a standard developed by DELOS, and currently managed by the International Well Building Institute (IWBI). It is a system aimed at measuring, certifying and monitoring the performance of building characteristics that directly affect the health and well-being of its occupants. It is currently in 67 countries, however it does not have certified buildings in Peru at present.

The WELL construction standard can be applied in commercial buildings, multi-family residential, education, restaurants and commercial kitchens, at the new and existing building level, new and existing interiors, or core and shell compliance to pilot standards.

The building certification pathway is aimed at the design, construction and operation phase of new and existing office buildings with a minimum of 90% of the total area occupied by the owner of the building and operated by the same administration.

It certifies the characteristics of buildings that impact human health and well-being through ten concepts: air, water, nutrition, lighting, physical condition, thermal comfort, sound, materials, comfort, mind and innovation. It combines best practices in design and construction with evidence-based scientific and medical research, leveraging the impact of buildings and communities on human health and well-being.

WELL v2 operates on a points-based system (WELL, 2021), with 110 points available, so in terms of achievement levels, the highest option can be achieved with the WELL Platinum Certification: 80 points, followed by Certification WELL Gold: 60 points and finally WELL Silver Certification: 50 points.

Regarding the evaluation of the water category, WELL covers aspects of the quality, distribution and control of drinking water within a building, includes characteristics that address the availability and contaminants of drinking water, as well as characteristics aimed at water management for Avoid damage to building materials and environmental conditions.

For example, it evaluates as a Prerequisite: Fundamental water quality which requires being within the parameters corresponding to sediments (turbidity level <1.0 NTU), microorganisms (no detection of coliforms including E.coli), in addition to the monitoring of fundamental water parameters.

The second prerequisite is to control Water Pollutants such as:

Metals (lead <0.01 mg / L., Arsenic <0.01 mg / L., Antimony <0.006 mg / L., Mercury <0.002 mg / L., Nickel <0.07 mg / L., Copper <1.0 mg / L., cadmium <0.005 mg / L), chromium (total) <0.1mg / L.)

Organic contaminants (styrene <0.02 mg / L., Benzene <0.005mg / L., Ethylbenzene <0.3 mg / L., Vinyl chloride <0.002 mg / L., Toluene <0.7 mg / L., Xylenes (total: m, pyo) <0.5 mg / L., tetrachlor-ethylene <0.005 mg / L.)

Disinfectant by-products (Total trihalomethanes (sum of dibromochloromethane, bromodichloro-methane, chloroform and bromoform) less than 0.08 mg / L., Total haloacetic acids (sum of chloroacetic, dichloracetic, trichloroacetic, bromoacetic and dibromoacetic acids) less than 0.06 mg / L.

Agricultural pollutants Fertilizers: Nitrate less than 50 mg / l (11 mg / l as nitrogen)

Red additives (Fluoride less than 4 mg / L., Chlorine less than 4 mg / L., Chloramine less than 4 mg / L.) (WELL, 2018)

Finally, the third prerequisite is to control Legionella where it is requested to present a Legionella control management plan, which consists of describing the following points: Formation of a team for the management of Legionella in the building, inventory of the system of water and production of process flow diagrams, risk analysis of water resources, identification of critical control points, etc.

Legionella or Legionellosis is a disease caused by the bacterium Legionella pneumophila, the spread of this disease can occur through contact with contaminated water vapor that usually comes from bathtubs or hot showers and air conditioning units in large buildings for example .

Also, consider other optional assessment requirements such as: Improved Water Quality, Drinking Water Quality Management, Drinking Water Promotion, Humidity Management, Hand Washing, Reuse of Non-Drinking Water on Site which can be read at the Version 2 manual.

HQE ™

Since 2013 the HQE ™ (Haute Qualité Environnementale) (High Environmental Quality) building certification is an internationally registered trademark and is the exclusive property of the HQE ™ Association in France covering construction, renovation and operation, as well as urban planning and development. It attaches importance to the analysis of the life cycle on a construction scale and the impacts of a project in 14 criteria distributed from 4 objectives: Energy, Environment, Health and Comfort. Five rankings are possible depending on the number of stars obtained on each topic. HQE Pass 14 PR targets HQE Good 1 to 4 Stars, HQE Very Good 5 to 8 Stars, HQE Excellent 9 to 11 Stars and HQE Exceptional ≥ 12 Stars.

The certification requires at least three categories in excellent level, four in superior and seven in good performance level (HQE, 2014).

The 14 evaluated criteria are: Site, Components, Worksite, Energy, Water, Waste, Maintenance, Hygrothermal comfort, Acoustic comfort, Visual comfort, Olfactory comfort, Spaces quality, Air quality, Water quality.

It is important to mention that in South America, in Brazil, the certification is also known as the AQUA process adapted from the original HQE model for the Brazilian version. (Vanzolini, nd)

HQE ™ not only evaluates the water from the environmental point of view (water efficiency), but also from the quality, where there are 2 prerequisites (mandatory): The first is to plan the washing and disinfection of all the pipes after giving it use and before the installation of the plumbing by the installation company. At this point it is required that there is a preliminary draft and design audit.

On the other hand, in a non-mandatory way, awarding 1 point for compliance is the following:

"For any contact with water intended for human consumption, the products are selected from the following materials: - Metals, alloys and metallic coatings based on copper, iron, aluminum and zinc - Materials based on hydraulic binders, enamels, ceramics and glass, - Organic materials with a certificate of compliance (equivalent to the Health Conformity Attestation validated by a recognized scientific body). " (HQE, 2014)

For countries where the water distributed by the network is intended for human consumption, it is requested, as a second prerequisite, that: Each house must be equipped with a retention system (backflow, non-return valve system, etc.) in the water supply cold water and, if necessary, hot water supply in the case of collective DHW, where a preliminary project and design audit will be required.

You can optionally perform a post-construction plumbing outlet water analysis, rinsing and disinfection. The ISO 147 standard is taken into account for this point.

The procedure is based on testing the home furthest from the building's water supply point, as well as a randomly chosen residence; On the other hand, for single-family homes, a sample must be taken that applies a rate of 5% to residences with a minimum of one residence.

As a tool, HQE ™ also provides a calculator in Excel format to predict consumption and a very detailed guide for its use (HQE, 2014)

PERUVIAN REGULATIONS THAT ARE IN CHARGE OF WATER QUALITY IN PERU

A quality regulation for human consumption of the Ministry of Health Peru / DS N ° 031-2010-SA is documented. of the year 2010 to manage water quality. (Ministerio de Ambiente, 2011)

This regulation establishes the general provisions related to the management of the quality of water for human consumption, in order to guarantee its safety, prevent health risk factors, as well as protect and promote the health and well-being of the population.

It is comprised of the following aspects: The management of water quality, the sanitary surveillance of water, The control and supervision of water quality; Inspection, authorizations, records and sanitary approvals regarding water supply systems for human consumption; The physical, chemical, microbiological and parasitological requirements of water for human consumption, and the dissemination and access to information on the quality of water for human consumption.

In this regulation it details which are the entities in charge of ensuring the quality of water in Peru, being in the field of construction at the national level; The Ministry of Housing, Construction and Sanitation, which is in charge of providing in the regulations of its sector the application of the provisions and sanitary requirements established in these regulations, Also establishing in the plans, programs and projects of water supply for human consumption the application of sanitary norms; Provide the necessary measures in your sector, as a result of the declaration of sanitary emergency of the water supply by the health authority of the jurisdiction; and generate the necessary conditions for access to water services at levels of quality and sustainability in its provision,

The regulation establishes the maximum permissible limits in terms of microbiological and parasitic parameters of organoleptic quality, inorganic and organic chemicals, radioactive that are shown below: (Ministerio de Ambiente, 2011)

Tables extracted from the Regulation of the Ministry of Health Peru / DS N ° 031-2010-SA translated into English Source: http://www.digesa.minsa.gob.pe/publicaciones/descargas/Regdamientos_Calidad_Agua.pdf

Table 1.

MAXIMUM PERMISSIBLE LIMITS OF PARAMETERS
MICROBIOLOGICAL AND PARASITOLOGICAL

Parameters	Unit of measure	Maximum limit permissible
1. Total Coliform Bacteria.	CFU / 100 mL a 35°C	0 (*)
2. E. Coli	CFU / 100 mL a 44.5°C	0 (*)
3. Thermotolerant or Fecal Coliform Bacteria.	CFU / 100 mL a 44.5°C	0 (*)
4. Heterotrophic bacteria	CFU / mL at 35°C	500
5. Helminth eggs and larvae, cysts and oocysts of protozoa pathogens.	Org / L no.	0
6. Viruses	CFU / mL	0
7. Free-living organisms, such as algae, protozoa, copepods, rotifers, nematodes in all their evolutionary stages	Org / L no.	0

CFU = Colony Forming Unit (*)
In case of analyzing by the MPN technique by multiple tubes = <1.8 / 100 ml

Table 2.

MAXIMUM PERMISSIBLE LIMITS OF PARAMETERS OF ORGANOLEPTIC QUALITY

Parameters	Unit of measurement	Maximum allowable limit
1. Smell	---	Acceptable
two Taste	---	Acceptable
3. Color	UCV Pt / Co scale	fifteen
Four. Turbidity	UNT	5
5. pH	PH value	6.5 to 8.5
6. Conductivity (25 ° C)	µ mho / cm	1,500
7. Total dissolved solids	mgL-1	1 000
8. Chlorides	mg Cl - L-1	250
9. Sulfates	mg SO4=L-1	250
10. Total hardness	mg CaCO3L-1	500
eleven Ammonia	mg N L-1	1.5
12. Iron	mg Fe L-1	0.3
13. Manganese	mg Mn L-1	0.4
14. Aluminum	mg Al L-1	0.2
fifteen Copper	mg Cu L-1	2.0
16. Zinc	mg Zn L-1	3.0
17. Sodium	mg Na L-1	200

UCV = True Color Unit
UNT = Nephelometric unit of turbidity

CONCLUSION

An overview has been shown of the approach to sustainability certifications in water matters that are certifying buildings in Peru and, on the other hand, other international certifications that go beyond the evaluation of water efficiency that could contribute to new standards or certifications in the Peruvian sociocultural context, with a focus on the quality of the inhabitant within the buildings, a human approach as well as a regulation on water quality for the Peruvian context of 2010. On the other hand, it is good to mention below that the Finding of a scientific article that is supported by others, where they analyze the category of water from a life cycle approach, for example Robert H. Crawford &Stephen Pullen (2011) analyzed the direct and indirect water consumption of a conventional Australian residential building and its occupants over a 50-year period, which is a benchmark for other research.

The study showed that direct water consumption is 6.4% of the use during the life cycle of a residential building and its occupants. The indirect incorporated water in the materials used for construction was 9.7% of the total, for which it shows little impact on total consumption, however, it is important to mention it.

Table 3.

Organic Parameters	Unit of measurement	Maximum allowable limit
1. Total trihalomethanes (note 3)		1.00
2. Dissolved or emulsified hydrocarbon; mineral oil	mgL^{-1}	0.01
3. Oils and fats	mgL^{-1}	0.5
4. Alachlor	mgL^{-1}	0.020
5. Aldicarb	mgL^{-1}	0.010
6. Aldrin and dieldrin	mgL^{-1}	0.00003
7. Benzene	mgL^{-1}	0.010
8. Chlordane (total isomers)	mgL^{-1}	0.0002
9. DDT (total isomers)	mgL^{-1}	0.001
10. Endrin	mgL^{-1}	0.0006
11. Gamma HCH (lindane)	mgL^{-1}	0.002
12. Hexachlorobenzene	mgL^{-1}	0.001
13. Heptachlor and heptachloroepoxide	mgL^{-1}	0.00003
14. Methoxychlor	mgL^{-1}	0.020
15. Pentachlorophenol	mgL^{-1}	0.009
16. 2,4-D	mgL^{-1}	0.030
17. Acrylamide	mgL^{-1}	0.0005
18. Epichlorohydrin	mgL^{-1}	0.0004
19. Vinyl chloride	mgL^{-1}	0.0003
20. Benzopyrene	mgL^{-1}	0.0007
21. 1,2-dichloroethane	mgL^{-1}	0.03
22. Tetrachloroethene	mgL^{-1}	0.04

Table 4.

MAXIMUM PERMISSIBLE LIMITS OF
INORGANIC AND ORGANIC CHEMICAL PARAMETERS

Inorganic Parameters	Unit of measurement	Maximum allowable limit
1. Antimony	$mg\ Sb\ L^{-1}$	0.020
2. Arsenic (note 1)	$mg\ As\ L^{-1}$	0.010
3. Barium	$mg\ Ba\ L^{-1}$	0.700
4. Boron	$mg\ B\ L^{-1}$	1,500
5. Cadmium	$mg\ Cd\ L^{-1}$	0.003
6. Cyanide	$mg\ CN^{-}\ L^{-1}$	0.070
7. Chlorine (note 2)	$mg\ L^{-1}$	5
8. Chlorite	$mg\ L^{-1}$	0.7
9. Chlorate	$mg\ L^{-1}$	0.7
10. Total chromium	$mg\ Cr\ L^{-1}$	0.050
11. Fluorine	$mg\ F^{-}\ L^{-1}$	1,000
12. Mercury	$mg\ Hg\ L^{-1}$	0.001
13. Nickel	$mg\ Ni\ L^{-1}$	0.020
14. Nitrates	$mg\ NO_3\ L^{-1}$	50.00
15. Nitrites	mg NO two L^{-1}	3.00 Short exposure 0.20 Long exposure
16. Lead	$mg\ Pb\ L^{-1}$	0.010
17. Selenium	$mg\ Se\ L^{-1}$	0.010
18. Molybdenum	$mg\ Mo\ L^{-1}$	0.07
19. Uranium	$mg\ U\ L^{-1}$	0.015

Table 5.

Organic Parameters	Unit of measurement	Maximum allowable limit
23. Monochloramine	mgL^{-1}	3
24. Trichloroethene	mgL^{-1}	0.07
25. Carbon tetrachloride	mgL^{-1}	0.004
26. Di (2-ethylhexyl) phthalate	mgL^{-1}	0.008
27. 1,2- Dichlorobenzene	mgL^{-1}	1
28. 1,4- Dichlorobenzene	mgL^{-1}	0.3
29. 1,1- Dichloroethene	mgL^{-1}	0.03
30. 1,2- Dichloroethene	mgL^{-1}	0.05
31. Dichloromethane	mgL^{-1}	0.02
32. Edetic acid (EDTA)	mgL^{-1}	0.6
33. Ethylbenzene	mgL^{-1}	0.3
34. Hexachlorobutadiene	mgL^{-1}	0.0006
35. Nitrilotriacetic Acid	mgL^{-1}	0.2
36. Styrene	mgL^{-1}	0.02
37. Toluene	mgL^{-1}	0.7
38. Xylene	mgL^{-1}	0.5
39. Atrazine	mgL^{-1}	0.002
40. Carbofuran	mgL^{-1}	0.007
41. Chlorotoluron	mgL^{-1}	0.03
42. Cianazina	mgL^{-1}	0.0006
43. 2,4- DB	mgL^{-1}	0.09
44. 1,2- Dibromo-3- Chloropropane	mgL^{-1}	0.001
45. 1,2- Dibromoethane	mgL^{-1}	0.0004
46. 1,2- Dichloropropane (1,2- DCP)	mgL^{-1}	0.04
47. 1,3- Dichloropropene	mgL^{-1}	0.02
48. Dichloroprop	mgL^{-1}	0.1
49. Dimethate	mgL^{-1}	0.006
50. Fenoprop	mgL^{-1}	0.009
51. Isoproturon	mgL^{-1}	0.009
52. MCPA	mgL^{-1}	0.002
53. Mecoprop	mgL^{-1}	0.01
54. Metolachlor	mgL^{-1}	0.01
55. Molinato	mgL^{-1}	0.006
56. Pendimethalin	mgL^{-1}	0.02
57. Simazine	mgL^{-1}	0.002
58. 2,4,5- T	mgL^{-1}	0.009
59. Terbutylazine	mgL^{-1}	0.007
60. Trifluralin	mgL^{-1}	0.02
61. Chloropyrifos	mgL^{-1}	0.03
62. Pyriproxyfen	mgL^{-1}	0.3
63. Microcystin-LR	mgL^{-1}	0.001

Table 6.

Organic Parameters	Unit of measure	Maximum allowable limit
64. Bromate	mgL^{-1}	0.01
65. Bromodichloromethane	mgL^{-1}	0.06
66. Bromoform	mgL^{-1}	0.1
67. Chloral hydrate (trichloroacetaldehyde)	mgL^{-1}	0.01
68. Chloroform	mgL^{-1}	0.2
69. Cyanogen chloride (as CN)	mgL^{-1}	0.07
	mgL^{-1}	0.07
70. Dibromoacetonitrile	mgL^{-1}	0.1
71. Dibromochloromethane	mgL^{-1}	0.05
72. Dichloroacetate	mgL^{-1}	0.02
73. Dichloroacetonitrile	mgL^{-1}	0.9
74. Formaldehyde	mgL^{-1}	0.02
75. Monochloroacetate	mgL^{-1}	0.2
76. Trichloroacetate	mgL^{-1}	0.2
77. 2,4,6- Trichlorophenol		

Table 7.

MAXIMUM PERMISSIBLE LIMITS OF
RADIOACTIVE PARAMETERS

Parameters	Unit of measure	Maximum allowable limit
1. Total reference dose (note 1)	mSv / year	0.1
2. Global activity α	Bq / L	0.5
3. Global activity β	Bq / L	1.0

Figure 1. Table extracted from Crawford and Pullen, 2011 showing the coefficient of incorporated water in kL / m2

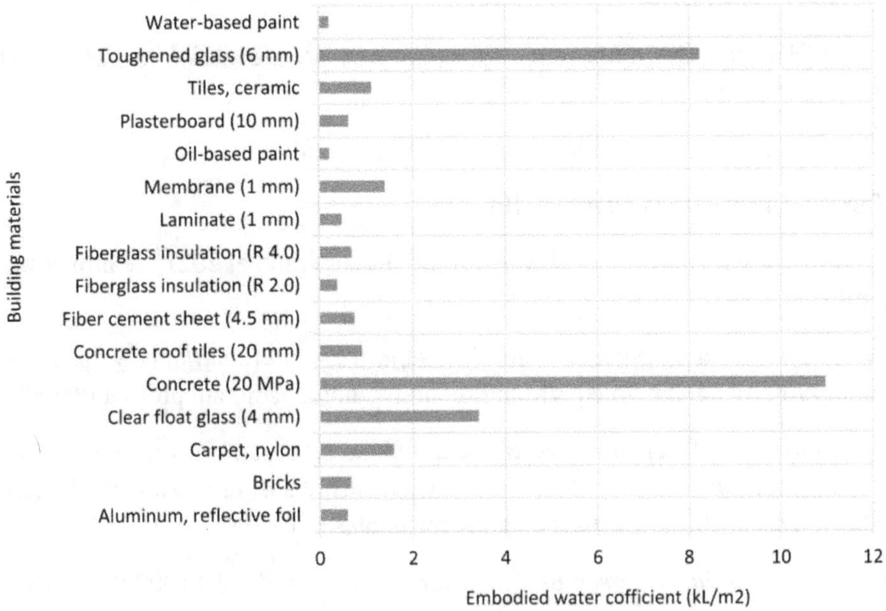

REFERENCES

Biondi, S. (2012, Noviembre 2). *Arquitectura Sostenible*. Retrieved from https://www.youtube.com/watch?v=wxIOK1V1joc&ab_channel=PUCPPUCP

Breeam. (2011). *Manual BREEAM ES VIVIENDA®*. Galicia.

Bunclark, L. (2020, Febrero 13). *Consideran al Perú en un nivel medio alto de estrés de agua*. Retrieved from https://rpp.pe/peru/actualidad/consideran-al-peru-en-un-nivel-medio-alto-de-estres-de-agua-noticia-1245508

Crawford, R. H., & Pullen, S. (2011). Life cycle water analysis of a residential building and its occupants. *Building Research and Information*, *39*(6), 589–602. doi:10.1080/09613218.2011.584212

Edge. (2021). *Guía del usuario de EDGE para todos los tipos de edificios Versión 3.0 BETA*. Recuperado el junio de 2021, de https://edgebuildings.com/wp-content/uploads/2021/02/201211-EDGE-User-Guide-for-All-Building-Types-Version-3.0.A-Beta.pdf

Edge. (n.d.). *Software EDGE*. Retrieved from https://edgebuildings.com/software/?lang=es

Fernández, A. (n.d.). *Aguas residuaes en Perú, Problemática y uso en la agricultura*. Retrieved from https://www.ais.unwater.org/ais/pluginfile.php/356/mod_page/content/128/Peru%20INFORME%20DE%20PAIS.pdf

Fondo Mivivienda. (2020). *Procedimiento de Certificación de proyectos del Programa Mivienda Sostenible.* Retrieved from https://www.mivivienda.com.pe/PORTALCMS/archivos/documentos/8586096294727711719.PDF

HQE. (2014). *HQE™Scheme Environmental Performance Residential Building*. Retrieved from https://www.behqe.com/schemes-and-documents

HQE. (2014). User's Guide to the Tool for Target 5 – Water. Author.

IFC. (2018). *EDGE User Guide Versión 2.1*. IFC.

Inca, H. (n.d.). *Hidráulica Inca Camino- Inca del Agua*. Recuperado el 2021, de https://hidraulicainca.com/cusco/tipon/

INEI. (2020). *Nota de Prensa La población de Lima supera los nueve millones y medio de habitantes*. Retrieved from http://m.inei.gob.pe/media/MenuRecursivo/noticias/notadeprensa006.pdf

Larios-Meoño, J., González Taranco, C., & Morales Olivares, Y. (2015). Las aguas residuales y sus consecuencias en el Perú. *Saber y Hacer*, 21-23. Obtained from https://pre-www.usil.edu.pe/sites/default/files/revista-saber-y-hacer-v2n2.2-1-19set16-aguas-residuales.pdf

Leed for Homes. (2011). *Guide to Green Building Rating Systems*. doi:10.1002/9781118259894.ch4

Ministerio de Ambiente. (2015). *Regionalización y Caracterización de sequias en Perú*. Obtained from https://www.senamhi.gob.pe/pdf/estudios/hidro_2015_Reg_car_seq_Per.pdf

Ministerio de Salud. (2011). *Reglamento de la calidad del agua para Consumo Humano*. Obtained from http://www.digesa.minsa.gob.pe/publicaciones/descargas/reglamento_calidad_agua.pdf

Miranda, A. L. (2018, mayo 28). *¿Agua o Energía?* (E. Samamé, Interviewer). Academic Press.

OXFAM. (n.d.). *OXFAM en Perú*. Retrieved from Entre 7 y 8 millones de peruanos no tienen acceso a agua potable: https://peru.oxfam.org/qu%C3%A9-hacemos-ayuda-humanitaria/entre-7-y-8-millones-de-peruanos-no-tienen-acceso-agua-potable

PérezC. J. (2017). fromhttp://repositorio.senamhi.gob.pe/bitstream/handle/20.500.12542/246/Causa-sequ%C3%ADas-severas-sur-Per%C3%BA_2017.pdf?sequence=1&isAllowed=y

PUPC. (2018). *Informe Puntoedu sobre estrés hídrico en el Perú*. Retrieved from https://puntoedu.pucp.edu.pe/noticia/informe-puntoedu-sobre-estres-hidrico-en-el-peru/

Revista peruana Geo-Atmosférica RPGA. (2010). *Recent droughts in the Peruvian Amazonas basin: Climate origins and.* Revista Peruana Geo-Atmosferica RPGA. Obtained fromhttps://web2.senamhi.gob.pe/rpga/pdf/2011_vol03/art5.pdf

Senamhi. (n.d.). *Eventos Climáticos - Fenómeno del Niño*. Retrieved from Senamhi: http://senamhi.gob.pe/?p=fenomeno-el-nino

U.S. Green Building Council. (2017). *LEED v4 for Homes design and Construction*. LEED.

Vanzolini. (n.d.). Obtained from https://vanzolini.org.br/aqua/certificacao-aqua-hqe/

WELL. (2018). *Well V2 tm*. WELL.

WELL. (2021). *WELL Performance Verification Guidebook*. Obtained from https://a.storyblok.com/f/52232/x/29668f7afb/well-performance-verification-guidebook_q2-2021.pdf

Chapter 6
Environmental Awareness:
An Improvement Strategy in the Education of Architects

Felix Aramburu
Universidad CEU San Pablo, Spain

ABSTRACT

University studies for the architecture degree in Spain give very little weight to considerations related to the design of a healthy interior environment. The low number of subjects related to interior comfort criteria may cause the student to underestimate the importance of environmental design of closed spaces in favor of aesthetic or merely functional aspects. However, there is a direct relationship between formal design decisions and environmental conditions in buildings, and future architects must understand those connections in order to make designs that combine efficiency and high aesthetic value. In this chapter, several pedagogical strategies are presented to get architecture students to learn and internalize the link between design and interior conditions, aiming at the acquisition of an adequate environmental awareness.

INTRODUCTION

Students of architecture in the 21st century face a colossal challenge. Whereas previous generations were required "only" to satisfy questions of habitability with artistic creations, future generations are asked to change the world. Function, Context, Construction, Economy and Beauty were the parameters required of architecture (Campo-Baeza, 1996) and now it is necessary to add the concept of Sustainability. Architecture must make human activity sustainable, from an energy consumer to a producer. It must change the environment, collaborate in reversing the planet's climate change. An ambitious and mandatory challenge for future architects, which is included among the sustainable development goals set by the United Nations for 2030 in its SDG 11: "Make cities and human settlements inclusive, safe, resilient and sustainable" and expected to be achieved by Spain (Boto-Álvarez & García-Fernández. 2020). Thus, during their education, architecture students must face an increasing variety of disciplines, which they will have to integrate appropriately in their future professional work.

DOI: 10.4018/978-1-7998-7279-5.ch006

Architecture students must learn to unify and interrelate the concepts of functional design, aesthetics, verification of regulations and urban planning together with the technological systems that allow buildings to function and be habitable: lighting, hydraulic, mechanical and environmental systems. In this document we focus particularly on technical studies, and specifically on those aimed at environmental comfort. During the student's training period, it is of utmost importance that all students acquire an environmental awareness, in order to understand that during the formal development of building projects, the variables of efficient design in terms of energy and air quality must be integrated. The aim of this chapter is to analyse the pedagogical strategies that encourage students to integrate environmental quality into building design. The aim is to highlight the strategies proposed by technical subjects to improve the environmental awareness of students, who will be responsible for the building designs that we will necessarily inhabit in the future. The strategies presented seek to involve students in one of the design variables that is rarely shown in architectural journals: the design of interior environments.

BACKGROUND

The Environmental Requirements of Nowadays Architecture

The increasing demands for energy efficiency in building have led to a paradigm shift in the architectural profession. While previous generations of architects were required to make buildings increasingly less demanding of fossil fuels, current generations will be required to make buildings collaborate in the reduction of greenhouse gas emissions, with a decisive integration of renewable energies in the building process. This is evident in the latest version of the " Technical Building Code, in its basic document on energy saving" (CTE HE), where strict compliance with its energy consumption targets means that at least 50% of the total primary energy consumption must come from renewable systems. Architects should be aware that this requirement is applicable to practically all the buildings they are going to design once they graduate, and that this requirement, far from being reduced, will be increased in subsequent years. In this sense, they should be aware of the European policies that will affect them in the immediate future, such as those included in the "Proposal of the European Commission Framework 2030 (EU Council 2014), or the "Roadmap to a Competitive Low Carbon Economy by 2050 (EU Commission 2011), published by the European Parliament and which will force them to reformulate their way of designing architecture.

Air renewal requirements are particularly in the spotlight nowadays, after the reflection on air healthiness that the SARS-COV 19 pandemic has forced us to reflect on. Before the SARS outbreak, it was not uncommon to find advocates for the non-obligation of mechanical ventilation systems in certain buildings such as schools. After the events of 2020, nobody has any doubt about the need for environmental systems that guarantee maximum quality and absence of pathogens in all types of buildings and particularly in dwellings (Domínguez-Amarillo et al. 2020). These ventilation systems should be re-examined in the design of new buildings; natural ventilation should be a viable option in all types of buildings, in addition to minimising air recirculation and promoting the use of effective and easy-to-maintain filters (Chirico et al, 2020). Working as an architect requires the integration of various disciplines under the same responsibility, so the professional must have knowledge of functional, structural and technical design, and be able to integrate them into a single object in an efficient way. This approach does not imply that the architect should be the sole author and designer of all the technical processes involved in construction. Collaboration with other specialists (engineers, structural calculators, technical architects) is vital and necessary. Collaboration must be interdisciplinary in such a way that this relationship with other technicians generates a new framework of knowledge in the architect's training and professional life (Borrego, 2008).

In the professional activity of an architect, innumerable technical requirements will be presented, both from general plans and building codes. They also have to face countless budgetary, constructive and even client relationship constraints (Stang & Hedegaard, 2018). But there is no aesthetic code, and in no case are limitations on the formal design of buildings acceptable. In other words, most of the requirements of municipalities and other governmental agencies are of a technical nature, and a minimal percentage are aesthetic. A study of the town plans and building regulations of the various municipalities is particularly revealing. As far as aesthetic requirements are concerned, the only requirement is restricted to appropriate integration within the already built or historic surroundings, while in terms of technical and environmental requirements they refer to a multitude of regulations and mandatory requirements.

In addition to all these regulatory requirements, the profession demands high aesthetic value in architectural creations, and here arises the tension between technique and design. The efforts required to obtain adequate thermal, energy and environmental conditions are often seen as an aesthetic hindrance, instead of an opportunity to improve the design. It is necessary to change this perception; these concepts must be associated as part of the integral design. The architect must, in short, have an environmental awareness.

The Environmental Footprint in the Architecture

It is interesting to briefly analyse how climatic variables left their mark on the architecture of the past, in order to understand the relationship between form and environmental comfort.

Environmental Approach of Vernacular Architecture

Traditional buildings, lacking cheap and easily accessible energy, had to be designed to be sustainable. Environmental considerations were an absolute priority, and building design had to provide the best level of solar control, ventilation, thermal stability and autonomy. This was inherited knowledge, the result of accumulated experience and necessity. Architecture was bioclimatic, understood as architecture that is consistent with the climatic conditions of its surroundings. In this way it is easy to understand the wooden architecture of northern Europe, the massive constructions of dry climates or the open designs of tropical buildings.

In general, vernacular architecture sacrificed form to obtain improved, but uncontrolled, interior conditions. The construction systems were not very hermetic, making thermal control difficult, but favouring air renewal. In cold climates, houses were built around the fire (oven, fireplace, hearth...). This heat producer "was the first thing to be built. From this point onwards, the house continued to be built, sometimes little more than a room, on other occasions of a more significant size" (Neila, 2020). The architecture of warmer climates was built around courtyards with fountains, also seeking shade and natural ventilation. This is the case of the Alhambra in Granada, with its lattice architecture that allowed solar control and ventilation, and the presence of water to favour evaporative cooling.

In short, as there were no technological systems to palliate possible environmental imbalances, the design was totally conditioned to the achievement of a habitable interior environment.

Figure 1. Alhambra – solar control.
Photo: Tama66

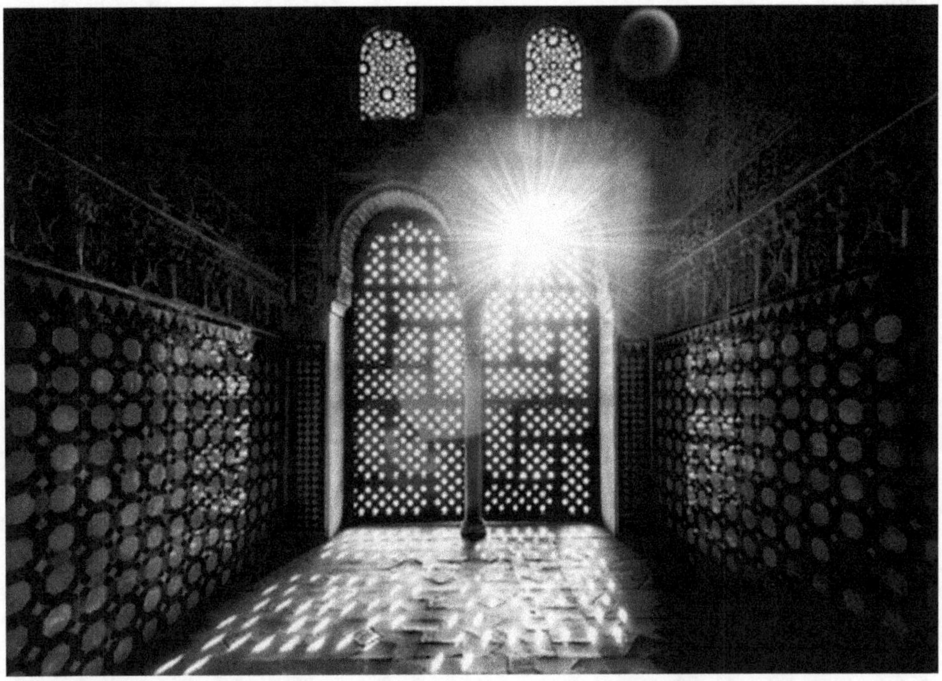

Environmental Design Factors in Post-Industrial Architecture

The improvement in the quality of building materials, mechanisation and improved access to energy curiously brought several problems associated with the indoor building environment. Having continuous thermal output increased indoor pollution, and at the same time more airtight building solutions made ventilation more difficult. Health problems associated with gas lighting in England were the beginning of an early stream of environmental awareness, led by doctors and engineers, but not by architects. This can be seen in some of the earliest modern buildings with mechanical ventilation systems (such as the London Parliament), where the first confrontations between the Architect and the Technician in charge of the air renewal systems could be registered (Sturrock & Lawson-Smith, 2006).

The incipient environmental awareness was understood to be relevant for certain buildings such as parliaments, hospitals or prisons, but had not yet been extended to all buildings. In buildings where the indoor environment was taken into consideration, the design was altered by incorporating ventilation chambers and ducts. Basements were fitted out as technical spaces to capture, filter and temper the ventilation air, as can be seen in the ventilation design for St Georges Hall by D.B. Reid. (Mackenzie 1964). –

The Environmental Approach in 20th Century Architecture

The technological advances of this century completely altered the design of buildings to such an extent that they gave rise to new architectural typologies. For instance, the Otis elevator enabled the Chicago school to promote high-rise buildings (Goodwin, 2001), and C.W. Carrier's artificial climate enabled office buildings to move away from cross ventilation set uses far from façades (Abalos & Herreros,

Figure 2. Mechanical ventilation and warming os St Georges Hall. Basement and cavities reserved for ventilation and heating
Figure: MacKenzie, W.

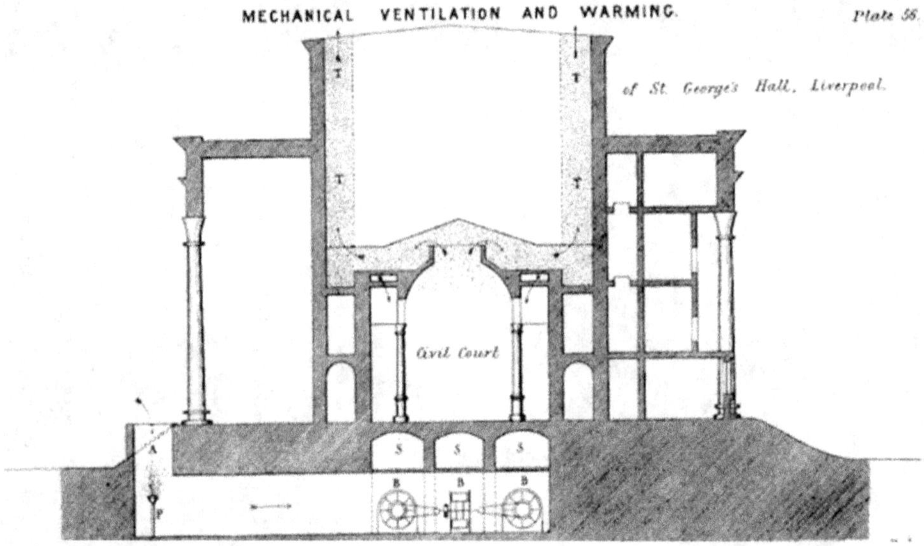

2000). Frank Lloyd Wright integrated a solar control system like the cantilever into his designs for the Prairie Houses, and incorporated ventilation towers into the Larkin Buffalo office building (1906). Some architects were determined to experiment with the relationship between form and environmental conditions, as Le Corbusier did, in some cases with less than favourable results, forcing him to redesign his own buildings (Banham, 1969). In his project for the "Cité de Refuge" (Paris, 1933) he tested the techniques of thermal stabilisation and ventilation of interior spaces (Mur neutralisant and Respiration exacte); these did not prove to be functional due to solar radiation, so the design was altered by incorporating the Brise-soleil (an element that became representative of his architecture).

Figure 3. Le Corbusier. Cite de refuge. Brise-soleil addition (source: Le Corbusier Foundation)

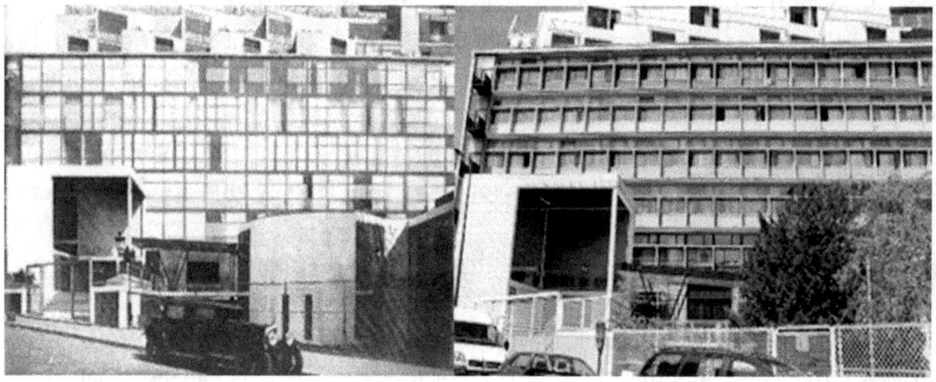

However, the ease of access to energy resources brought about by modern technology led to an inefficient way of constructing. The abuse of glazed surfaces led to an architecture dependent on mechanical systems beyond what was reasonable. The architect's general perception was that it was possible to design independently of the weather or solar radiation, because air conditioning would save us from a bad indoor environment.

Environmental Architecture in the 21st Century

At the beginning of the 21st century, architects have inherited the training of the 20th century. It is beginning to be understood that in order to achieve indoor environmental comfort, appropriate design guidelines must be adopted from the very beginning of the design phase. But the idea that technology can make an inefficient architectural design feasible from the outset is still very common. This is where the energy parameter, efficiency and the environment come into play. Architecture that is designed without regard for its surroundings could achieve acceptable indoor environmental conditions at the cost of high energy consumption. And this conception of architecture, although it may have been an option in part of the 20th century, is no longer acceptable in the 21st century. Environmental comfort must be efficient, and it must be based on an environmental architectural design from its conception.

The balance between design and environmental considerations can be seen in various projects such as the "Hemiciclo Solar" residential building by Cesar Ruiz-Larrea, (Madrid, 2009), the 8-house building by Bjarke Ingels Group BIG (Denmark 2009) or the Greater London Authority Headquarters by Norman Foster (London, 2002).

Figure 4. London Greater Authority by Norman Foster. Photo by Simone Hutsch

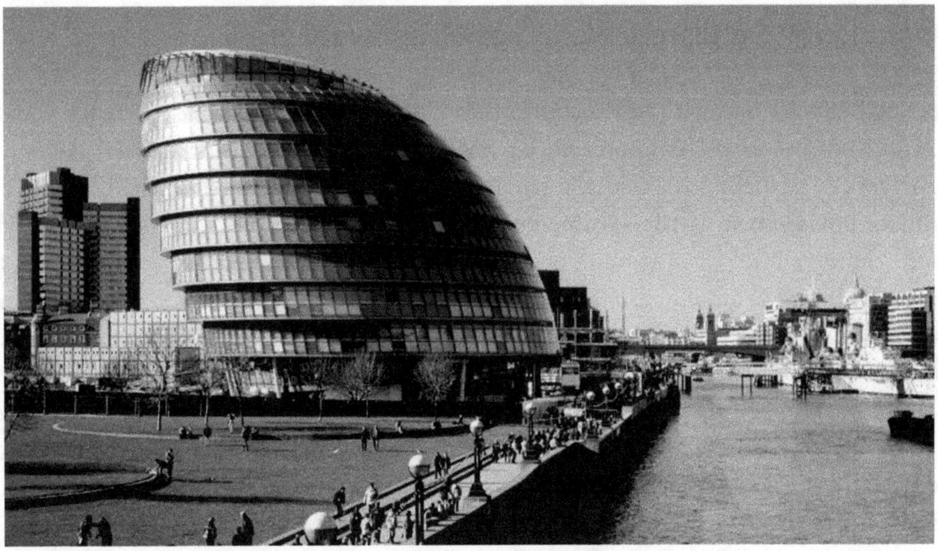

THE ENVIRONMENTAL EDUCATION OF ARCHITECTS

Background on Environmental Education

In the first architecture curricula in Spain there were no subjects related to environmental comfort, and it was not until the 1875 plan when concepts related to ventilation and air conditioning were mentioned (García 2016). But its weight in the studies was minimal, to the point that in later developments -Plan 1964- two specialisations were established called "Urbanism" and "Building"; the specialisation in urbanism did not have any subject related to environmental comfort. In 1996, the specialisations were eliminated, and subjects related to Environmental Conditioning were established as core or compulsory in most of the faculties of Architecture in Spain. This situation means that a high percentage of current practicing architects over the age of 40 may have obtained the title of architect without having taken any subject related to environmental comfort.

Since then, curricula have incorporated subjects related to environmental criteria, but these had been accompanied by minimum regulatory requirements that were difficult to control. In practice, regulatory standards were hardly met and there were no efficient systems for monitoring compliance. Traditionally, architecture has been taught by architects, and this lack of requirements was passed on to the students.

In consequence, the lack of requirements in the profession was translated into a low presence of environmental subjects in the architect's training. There was a misconception that complying with climate standards did not affect building design, and so building design began to be disassociated from environmental design.

Architects at the beginning of the 21st century have been educated in that period of the 20th century, where indoor environment quality standards were very low (let's not forget that it was not until the 1990s when air conditioning became widespread, and that until 1999 it was possible to smoke in an aeroplane).

The Environmental Education of Architects Nowadays

Usually, studies focus on optimal indoor comfort conditions in buildings based on three determining factors: thermal comfort, visual comfort and air quality (Castilla et al, 2010; ASHRAE 1992, 2005). These parameters can be extended to include environmental quality, a concept that combines conditions in healthy indoor environments with possible concentrations of toxins from outside or inside the building (Vargas & Gallego, 2005). Some authors exceed the minimum regulatory requirements for indoor comfort, generally linked to air temperature and humidity (hygrothermia), two parameters whose weight is undoubted but cannot be unique. Thus, surface temperature, air movement and air quality are variables that must be taken into consideration, in addition to other acoustic and visual conditioning factors. These parameters have been joined by sustainability and energy efficiency as indispensable requirements in the design of buildings, not only as a means of lowering electrical energy consumption and minimising greenhouse gases, but also as a method of improving people's life quality and constituting a place to live in (Gallardo, 2013).

As already stated in the White Paper on the Bachelor's Degree in Architecture (ANECA, 2005), the continuous evolution of technical regulations implies the appearance of "new requirements to be included in the projects, including all aspects related to building technology (Energy Evaluation, Environmental Assessment,...)". This regard it also indicates "...that only the architect can carry out from his competence in the drafting of projects, where all the aspects to be considered in the building are included in an integral way, both design (adequacy, integration, innovation, ...) and technical (calculation of structures, building services, ...) as well as in the subsequent construction management". The text itself states that one of the objectives of the current Architecture studies is to "maintain the current technical capacity of the Spanish architect to carry out the functions of the building profile in its entirety". However, this high level of technology and regulatory requirements has not been reflected in a significant alteration in the syllabuses. The way architecture syllabuses are structured in Spain, the first years are dedicated to basic training, core contents that in the first year are even homologated or identical to those of other engineering courses or specialities. From the second cycle onwards, environmental and technical contents are taught, usually under the subjects known as "installations". These constitute between 5 and 12% of the degree programme (it varies according to the study plans of each faculty), as stated in the aforementioned White Paper on the Bachelor's Degree in Architecture (ANECA, 2005).

According to the teaching guides, the theoretical content relating to environmental conditions and air conditioning systems represents between 3 and 6% of the ECTS credit load of the Bachelor's Degree in Architecture. This percentage is increased by the only workshop-type subject dealing with technical issues, which is taught in the final year. In this subject, and mainly in the Final Degree Project, students can - and should - take a multidisciplinary approach that anticipates what will be a professional work in the field of building.

Current Environmental Education Issue

The holistic approach that integrates environmental aspects is difficult to perceive when a student reads architectural magazines or analyses building pictures. Environmental comfort is not perceived in photos, and because of this it is difficult to establish a link between graphic subjects and these parameters necessary to make a building habitable, which are mainly studied in the so-called "building services" subjects.

Traditional training in schools of architecture has given priority to compositional, aesthetic and artistic criteria, leaving behind methods that aim to generate habitable spaces of environmental quality. Professionals can even be seen to shift the responsibility for creating well-ventilated, temperature-controlled and energy-efficient spaces to engineers or collaborators specialising in building services. Or even worse, as could be heard in a Final Degree Project session from a teacher of the design branch: "...you design as you like, the engineers will come along later to solve the efficiency issue...". And the fact is that in many cases the seed of this dichotomy between technique and design lies in the syllabuses and subject contents themselves. It is not uncommon to see thematic sessions and parts of subjects such as "Bioclimatic Architecture" or "Efficient Architecture", implying that this is a special type of construction design or building typology. But can there be architecture that does not take the climate into account, or architecture that is not efficient? Can there be architecture whose sole purpose is mere observation, disregarding the achievement of a healthy and comfortable indoor environment? It is obvious that it is not possible to separate these concepts, but year after year, students still come to the Air Conditioning Techniques course with the same prejudice: this is about installing heating and cooling systems; the design is done in the "Project" subjects (as all those subjects oriented towards the design of building solutions are called at university circles). Contributing to this lack of attention to technical issues are the various publications specialized in architecture. Their analyses, plans and photographic reports rarely deal with installation, environmental and climatic issues. Technical floor plans or installation plans are ignored, and in some cases even deliberately erased or removed, giving the observer the false impression that "good architecture is not about that". In this way, the concept of architecture is systematically simplified from a complex object that must function structurally, environmentally and functionally to an aesthetic response. Such a situation is the legacy of a purely aesthetic approach to architecture that sees mechanical systems as a toll to be borne, rather than the tool that enables the buildings to be used. It should not be forgotten that "the house is a machine to be inhabited" (Le Corbusier, 1923), and the fact that incorrect environmental design can result in an 'uninhabitable habitat'. In that case, however fortunate the aesthetic design may be, the building will be unusable, and the architecture loses its purpose of providing shelter for people.

SOLUTIONS AND RECOMMENDATIONS

The Environmental Awareness

The multidisciplinary teaching approach is key in the training of the future professional. It is vital that the teacher tries to recompose a holistic vision of architecture, raising students' awareness of the importance of these energy and environmental variables from the early stages of building design. They must be able to visualize the relationship between all environmental parameters and building design. They must understand the urgency and importance of adequate environmental conditions but without having high energy consumption. And they must internalize that achieving low energy consumption must be done with design as the starting point.

There is a broad consensus in academia on the suitability of the multidisciplinary approach in the training of technical disciplines (Graham 2018), and on the particular benefits of this approach in so-called "environmental education" (Oliveira et al 2021). Similarly, project-based learning has been found to be largely positive in the studies of architects, environmental designers and engineers (Dym et al 2005), as the most recent pedagogical strategies focus on "Design thinking" and "Project based learning" as the cornerstone of technical career education. It is important to keep in mind the focus given by the Bologna process (Bologna Declaration, 1999) to the professionalising character of university education, with the aim of "promoting the 'employability' of European citizens and competitiveness...". Despite the fact that architecture studies have various professional prospects, building is the field that the majority of graduates choose, 91.2% (Puig-Pey, 2017), so it is reasonable that the curricula in schools of architecture give priority to training in the field of construction.

It is in this field where interdisciplinary training acquires added value, as an architectural project requires the integration of various disciplines and knowledge of different technical fields that must be applied to a single element, the building.

The teaching objective is twofold in this case; students should be trained in the environmental concepts that affect architecture and an Environmental Awareness should be instilled in order to alter the way they understand their future architectural designs. Strategies should be multiple, combining conventional lectures with relevant examples and a high level of personal experimentation.

The experimental area is part of the Conditioning Techniques and Installations Project subjects, taught in the third and fifth years of the CEU San Pablo Faculty of Architecture, as well as the Final Degree Project projects of the same students over the course of a decade. As these are second cycle subjects, one at the beginning and one at the end of the cycle, they allow us to observe the evolution of the students' environmental awareness, monitoring the evolution of the students' commitment to environmental and energy parameters.

Formative Strategies for Environmental Awareness

The solution to this problem consists of adopting measures within the subjects that encourage this broader vision in students. The relationship between environmental quality and the design of the above spaces must be understood and internalized by future architects. To do so, teachers must have strategies that allow them to emphasize and relate these key concepts.

However, environmental awareness cannot be acquired if it is only addressed in technical subjects. The measures outlined here can be applied in whole or in part throughout all subjects, and only this can ensure their success. It is not necessary to alter the teaching program of the faculties; it is enough to extend the integrative vision of architecture to all compositional and technical subjects.

The measures described here have been effective in achieving the aforementioned environmental awareness objective:

- Visualization measures
- Measures of association
- Assessment measures.
- Analysis measures
- Reconstruction process.

Visualisation Measures

The first pedagogical task undertaken in the technical subjects is to recompose the relationship between design and technology, between form and environment, between envelope and thermal control. Students arrive in the third year with a fragmented vision of architecture, with unconnected concepts that are barely related to each other. Visualisation and association techniques are highly effective at this early stage. In the initial phases it is the teacher who must establish the points of relationship.

In a first association technique, the aim is to break down one of the prejudices that architecture students bring to the classroom: the idea that the most relevant architecture is not influenced by environmental variables. At the beginning of the training course, the students are shown images of "famous" projects or projects that are well known for their aesthetic values. From these images it has been sought those plans or pictures where the systems or strategies involved in environmental performance can be understood, and how good architects have incorporated them into the building design. Emphasis is placed on those in which the same environmental criteria have had a decisive weight in the final project configuration. The aim of this approach is to ensure that the student, from the initial phases of the study of environmental technology, perceives that it is possible to create good and prestigious architecture without renouncing adequate formal integration. It is vital to emphasise the effort made by the architect himself to treat environmental systems as part of the building design from the initial phases of the project, so students perceive that it is a task inherent to the conception of the architectural proposal.

In this first approach, students start to perceive that building design has a link with the environment, and that it can be the environmental conditions that define shapes and volumes.

It is at this moment when it becomes interesting to advance in the formation of Bioclimatic Architecture. This brings a range of environmental design strategies that came to define traditional architecture according to local climatic conditions. Images of traditional architecture show that most of the formal choices made in vernacular architecture were a response to local climates.

Measures of Association

The student should be able to understand in a deeper way the relationship between design decisions and environmental variables. They should be able to identify at each step of the project development the environmental and energy implications that are linked. Associating project phases with energy issues allows the student to internalise the link between project decisions and thermal issues, to link them to the design process.

Throughout the design process, decisions involve or depend on parameters related to energy or environmental variables. It is useful to review the development phases of architectural projects, particularly if students are still in their first years and are not aware of the complete process leading to the execution of a building project. This detailed process brings all the points of contact between design and environmental issues to the attention of future architects. The design process usually includes the following project stages:

Table 1. Project stages

Phase	Objective
Project location	Set geographical settlement. Usually fixed by client.
Site placement	On the selected plot, the position of the building is decided according to urban planning, formal criteria, views etc.
Functional programme	based on the client's criteria, the interior uses are adapted within the available area per site.
Interior design	Aesthetic and formal adaptation that responds to the functional programme.
Exterior design	Definition of facades and roofs.
Construction design	Establishes the materiality of the building envelope.

Source: Aramburu, 2021 (own elaboration)

The order described for the project phases is not intended to be chronological, but it does represent a common development in architectural projects. Particularly the last three phases (interior, exterior and construction design) can be arranged in a very different order, or even overlap.

During the development of the aforementioned project phases, decisions are made that, consciously or unconsciously, are directly related to environmental variables. These variables affect the thermal and environmental performance of the building. If we are aware of them, we can make design decisions that generate a passive architecture that is sensitive to the environment and much more sustainable and efficient. On the other hand, if the influences of environmental variables are ignored and a project is developed without taking into account external and internal conditioning factors, the resulting architecture will be clearly inefficient. At the time of the environmental assessment, the absence of control over the aforementioned parameters could result in architecture that exceeds regulated parameters, such as energy demand and consumption. It should be remembered that the current energy saving regulations prevent the construction of buildings that do not have near-zero energy consumption (NZEB), so that in the event of an unfavourable result, the process would have to be repeated from the design phase.

It is important that the student handles the regulatory documents directly, becoming familiar with them and understanding that they are laws. Compliance with them must be associated with the viability of the projects, so that they understand that in the future they will not be able to build architecture that is not efficient and sustainable

Figure 5. Design processes
Source: Aramburu, 2021 (own elaboration)

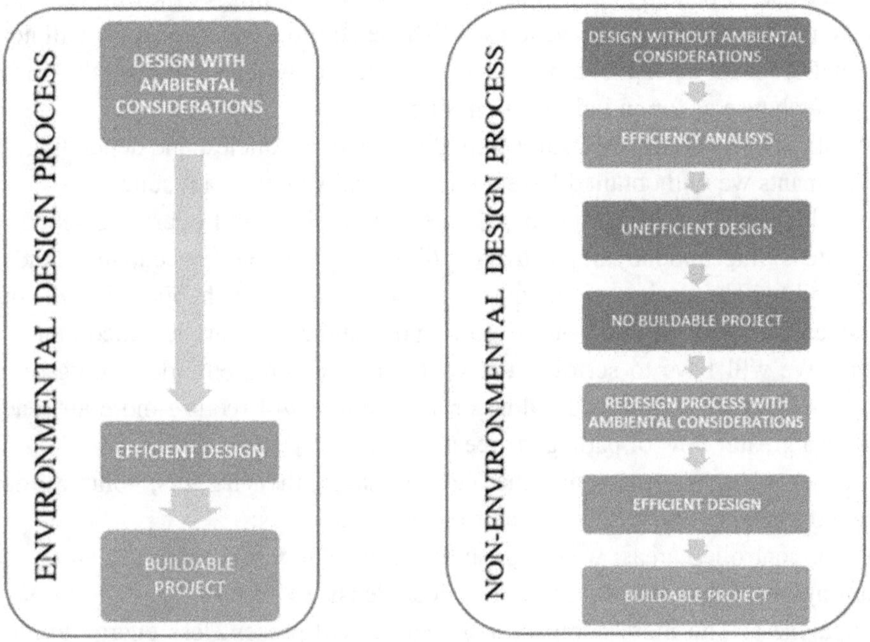

Each stage of the process is affected by environmental variables, which provide us with data related to thermal behaviour and ventilation (ENVIRONMENTAL INPUT), From these variables we can extract data that will affect the environmental quality of the building (ENVIRONMENTAL OUTPUT):

- Location Stage: When the building's location is being decided, it is affected by the Local Climatology variable. This provides us with information on outdoor temperature, relative humidity, hours of solar radiation and solar azimuth. From this data we can obtain temperature differences, absolute humidity values, incident solar energy and facades that will receive this radiation.
- Site Stage: When setting the location of the building within the plot we must take into account the influence of the following variables:
    - Position relative to the surroundings: this variable conditions the façade orientations and will present us with different solar exposure values.
    - Obstacles to solar radiation: shadows cast by the surrounding elements are generated, with regard to those elements we can analyse the distances at which we must remain depending on the cooling or air conditioning objectives we establish.

- Availability of energy resources: the location on the plot determines the availability of supplies and exposure to possible renewable energy sources (wind, solar, geothermal, etc.).
- Water masses: the proximity to water masses conditions the local microclimate, indicates the possibility of passive humidity supply and can facilitate evaporative cooling strategies.
- Type of terrain: Certain types of terrain may prevent excavation, making it difficult to exploit the thermal inertia of the terrain or to exploit geothermal energy.

- Implementation stage of the functional programme. During this phase, decisions are made about the operation of the building, which affect the following variables:
    - Intended use: depending on the intended use of the building, or the different uses that we decide to implement, we will have to establish the comfort conditions; we will not set the same thermal needs for a hospital as for a sports centre, nor will we establish the same temperature for a warehouse as for an indoor swimming pool.
    - Intensity of use: certain enclosures have different occupancies, and depending on the number of occupants we will obtain different internal load values as a result.
    - Schedules: The design can facilitate access limitations and operating schedules. This can generate an intermittency of use that conditions us to variable occupancy loads.
    - Habitability: The design of enclosures can condition their habitability. A corridor can be considered a habitable enclosure if waiting or lounge areas are installed in it.
    - Users: We will have to set different ventilation requirements depending on the users for whom a building is designed. Older or sick people will require more air renewal and will require a greater flow of pathogen-free air.
- Interior design stage. When defining the interior spaces, their heights, volumes, depth, etc., the result is conditioned by the following environmental variables:
    - Climate-controlled areas: we establish the surface area susceptible to energy consumption, resulting in spaces with higher or lower load densities per m^2.
    - Compactness: The more compact architecture will present less energy exchange with the environment, as it has fewer surfaces per unit volume.
    - Volumes: The volumetric design conditions the amount of air that will need to be renewed to ensure air quality in the enclosures.
    - Height: Higher spaces can generate problems with air stratification, conditioning the system chosen for the diffusion of thermal energy.
    - Normal exposure to solar radiation: when designing more extensive architectures, or when establishing the inclination of the walls, we condition the angle at which solar radiation falls on the buildings.
    - Own shadows: by establishing overhanging bodies or bodies of different heights, we generate shaded spaces, with the shape of the building itself providing protection from solar radiation.
    - Double orientation: if, when defining the occupied spaces, we establish a double orientation for the enclosures, we will be facilitating the existence of different external pressures, making cross ventilation possible.
    - Lighting requirements: the design of deeper enclosures with areas away from windows forces the use of artificial lighting, increasing energy demand and overheating these spaces.
- Exterior design stage. Although in many cases it is the result of interior design decisions, there are a number of environmental variables at this stage of design:

    - Thermal envelope. The external surfaces are the point of passage of the energy that the building exchanges with the environment, conditioning the building envelope load.
    - The surface of openings, understood as solar capture areas, the points through which solar energy enters the building's interior environments. Their design, size and geometry are key to the thermal performance of buildings, as well as allowing for natural ventilation.
    - Solar shading: the design of façades must allow for solar control systems, whether fixed, movable or seasonal. They allow for solar load management.
    - Exterior colour. The albedo coefficient associated with different façade colours alters the temperature of the exterior surfaces, which can be used to enhance or reduce the heat flow through the envelope.
    - Location of equipment: some air conditioning and ventilation equipment requires external locations or at least ventilation intakes and extraction stacks should be located in the design. Incorrect location of these items can alter the performance of the systems.
- Construction design stage. Particularly with regard to the selection of the materials that make up the envelope, it affects the following environmental variables:
    - Insulation: Both the material and the thickness of the insulation, and even its position in relation to the rest of the layers of the envelope, will influence the energy that passes through the envelope and the presence of thermal bridges.
    - Permeability of materials: a proper selection of materials will prevent the presence of condensation, which reduces indoor air quality.
    - Ventilated chambers; building design with the presence of ventilated chambers can encourage passive ventilation strategies, as in the case of ventilated façades or double roofs.
    - Type of windows: the appropriate selection of window materials has a very high influence on the thermal performance of buildings. Their transmissivity, emissivity and solar control characteristics condition the transmission of solar radiation and energy demand.

The following table summarises the environmental variables that influence each of the project's development phases.

Assessment Measures

Based on the constructivist model of education, it aims for an active generation of knowledge by the student, for which the use of technological tools is favourable (Hernández, 2008). It is vital to give students the tools to create their own learning. No matter how many lectures or master classes are given, the way to consolidate their knowledge is through their own experimentation. To do this they must learn to apply systems and processes that enable them to discover the intimate relationship between architectural configuration and energy. The evaluation processes must go from the particular to the general, starting with the inherent characteristics of materials (conductivity, thermal inertia, resistance, transmittance, etc.). In this aspect, it is interesting to get the students to see the relationship between the thicknesses of the construction elements and their thermal and energy functions; at this point, they can make a very simple evaluation on a plan of a real execution project, discovering how the thicknesses adapt to the thermal and energy requirements. The analysis of different projects enables them to make a comparative assessment relating locations, climatic conditions and requirements in terms of the efficiency needed for each geographical location.

Table 2. Design process and environmental variables

PROJECT STAGES	ENVIRONMENTAL VARIABLE	ENVIRONMENTAL INPUT	ENVIRONMENTAL OUTPUT
LOCATION	Climatology	Temperature Relative humidity Radiation hours Azimuth	Thermal difference Absolute humidity Incident solar energy Façade gains
SITE	ON-site placement Obstacles to solar radiation Energy sources availability Water masses Terrain type	Orientation Thrown shadows Available energy Humidity supply Excavation possibilities	Solar exposition Distance from obstacles Alternative sources Evaporative cooling Geothermia
FUNCTIONAL PROGRAMME	Intendede use Intensity of use Schedules Habitability Usuarios	Comfort conditions Occupancy Operating hours Climatised areas Requisitos ventilación	Heating cooling necessity Internal load Occupancy loads Operative temperatures Air flow and quality
INTERIOR DESIGN	Climatised areas Compactness Volumes Height Normal exposure to solar radiation Own shadows Double orientation Lighting requirements	Calculation areas volume-surface relationship Volumetric design Stratification Solar angle Protected areas Pressure difference Lighting energy	load density thermal exchange surfaces Air flow rate Energy system Solar energy received Solar auto-protection Crossed ventilation Ilumination loads
EXTERIOR DESIGN	Thermal envelope Windows areas Solar protections Colour Machine placement	Exchange areas Solar caption areas Shadow factor Albedo Machine selection	Envelope loads solar loads Solar load control Exterior surfaces temp Performances
CONSTRUCTIVE DESIGN	Insulation Permeability Ventilated chambers Windows type	Layer position Used materials Passive energy Solar factor and emissivity	Thermal transmittance Condensations Enhanced ventilation Radiation transmission

Source: Aramburu, 2021 (own elaboration)

Solar analysis tools should be part of the training process in any energy assessment. The geometry, size and layout of openings should be studied, learning the variables that affect the passage of energy through the perforations in the façades. In this case the relationship between exterior building configuration and environmental comfort is easy to be shown.

It is essential that they understand the process of assessing the different parameters independently before moving on to more complex procedures. From the most basic assessment tools, they should move on to more complicated systems, combining parameters of envelope, ventilation, water heating, internal load, etc.

It is particularly formative for students to generate their own evaluation tools. They should not be required to have programming knowledge, so a simple calculation table is a very powerful learning tool. The integration of calculation routines requires them to apply complex formulas, data relationships and organisation. It also allows them to experiment by varying the input data and checking how the output data is altered, which sets in motion processes of metacognition about the learning received.

Teachers must emphasise that the thermal calculation and ventilation processes will be part of the student's performance in subsequent courses and in their professional careers. It is common to find that final year and end-of-degree students who have generated their own tools keep them and apply them in the different phases of their learning, a sign of the intrinsic value that the students themselves give to these instruments.

Analysis Measures

Learning all the tools mentioned above becomes a useless effort if they cannot be applied to a real building project. Particularly if it is in the intermediate courses of training as architects, where they have not yet acquired all the constructive knowledge for their own design at the level required. This part of the process encourages their ability to search and analyse, which is vital in this age of over-information. It is a strategy to promote the link between previous knowledge and the new information to be learned (Díaz, F 1999).

The search in a real project for all the information that is going to be energetically relevant forces them to summarise and concentrate the parameters that they will need to analyse. It is usual in this phase that students discover and learn that in digital sources there is a lot of image, but little construction; discovering their own sources, filtering and analysing whether the available information is sufficient for environmental analysis is a high-level learning process.

The analysis process should go alongside the tool discovery process, so the understanding of the relationship between construction decisions, elements and the associated thermal energy is complemented and completed. If any of the parameters to be applied in the evaluation are not available in the documentation obtained, the student becomes aware of the weakness of his analysis. He also discovers which elements are relevant when representing architecture with an environmental approach, which will enable him to generate his own graphic documentation. It is often at this point that students begin to understand the reasons for the position of many of the elements that make up the thermal envelope, knowledge that is of great use to them when faced with construction design tasks in other subjects.

This way, architecture students can understand the thermal function of the opaque elements of the envelope, learning the reason for their implementation in buildings and the reasons for their position, thickness, spacing, etc. At the same time they understand the effect of the location, size and protection of openings, which combined with the right orientation has an extraordinary relevance on the thermal behaviour of buildings.

Reconstruction Process

This is a training strategy based on the application of reflection on practice as professionalisation, or as it has also been defined as "science-action" (Fernandez, 2009). Obtaining data from a real project and awareness of the variables involved must be complemented by knowledge of the standards and target values that a well-designed project should meet. For this purpose, the Technical Building Code is of extraordinary help, as it sets ratios and figures that the project should respect.

The constant revision of the energy targets forces the publication of successive updates of this document of the CTE, so trying to achieve the objectives of this document is a guarantee of high energy efficiency standards. Such is the frequency of the advancement of the requirements that it is rare to find a real project already built that complies with all the minimum values required by the energy saving document. The process of reflection on the lack of compliance with the parameters, and how to face a process of reconstruction (energy rehabilitation) to improve the thermal performance of the building is highly formative.

At this point the students must apply the acquired knowledge, a deep level of learning as it implies a deep understanding of the environmental variables involved. It is no longer just a matter of evaluating or calculating energy or ventilation parameters. Knowing which variables are involved, their relative weight in the behaviour of the building and how to alter them to improve environmental conditions represents the acquisition of second level knowledge. This relational learning involving a reconstruction of a building to improve it environmentally (followed by a reassessment) allows the student to understand and internalise the link between design, form and sustainability.

During the final years of the degree course, there are workshop-type subjects where the student must apply the knowledge acquired with a multidisciplinary approach. In the final degree project, all knowledge must be incorporated with the integration of all energy parameters in a complete project, so that the consolidation of environmental awareness is effective. The tutors must demand it and the examining board must assess it so that the student can consolidate it as significant knowledge.

CONCLUSION

Environmental awareness is slowly penetrating into society, but it is still a slower process in the training of the architect. This renewed approach to architecture must begin in the first years of the degree course, be reinforced in the intermediate stages and consolidated in the final years and in final degree project. And it is vital that during this process of knowledge consolidation the student understands that indoor comfort and air quality are not alien to their design. They must be prevented from perceiving the environmental qualities in their buildings as a problem whose solution does not depend on them; they should not perceive that technology or other technicians are responsible for ensuring that their buildings are efficient.

It is difficult to change the educational inertia of architecture faculties. Training focused on aesthetic constraints must give way to training that balances environmental awareness and design.

Teachers must establish systems that do not only explain the subject matter contained in the teaching guide. They must establish systems that prepare students for the multidisciplinary work they will face in their professional life. Although the curricula establish systems that compartmentalise the areas of study, it is the task of the teacher to establish the links that exist between the different branches of knowledge applied to architecture. It is complicated from certain technical disciplines to show the link that should exist between environmental conditions and design, and the effort is greater when learned stereotypes and acquired prejudices must be changed. The idea that technical and environmental issues are not the architect's job must be banished. They must be considered from the earliest stages of the architectural project, and only then can results be achieved that seamlessly integrate all the requirements of good architectural performance.

The methods, processes and strategies presented here are useful tools for generating a genuine environmental awareness in future architects. This will contribute to achieving one of the essential objectives of architecture in the 21st century, a commitment to the environment.

REFERENCES

Abalos, I., & Herreros, J. (2000). *Técnica y arquitectura en la ciudad contemporánea. 1950-2000*. Ed. Nerea.

ASHRAE. (1992). *Thermal environment conditions for human occupancy*. American Society of Heating, Ventilating and Air Conditioning Engineers.

ASHRAE. (2005). *ASHRAE Handbook - Fundamentals. Refrigerating*. American Society of Heating and Air-Conditioning Engineers.

Banham, R. (1975). *La arquitectura del entorno bien climatizado*. Infinito.

Borrego, M., & Newswander, L. (2008). Characteristics of Successful Cross-disciplinary Engineering Education Collaborations. *Journal of Engineering Education*, *97*(2), 123–134. doi:10.1002/j.2168-9830.2008.tb00962.x

Boto-Álvarez, A., & García-Fernández, R. (2020). Implementation of the 2030 Agenda Sustainable Development Goals in Spain. *Sustainability*, *12*(6), 2546. doi:10.3390u12062546

Campo Baeza, A. (1996). La Idea Construida; La arquitectura a la luz de las palabras. *Colegio oficial de arquitectos de Madrid*, 29.

Caraiscos, C. (2009, August). Advanced control systems engineering for energy and comfort management in a building environment - a review. *Renewable & Sustainable Energy Reviews*, *13*(6-7), 1246–1261. doi:10.1016/j.rser.2008.09.015

EU Commission. (2011). *Hoja de ruta hacia una economía hipocarbónica competitiva en 2050, Comunicación de la comisión al parlamento europeo, al consejo, al comité económico y social europeo y al comité de las regiones*. Author.

Corbusier, L. (1923). *Towards architecture*. Éditions Crès, Collection of "L'Esprit Nouveau", Paris. http://www.fondationlecorbusier.fr/corbuweb/morpheus.aspx?sysId=13&IrisObjectId=6463&sysLanguage=en-en&itemPos=46&itemSort=en-en_sort_string1%20&itemCount=47&sysParentName=&sysParentId=25

EU Council. (2014). *2030 climate and energy policy framework*. General Secretariat of the European Council.

Council of Europe. (2002). The European Higher Education Area. Joint Declaration of the European Ministers of Education (Bologna Declaration). Bologna, Italy, June 19, 1999. In *Compendium of Basic Documents in the Bologna Process: Steering Committee for Higher Education and Research (CD-ESR), 1st plenary session, Strasbourg, 3-4 October 2002, Item 7* (pp. 3-6). Academic Press.

Díaz, F. (1999). *Estrategias docentes para un aprendizaje significativo*. McGraw-Hill.

Fernandez, E. (2009). Aprendizaje experiencial, investigación-acción y creación organizacional de saber: La formación concebida como una zona de innovación profesional. *REIFOP*, *12*(3), 39–57.

Gallardo Frías, L. (2013). Ser humano, lugar y eficiencia energética como fundamentos proyectuales en las estrategias arquitectónicas [The human being, place and energy efficiency as a projective basis in architectural strategies]. *Revista de Arquitectura, 15*(1), 62–69. doi:10.14718/RevArq.2013.15.1.7

García Gener, P. (2016). *La docencia de la ETSAM en su contexto histórico*. TFG. Archivo digital UPM.

Goodwin, J. (2001). *Otis: Giving rise to the modern City. Ivan R.* Dee Publisher.

Hernández, S. (2008, October). El modelo constructivista con las nuevas tecnologías: Aplicado en el proceso de Aprendizaje. RUSC. *Universities and Knowledge Society Journal, 5*(2), 26–35.

Mackenzie, W. (1964). On the mechanical ventilation and warming of St. George's Hall, Liverpool. *Proceedings of the Institution of Mechanical Engineers Conference Proceedings.*

Neila, J. (2020). *Diferencias entre dos cabañas de madera: la isba rusa y la vivienda popular rumana.* http://sostenibilidadjavierneila.blogspot.com/

Oliveira, S., Olsen, L., Malki-Epshtein, L., Mumovic, D., & D'Ayala, D. (2021). Transcending disciplines in architecture, structural and building services engineering: A new multidisciplinary educational approach. *International Journal of Technology and Design Education*. Advance online publication. doi:10.100710798-020-09645-3

Palacio, B. (2016). La enseñanza integral de la Arquitectura, desde la perspectiva de la sostenibilidad ambiental. *Módulo Arquitectura CUC, 16*(1), 35–58. doi:10.17981/moducuc.16.1.2016.02

Puig-Pey Clavería, A. M. (2017). El Arquitecto: Formación, Competencias Y Práctica Profesional. *ACE: Architecture, City and Environment, 12*(34), 301–320. . http://hdl.handle.net/2117/106075 doi:10.5821/ace.12.34.5296

Stang, M. & Møller, C. (2018). Between regulation mechanisms and professional essentials: Exploring current challenges in architectural education. *Artifact: Journal of Design Practice, 5*(1). doi:10.1386/art.5.1.3.1_1

Sturrock, N., & Lawson-Smith, P. (2006). The Work and Influence of David-Boswell Reid, Physician, Chemist, Engineer (1805-63). *Proceedings of the Second International Congress on Construction History*, 3, 2981-2998.

Vargas Marcos, F., & Gallego Pulgarín, I. (2005, March-April). Environmental quality: Wellfare, confort and health. *Revista Espanola de Salud Publica, 79*(2), 243–251. doi:10.1590/S1135-57272005000200011 PMID:15913058

Chapter 7
Evalutation of the Roof Garden Design Criteria in the Example of Istanbul Marmara Forum Mall

Gökçen Firdevs Yücel Caymaz
Istanbul Aydın Unıversity, Turkey

Selim Şükrü Gündüz
İstanbul Aydın University, Turkey

ABSTRACT

The aim of this study is to create a checklist of roof garden design criteria. This scope of work includes an encompassing review of international standards studies such as German Landscape Research, Development, and Construction Society; the American Society for Testing and Materials; the U.S. Green Building Counci; and Green Roofs for Healthy Cities, whereas the generated checklist was evaluated in the Marmara Forum Mall. As a result of the study, an answer was sought to the question, "What are the prerequisites for a roof garden serving the needs of users in today's conditions?" whereas on-site detection, observation, and photography were used as working methods. As a result, in considering the evaluation of the checklist on a scale of the Marmara Forum Mall, climatic data, activities with its hard structure, promenade areas, and designs of plantlife and water elements in soft structure are moderately sufficient, whereas it was determined there is no problem in the roof furniture design and maintenance.

INTRODUCTION

The terms 'green roof,' 'living roof,' 'eco-roof,' 'planted roof' and 'roof garden' have been used to describe two types of green roofs, naturalistic, or a large, dense type of roof with self-settled vegetation. Green roofs are a layered combination of foliage and membrane on a building; It can help ensure water management and isolation. Since the roof structure and waterproofing are integrated to building subsequently, making sure that the roof is waterproof and protecting the waterproofing from mechanical damage are responsibilities of architect as well as insulating the roof for energy concerns. Until the middle

DOI: 10.4018/978-1-7998-7279-5.ch007

of the 20th century, green roofs were seen mainly as a local building practice. In the 1960s, however, the growing concern about the deterioration of the urban environment and the rapid decline of green spaces in urban areas revived interest in green roofs as a "green solution" in Northern Europe (Velazquez, 2005). New technical research has been done from studies on root repellent agents, membranes, drainage, light growing environment to plant suitability (Peck and Kuhn, 2003). Today, roof gardens (green roofs) with similar details continue to be designed for high-profile international hotels, business centers and residences. These green roofs are known as dense green roofs due to the deep-growing environment and the variety of vegetation. While they look like traditional ground-level gardens, they can increase living and recreational spaces in densely populated urban areas (Oberndorfer et al., 2007).

More recently, many European municipalities have required the inclusion of green roof systems as standard building practice. Legal authority notwithstanding, landscape architects and architects have designed a large number of green roofs as comfortable, accessible, open spaces over building and rainwater management systems with the personal will and authority of their customers. It stemmed from the fact that most of these areas were imperceptibly integrated with the architecture and surrounding urban fabric, and perhaps most of the things that sustained functionality of the green roof were invisible to most users (Weiler and Scholz-Barth, 2009).

There are many international studies available that show that environmentally, economically and socially beneficial roof gardens can be created with the right decisions made during the design phase. As for a guide to roof garden design, guidelines and standards such as German, Landscape Research, Development and Construction Society (FLL) (Landschaftsentwicklung, 2008). [Landscape Development and Landscaping Research Society], American Society for Testing and Materials (ASTM E 2400, 2006) as well as U.S. establishments and associations, like Green Building Council (Council, 1998), Green Roofs for Healthy Cities (2021) are the leading organizations. The principle these institutions derive from is to create a roof garden with a design suitable for both the region and the structure. For this reason, it is important to design roof gardens with the right design decisions at the design stage.

The scope of this study is aimed at determining the design criteria of roof gardens *in respect of the more recent techniques for improving sustainability with the incorporation of gardens and green areas on the rooftops of buildings*. Standard guidelines such as FLL, ASTM, USGBC, GRHC have been taken into consideration in determining design criteria. In spatial design practices; For roof garden design criteria with topics such as climatic criteria, flooring and structure bearing, roof slope, function and location selection, accessibility and security, roof equipment, hard floor material selection, irrigation, activities, walking areas, roof furniture, plant, water elements. An appropriate, comprehensive checklist has been established. It is aimed to evaluate the criteria of roof gardens and recommend improvement suggestions for inadequate points with this checklist, which has been evaluated in the example of the Marmara Forum Mall.

LITERATURE REVIEW

Roof gardens or green roofs refer to roofs supported by vegetation (Werthmann, 2007). As one of the modern advocates of green roof technology, Le Corbusier promoted roofs as an alternative for urban green space; Another was Frank Lloyd Wright, who used green roofs as a means to integrate his buildings more closely with the landscape (Peck and Kuhn, 2003).

The creation of roof gardens in pedestrian shopping malls, plazas, courtyards and roof gardens has expanded the functional landscape towards the built up environment and enriched the visitor experience significantly. Roof gardens located at the top of a built structure, below, at the same level or above the surrounding ground plane, provide longer life of the roofing material, better water retention after a rain event, reducing urban heat island effects. Many studies have supported that the presence of planted areas increases people's comfort (Kaplan and Kaplan, 1989; Ulrich et al., 1991; Ulrich, 1998; Bass and Baskaran, 2003). Roof gardens increase the quality of space with their presence in the building environment, providing users with green space and recreation opportunities (Pouya, 2019) physical and social (Wang and Pryor, 2019); economic (Lazzarin, Castellotti and Busato, 2005; Acks, 2006; Peck et al., 1999), psychological (Herzog, Maguire and Nebel, 2003; Laumann, Gärling and Stormark, 2003), and physiological (Tooke et al., 2011; Knaus and Haase, 2020; Wong et al., 2003; Köhler et al., 2002; Sailor, 1995) benefits (Oberndorfer, 2007; Wang and Pryor, 2019; Davis, 2011; Dunnet, 2006; Yuen and Hien, 2005; Liu and Baskaran, 2003). They increase the aesthetic values and land values of their environment, biodiversity (Brenneisen, 2003; Gedge, 2003; Brebbia, 2017) and food production in urban environments (Jafari et al., 2015; Dorr et al., 2017; Sanye-Mengual et al., 2015).

Climatic factors in the design of roof gardens including matters such as wind, shading, building height will have an impact on issures like flooring and structure support, roof slope, function and location selection, accessibility and security, which encompasses subjects like fire prevention, solar equipment, roof equipment including ventilation and chimneys, hard ground material selection and irrigation issues.

The height of the roof from the slope, exposure to the wind, the orientation of the roof to the sun, and the shading of the surrounding buildings at certain times of the day will be effective. The general climate of the region and the specific microclimate on the roof should also be taken into account. Views towards and from the roof can also determine where certain items are located for maximum effect. Luckett (2009), when the plant selection is also taken into consideration that the plants in winter and attention should be paid to the performance and hydration requirements against the summer, covering the green roof and which protects geo-textile material and the wind surface of the growing medium has indicated the importance of the use of wind blankets. Osmundson (1999) defined the importance of using wind breakers on roofs and emphasized the resistance of shatterproof glass to fierce winds. The importance of the roof's support system has been emphasized by various researchers, such as Luckett (2009), Hopper (2012), Snodgrass and Snodgrass (2006). In mentioning that costs will be lower if the green roof is included in the design plan earlier, they say that reinforcing an existing building would be much more expensive than a new design with a green roof. While green roofs supported by a reinforced concrete structure should have a minimum 2% slope, the minimum roof slope for green roofs supported by other structural systems is 3%. A slope of more than 40% is not recommended for an erosion-resistant green roofs (FMIC, 2007).

The roof garden design criteria can be taken up under two main headings; the first hard and the second, a soft structure design. Luckett (2009) defines the activities that can transpire in the roof garden as gardening, social, physical, scenic viewing and promenade or children's playgrounds. Social activities to be conducted in the roof gardens can be listed thusly; meeting and gathering areas, public spaces, recreation and sports areas, commercial areas and food production. Suitable sports fields can be designed according to age groups. Areas equipped with sports equipment or places for walking, jogging and swimming will provide opportunities for physical activity. Roof gardens with views and sightseeing activities should allow their users to wander about safely, interact with the environment and exercise comfortably.

Figure 1. Types of roof gardens (Olson Family Garden, 2021; Srenco, 2007; Bayhan, 2015; Ajuntament de Barcelona, 2018; Eckert and Koop, 2012).

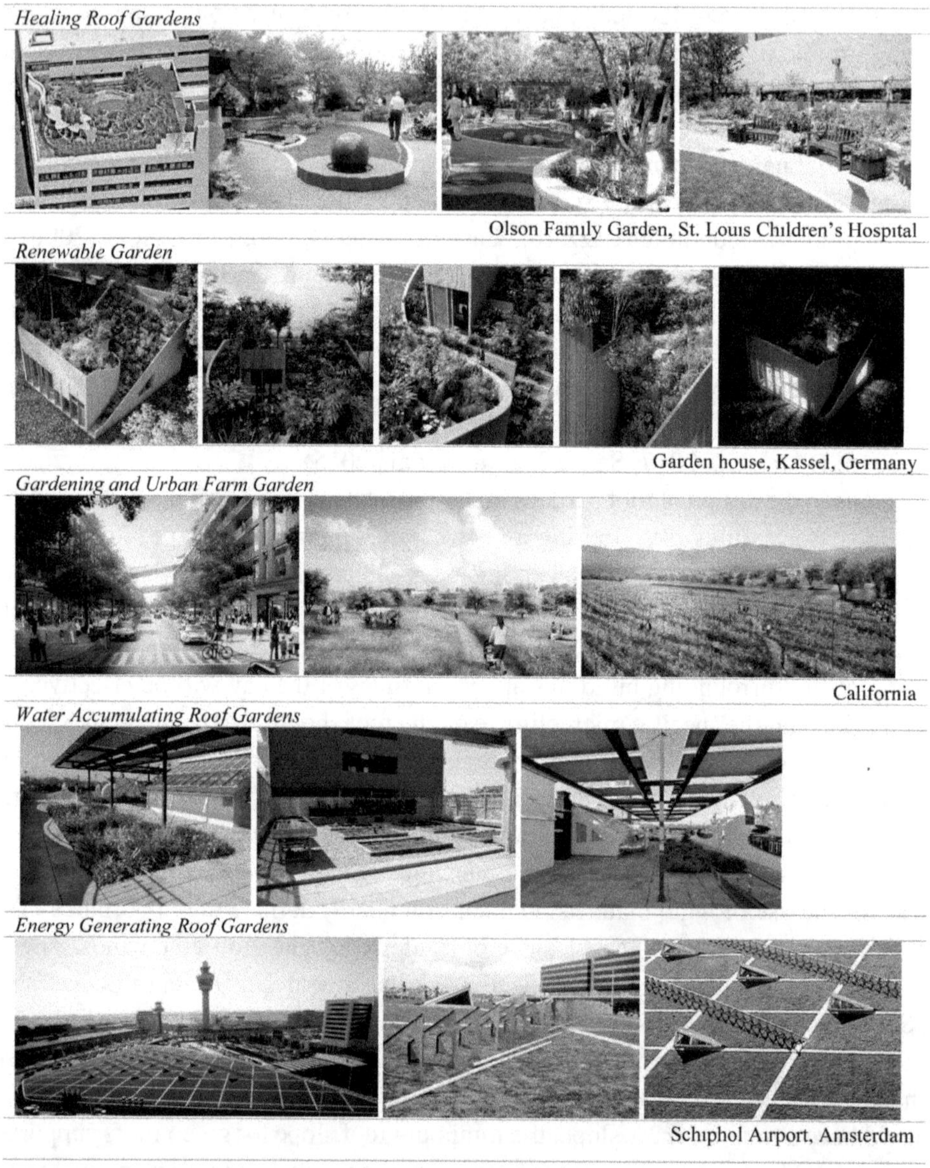

Tolderlund (2010) defined the types of access for roof gardens in the manner of elevators, stairs, stairwells with an entrance or a warehouse. When planning walkways on roofs, the weight of the structure and the required building height should be taken into account from the very start. Moreover, pressure resistance of the thermal insulation should be sufficient for walkway design. As with more traditional landscape designs, rooftop garden walkways will have many functions, offer aesthetic benefits, control traffic and prevent people from walking on plants. Concrete or asphalt surfaces require a minimum 1.5% slope while finisher surfaces must have a minimum 2%. Lightness and durability are the main mechanical properties while determining the suitable materials for the application. Among the other candidates, non-reflective brick, paving stones and tiles, textured wood flooring (considering the local laws and weather conditions) and colored concrete are eligible materials according to Harris & Dines (1998). In-situ cast concrete curbs, flowerbed boxes, aluminum and wooden edges partition the planting areas from walls, canals, skylights and walkways. Unlike landscaped roofs, where water will be kept back and flow delayed, walkways need most rainwater drained off the surface quickly. For this reason, it will require two drainage levels, the drainage points at the surface level as well as a lower drainage level.

Permanent roof landscape structures such as walls for privacy and space partition, parapets for security, windscreens, shades, furniture and play structures should be properly anchored at the roof level to order to avoid damage caused by strong winds (Harris and Dines, 1998). Utilizing heavy metal or wooden furniture as materials will reduce wind exposure. Restrictions for both safety and wind protection with higher opaque or transparent materials may be installed at these same locations. Measures must be taken to prevent people working within three meters of the roof edge from falling over. Care should be taken to ensure that the roof and parapet walls are at least 1 meter high (Luckett, 2009). In order to prevent grass fires, it is recommended to integrate the fire breaker at regular intervals around the perimeter of the roof and all roof protrusions along the roof. These fire breakers should be made of non-combustible materials such as gravel or concrete and placed 60 cm wide and 40 meters apart in all directions. Another option for ensuring safety is the use of fire retardant stonecrop. Hard floor materials to be used should be light, durable and permeable (Anderson, 2012). One of the security elements, handrails have border defining features as well as security features. Thus, they play an effective role in the formation of spaces. Game elements should be separated from the vicinity of the seating arrangements by means of a slight level difference or divider so as to provide subjectivity, spatial definition, physical and psychological protection. Seating elements can be listed according to their shape and usage purpose, as chairs, armchairs, couches, stools and sunbeds. It is important seating is ergonomic and positioned in a manner so as not to interrupt the flow of the road. Sculptures to be placed so as to increase the comfort of the space should be positioned in gardens as per their weight. Lighting systems' timing devices are electrically operated or controlled by photocells which are additional conveniences for gardens illuminated at nights, regularly. Waste storage area should be located in an easily accessible area for waste collection, service and deliveries. Marker plates must comply with standards and be found in the right places. Umbrellas, awnings, glass ceilings, pergolas, composite shades can be roof cover examples of roof gardens.

Figure 2. Parapets, walls and screens are required along the building (Lee, 1982)

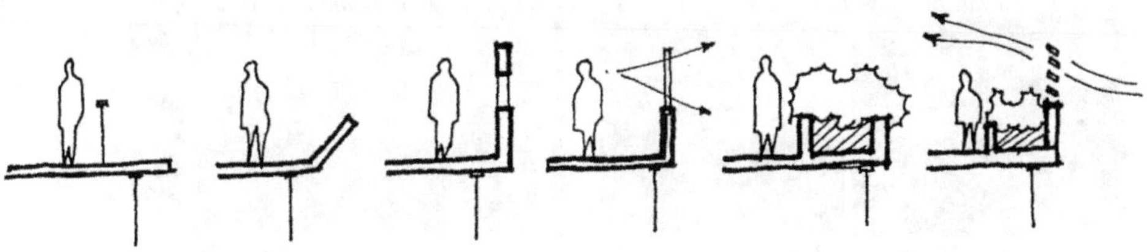

As Francis and Lorimer (2011) pointed out, heterogeneous designs can serve to maximize the biodiversity potential of green roofs and to make urban consensus ecology successful. Proper planning of flowering calendars can improve the evaluation of green roofs (Fernandez-Cañero et al., 2013). Factors such as aesthetic appeal, local climatic conditions, plant characteristics, and depth of the growing environment will be effective in the selection of plants for roof gardens (Getter and Rowe, 2006). Dry winds and excessive resin residue during the winter season bring a dramatic damage to coniferous trees and shrubs which is the reason why they should be protected from these environmental factors. Roof gardens will be exposed to high amounts of sunlight if there are no overhanging trees or tall structures

Figure 3. Roof garden designs and their components (Priority Zone, 2021; Proxima, 2021; Groundhog, 2021; Shuang, 2021; Future Green Studio, 2021; AFineLyne, 2019; WorldPress, 2021; LIGHTDESIGN, 2021; Mairs, 2017; GVL, 2021;National Park Service, 2021)

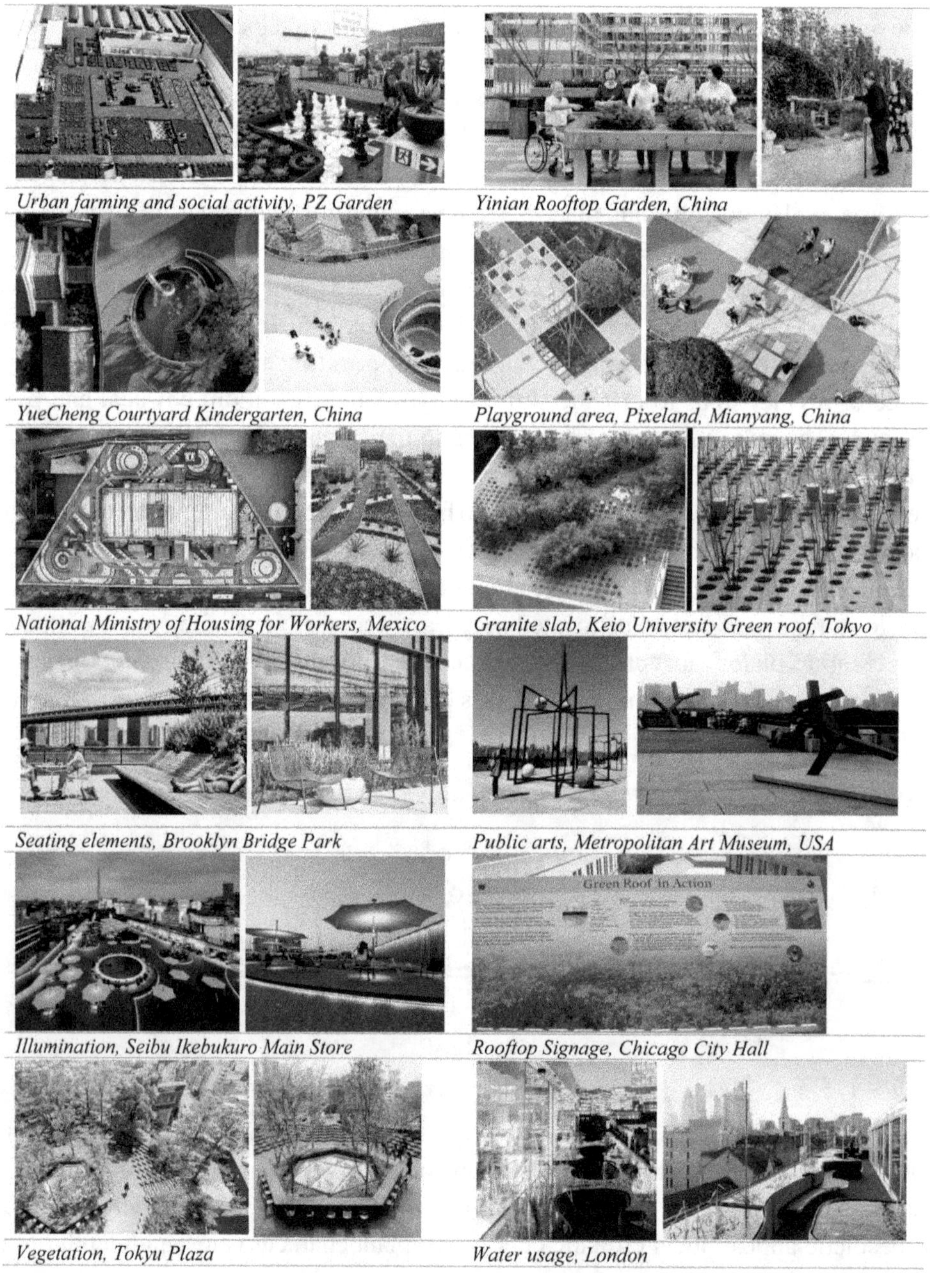
Urban farming and social activity, PZ Garden
Yinian Rooftop Garden, China
YueCheng Courtyard Kindergarten, China
Playground area, Pixeland, Mianyang, China
National Ministry of Housing for Workers, Mexico
Granite slab, Keio University Green roof, Tokyo
Seating elements, Brooklyn Bridge Park
Public arts, Metropolitan Art Museum, USA
Illumination, Seibu Ikebukuro Main Store
Rooftop Signage, Chicago City Hall
Vegetation, Tokyu Plaza
Water usage, London

around the garden (Willem, 2005). The steeper the roof, the faster water will flow off it, thus increasing the risk of drought. Stonecrop species are widely used on green roofs due to their ruggedness and drought tolerance. There should be a sufficient and appropriate water source for successful planting in roof gardens; adequate drainage; adequate environment for plant growth; as well as a periodic spray application for nutrition and reducing evaporation. It is recommended to create 12-inch vegetation-free zones around a green roof, around drainage zones, around glare areas and other penetration areas (rooftop structures, skylights, playground equipment, etc.) (Tolderlund, 2010). The intensity and exposure time of natural light can be affected by surrounding structures, so understanding local lighting conditions is important while selecting the right vegetation to plant. Additional specially designed grow lights can be installed for plants requiring more light, especially indoors (National Park Board, 2017). The use of drought tolerant plants would be a better choice for areas that don't get much rain.

Creating puddles on the roof brings special waterproofing worries to prevent leaks to the roof. The edge of a large body of water, such as a reflecting pool, can be constructed in a variety of ways using shaped concrete border walls (Baker, 1980). While using water elements in roof gardens, total weight contributed by water and its container and possibility of leakage into the structure lying under are the factors to be considered. The heaviest water elements should be placed on top of the support columns, if possible. By using dark colors or black for painting of the bottom and sides of the pool, a greater perception of depth is built up. At the shallow depths of 100-400 mm (4-16 inches), satisfactory water effects might be attained.

Most roof gardens require continual maintenance. Continual maintenance is the essential requirement for most of the roof gardens including irrigation, fertilizing, cutting, pruning, supporting, raking, replanting, sweeping, debris removal, repair and adjustment of irrigation and lightning equipment as well as clearing obstructions in the drainage system. In terms of cost, using this application for irrigation rather than using electricity to cool the building can further increase the sustainability of this practice (Austin, 2014). The irrigation system, growing environment and plant selection are critical factors that determine long-term maintenance needs and the survival of green roof vegetation under hot, dry conditions; otherwise, the vegetation may need to be replanted and/or the irrigation system changed. Access to flush out the drainage systems, i.e., the lower drainage system, flash flood drains, etc. is very important. Particular attention should be paid to pruning trees and shrubs in order to maintain a balance between branching and root expansion. Regular maintenance not only extends the life of plants, but also helps prevent overweight plants from toppling over due to strong winds.

METHODS AND MATERIALS

Research Questions

Main research question

- How can roofs be designed to increase community interaction and support a livable environment?
- Subheadings
- How do climatic factors, flooring and structure support, roof slope, function and location selection, accessibility and safety, as well as the use of roof equipment all affect the design of green roofs?

- What are the structural design issues in roof garden design?
- What are the planting design issues in roof garden design?
- What are the maintenance issues in roof garden design?

Reserach Area

While choosing the study area, an effort was make a preference amongst buildings with the highest user circulation at three different points of Istanbul Province. These structures are; the Marmara Forum Mall located in Bakırköy District, Özdilekpark Mall in Beşiktaş District as well as Meydan Mall in Ümraniye District. Amongst the three structures, the primary reason Marmara Forum AVM was preferred as a study area is its ability to meet the aforementioned criteria.

The Marmara Forum was brought to life in Bakırköy by the Investment Multi Development Turkey within the 'Forum' scope of the shopping mall concept. With a construction area of 375,000 m^2, the project is located in a densely populated area of the European side of Istanbul. The project is comprised of two main buildings, the Shopping Center and Garden Offices. Measuring 4500 m^2, the green roof on the shopping mall roof serves an important social venue need in the region with open seating spaces such as cafes, pedestrian paths, playgrounds for children, ponds and canals. At the same time, it provides a pleasant atmosphere with different plant species and a view of the Marmara Sea. As for the 2500 m^2 of garden office space, they all open into a few green courtyards that feature the green roof concept.

There are also two exterior terraces in front of the offices. As the region's green areas have been replaced by concrete buildings and highways due to the dense housing and population, the project aims to provide a natural environment for shopping center visitors and office residents with its huge green roof area.

Offering convenient access to public transportation, Marmara Forum is situated adjacent to the E-5 Highway in Bakırköy, near the coastal road.

The Bakırköy District, where Marmara Forum Shopping Mall is located, is affected by maximum and minimum temperatures of 30°-40° C. and -5°-+ 10° C., respectively, with generally mild and cloudy weather throughout the year. As observed, the warmest month is July, whilst the coldest month is January. Temperature values are measured above +10° between May and October and below +10° between November and April. The annual amount of rainfall in Bakırköy District is listed in the following table. The values obtained from the table are observed as Bakırköy District has mainly arid days during the annual timeframe. The average wind speed throughout the year was measured as 19 km/h in Bakırköy District. As the prevalent wind of Istanbul Province, the northeasterlie that blows from the northeast is the wind the Marmara Forum Shopping Mall is exposed to throughout the year (Meteoblue, 2021).

Method

In determining the design criteria for roof gardens, an attempt to create a comprehensive checklist which takes international standards into consideration has been made in order to test the adequacy of the spatial design principles of the roof garden. In the creation of the checklist, guidelines and standards such as FLL, ASTM and the studies and academic studies of organizations and associations such as AIA, ASLA, GHRC, IGRA, NRCA, USGBC were taken into consideration.. For analyzing the created checklist in the selected mall example, it was ensured that data, including images, satellite images, detection and measurements, project analysis and on-site observation of the topics in the control list, was collected

Figure 4. Views of Marmara Forum Mall (Pintps, 2021; Çalışkan, 2017; DS Architecture, 2021; Costerdesign, 2021)

Project Location	Istanbul Bakırköy
Project Type	Public Building
Project Type Group	Commercial Building
Employer	Multi Development Turkey and Area Property Partners
Designer	Tabanlıoğlu Architects
Prime Contractor	Yapı Merkezi Holding
Construction Area	375.000 m^2
Construction Years	2005-2011

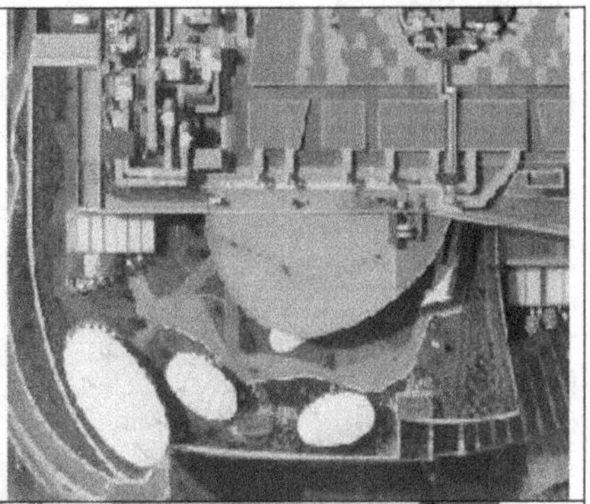

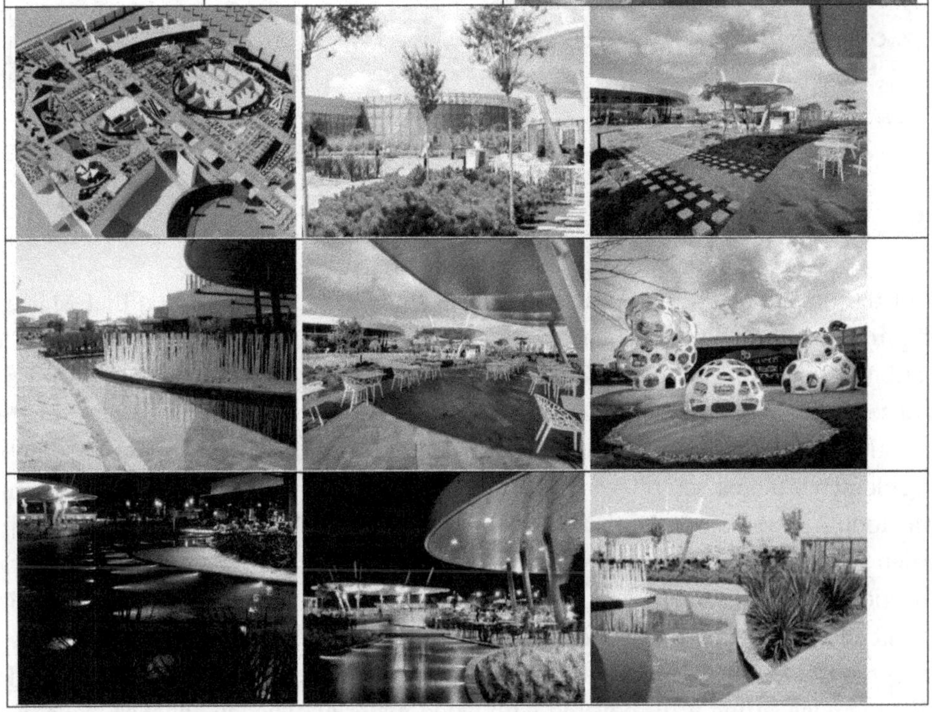

through on-site studies. An analysis of the subject headings found in spatial design practices, such as; climatic criteria, flooring and structure supports, roof slope, function and location selection, accessibility and security, roof equipment, hard ground material selection, irrigation, activities, walking areas, roof furniture, plants, water elements that comprised of the checklist was conducted. By evaluating the sample area analysis selected as a result of the study, it has been tried to determine the important subjects to increase the quality of the roof garden design.

Figure 5. Research methodology flowchart

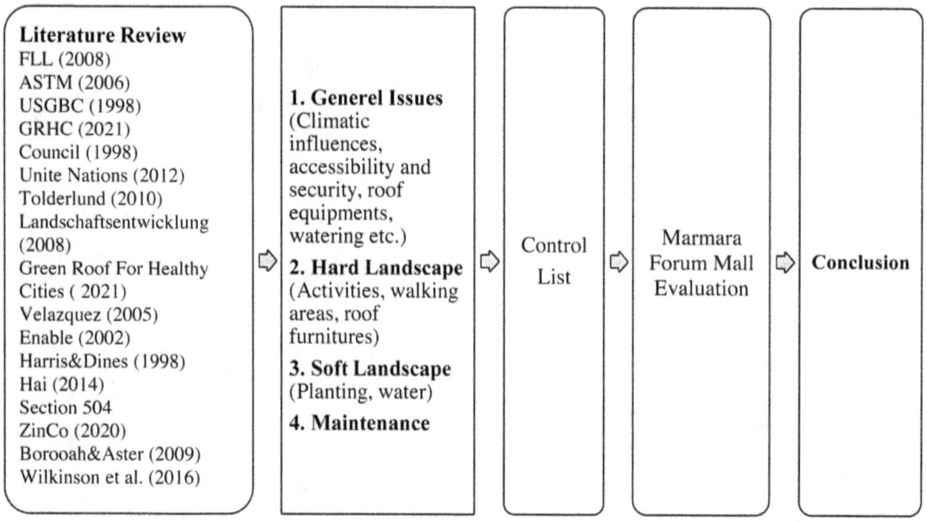

RESULTS

As a result of the on-site determinations made in the study area, it is observed that Marmara Forum AVM Roof garden is accessed from 4 entry points; It has been determined that the entrances comply with international standards and there are non-linear walkways with different widths around the roof. It has been observed that stone material was used as a floor covering on the walkways. There are many different activities in the roof garden; In these areas, furniture such as border elements, playground equipment, seating elements, tables, sculpture art structures, lighting elements, trash bins, signing, and shading elements was found. It was observed that there was a 1 meter high parapet wall at the outer border of the roof garden and a plant wall in front of the wall. At certain points of the walking path, borders were used as restrictions; It has been determined that there is a 400 m^2 playground area in the garden, and the play equipment such as climbing and slides in these areas appeal to different age groups. Around the area; It has been observed that there are different seating elements such as sitting poufs made of textile material, planting edge sitting walls covered with wood material, wooden benches made of wood, and sun loungers. There is no use of sculpture around the area; It has been observed that it is adequately illuminated by the lighting elements on the sides of the roads. In addition to standard waste receptacles, the use of recycled bins has been identified. In the roof garden, there are top cover elements that protect the users from the harmful effects of sun and rain. It has been observed that sedums, perennial plants and tall trees are used in the planting design, which define the feature of the dense roof garden. It has been determined that the pool is used as a water element in the roof garden in order to increase both visual and psychological effect.

In the second stage of the study, the criteria that were created as a result of the literature study were evaluated under two main headings: Hard structure and Soft structure. Prior to this, Climatic data, which is thought to be effective in the design phase, flooring and structure support, roof slope, function and location selection, accessibility and security, roof equipment, hard ground material selection and irrigation matters were closely examined.

In regards to the matter of exposure to climatic effects in the Marmara Forum area, which was the chosen sampling area, no problem other than orientation to sun in the direction selection was observed, whereas there was a moderate level of competence in terms of exposure to rain and providing sufficient daylight for plants. As for accessibility and security issues, it has been determined that the vegetation and flooring zone around the roof is insufficient. Looking at the roof equipment, the water, electricity and drainage systems are adequate and it has been determined that gravity is not used in irrigation in order to reduce energy consumption.

As a result of the examination of the rigid structure of the roof garden, while it has been determined that the activities in general are sufficient, the agricultural uses around the garden, the interactive game elements, the barbecue and observation areas and especially the passive activity opportunities offered to the users are deemed insufficient.

In the design analysis regarding the entry point of the roof, entry points are sufficient. It was ascertained that manholes are not provided for outside the flooring, 914 mm standard door fence is not used, access is not provided by fixed stairs, and more than one transport hub is not provided to ensure access in road designs. Again, protection is not ensured with 20-40mm rounded tiles or concrete floor plates along the roof, ramps are not available, ramp slopes do not comply with standards, whereby it observed the flooring is not of non-slip material and that permeable flooring material is not used.

Regarding the roof furniture, it was determined that the constraining elements were insufficient, the top cover elements and seating designs were sufficient. It was determined that the playground is not separated from other areas by a level or a divider, and there was no use of sculpture in the area. As for the lighting issue, while it is observed photocell illumination elements are not used, the design of the garbage bin is sufficient, but no marking plate is used.

No serious problems pertaining to the soft structure analysis were determined. The use of cages around the plants for cooling and humidification for hot days, and plant varieties hanging over the road surface was observed. The use of perennial and evergreen plants, sufficient water resources, flowering and scented plants was determined to be sufficient.

In regards to water usage, which is evaluated within the soft structure, the use of rainwater and mechanical cooling, the presence of fountains, and the provision of water accumulation with reservoirs were all deemed inadequate.

DISCUSSION

By focusing on the roof garden of Marmara Forum Mall in Istanbul, and creating standards in design, the objective of this study was to come up with roof garden design criteria in order to improve the quality of life and generate roof garden strategies. The roof garden was launched and put into service for it users in 2011. As a result of the layout and design stages, the roof garden has achieved a nearly perfect result. While its positioning according to the northern hemisphere was made incorrectly due to the design, it does not constitute a major problem in terms of use. Having both open and enclosed areas in the roof garden allows it to be used comfortably in inclement weather conditions as well as during the summer and winter.

When the project was new, the engineer designed the structure to meet the total load (Luckett, 2009). The construction is in the steel carcass-reinforced concrete framed structure building class. The mall is a 5-storey building comprised of 2 basement floors, 1 ground floor and 2 normal floors. The building is 10

Table 1. Evaluation of the Marmara Forum Roof Garden

DESIGN CRITERIA	POOR	AVERAGE	GOOD
GENERAL DESIGN ISSUES			
CLIMATIC INFLUENCES			
Exposure To Rain		√	
Exposure To Wind			
The use of wind-resistant plants, soil and supporting structures			√
Hindering the wind with the use of plants that are taller and upward on the roof edges			√
Orientation And Shading Towards The Sun			
Located in the part facing north in the southern hemisphere and facing south in the northern hemisphere.	√		
Having enough daylight that is not too much for the plants to grow		√	
FLOORING AND STRUCTURE SUPPORT			√
ROOF SLOPE		√	
FUNCTION AND LOCATION SELECTION			
Position Of The Roof			
Not in shade (good).			
Partially in shade (maybe okay).		√	
It has been overshadowed (May not be okay).			
ACCESSIBILITY AND SECURITY			
FIRE RISK			
No flammable materials are stored on the roof or near the building			√
Use of non-flammable materials around the roof		√	
Choosing the right place for the natural gas line		√	
Fire-fighting vehicles, adequate water supply and fire hoses		√	
The presence of a planting border comprised of 20-40 mm wide pebbles or 500 mm-wide concrete floor around the roof	√		
The presence of a minimum 1 m-wide gravel or concrete floor or a 300 mm-high firewall every 40m of planting	√		
Routine maintenance of planting borders			√
ROOF EQUIPMENT			
SERVICES			
Presence of water, electricity and drainage system			√
Spots where the drainage system can be checked and flushed out regularly			√
POWER USAGE			
Minimizing power usage for the sake of sustainability goals		√	
Considering access to natural light			√
Using gravity, not pumps, in the watering system where possible for less energy consumption	√		
SOLAR THERMAL AND PHOTOVOLTAIC PANELS			
The panels are not shaded by the planting on the roof; preferably A-shaped ones	√		
Placement of planting behind solar equipment areas	√		
HARD GROUND MATERIAL SELECTION	√		
WATERING			√
HARD STRUCTURE			
ACTIVITIES			
Existence of different user groups (children, senior citizens, tourists etc.)			√
Presence of the physically challenged		√	
AGRICULTURAL USES (CONTAINER GARDENING, SOIL-FREE GARDENING, etc.)	√		
PHYSICAL RECREATION			
Interactive game elements, barbecue and observation areas	√		
Children's playgrounds			√
Reading areas		√	
Youth venues (sports pitches etc.)		√	
SOCIAL FUNCTIONS			
More elements that encourage social communication, such as playground equipment, meeting areas and seating areas		√	
Presence of food & beverage activities			√
More educational opportunities and opportunities		√	
PASSIVE ACTIVITIES			
Scenery and excursion activities	√		
Presence of surrounding scenery	√		
Covering the unpleasant view with special planting			√
Suitable for use in intergenerational groups		√	
Suitable for container gardening	√		
Suitable for roof hydroponics	√		
WALKING WAYS			
ENTRY POINTS			
At least one, ideally two entry points (one as the emergency exit)			√
Lack of steps and stairs at the entrance			√

continued on following page

Table 1. Continued

DESIGN CRITERIA	POOR	AVERAGE	GOOD
Having a wide enough landing in front of the entrance			√
Leveling of the landing and non-slip flooring			√
Can the entrance doors operate independently?		√	
Min. 90 cm door width			√
Roof door not remaining permanently locked		√	
PATH DESIGN			
The presence of a minimum of 1.83 m uncultivated area around the roof garden connected with paths			
Paths clear of obstacles			√
Paths without steps and stairs			√
Paths are perceptible			√
Manholes are beyond the flooring	√		
Grid openings not more than 13 mm			√
Adequate drainage			√
Adequate width for easy access			√
Drainage element presence at a fixed edge			√
The landing is not constrained with a fence unless necessary			√
If necessary, use of a 914mm standard gated fence that opens inward	√		
The existence of a min. 2743 mm long x 1829 mm horizontal wide path from the front to the back of the building			√
Roof width and depth of 30480 mm from one side of the building to the other			√
Making the path through a 914 mm wide door in fenced areas	√		
When the main building rooftop has more than one level, access is provided via a fixed ladder when the floor level is between 1829 and 4077 mm.	√		
On an "H"-shaped building or other buildings whose irregular configuration renders a single clear path inadequate to provide access to each wing of the building or other rooftop area.	√		
UPSTAND DETAILS			
All up-stands, roof perimeters, outlets and protrusions through the roof should be protected by a non- planting barrier such as 20-40mm rounded shingle or concrete paving slabs.	√		
The depth of the substrate should not be less than 500 mm.			
The presence of constraints separating paths from planting, ponds and other landscape views			√
Ramps located outside the pedestrian flow	√		
Max. ramp slope of 8.33%			√
FLOORING MATERIALS			
The presence of non-slip flooring			√
The use of permeable flooring	√		
The use of light, durable materials	√		
ROOF FURNITURE			
CONSTRAINING ELEMENTS			
The use of tall plants along the outer border of the roof		√	
The use of handrails for height differences higher than 60 cm and slope greater than 50%	√		
Use of constraints of no less than 1070 mm around the roof			√
The presence of additional protective measures for parapet walls less than 100 cm high	√		
The use of strong, durable fencing		√	
The minimum height of the perimeter fence should be 1.8 meters	√		
Presence of wind protector at least 1m parapet wall			√
Mounted into the floor			√
TOP COVER ELEMENTS			
The presence of shading elements			√
Adequacy of shaded areas			√
Mounted into the floor			√
SEATING ELEMENTS			
Seats at a distance of at least 1 m from the roof border and guardrails			√
Provision for rest facilities at certain distances			√
Finding space next to the seating elements for wheelchairs			√
45-50 cm seat heights			√
The top point of the tables is between 75-90 cm.			√
Mounted into the floor			√
The presence of seating in the shade			√
The presence of seating in the sun			√
Availability of individual seating			√
Availability of group seating			√
PLAYGROUND ELEMENTS			
The use of safe equipment			√
The use of certified material		√	

continued on following page

Table 1. Continued

DESIGN CRITERIA	POOR	AVERAGE	GOOD
Proper drainage			
Mounted into the floor			√
Partition of playgrounds with level difference or divider	√		
Game elements suitable for all age groups		√	
STATUES AND FINE ARTS STRUCTURES			
Mounted into the floor	√		
LIGHTING ELEMENTS			
Roof gardens are often exposed to maximum sunlight if there are no overhanging trees or tall buildings in the area.			√
The presence of 110-120 volt electrical power			
Sufficient path illumination			√
Sufficient illumination of design elements			√
Mounted into the floor			√
Aesthetic lighting elements			√
Technological lighting elements		√	
The use of standby lighting elements		√	
The use of emergency lighting elements		√	
The use of photocell lighting elements	√		
TRASH RECEPTACLES			
Mounted into the floor			√
Do not interrupt pedestrian flow			√
Impact resistant			√
The presence of recycling bins			√
SIGNAGE ELEMENTS			
Identification of accessible areas with the international accessibility symbol	√		
Identification of accessible activities locations with direction signage	√		
Maps, information panels and wall-mounted signage between 90-180 cm	√		
Clear, simple and legible signage	√		
Distinct signage colors	√		
Non-glare signage surfaces	√		
Signage visible from a distance	√		
Mounted into the floor	√		
SOFT STRUCTURE			
PLANTING			
At least 70% of the roof area should have planting to achieve maximum benefit for SUDS, building energy performance and biodiversity.	√		
The use of perennial planting			√
The presence of 12-inch planting -free zones around the perimeter of a green roof, particularly around drainage or game equipment			√
Use of a cage around the planting for cooling and moisturizing on hot days	√		
The use of planting with low nutrient requirements		√	
The use of planting with low maintenance requirements		√	
Light weight of maturation		√	
Extreme cold and heat resistant mature planting		√	
Wind resistance		√	
Low, compact, spreading growth type		√	
Use of evergreen plants		√	
Planting varieties obstructing pathways			√
The presence of hazardous planting varieties	√		
Are the planting varieties used harmful to the path surface?	√		
Planting that is inherently non-flammable, such as succulents or others that store water.		√	
Green roof substrate does not contain a high volume of organic content)		√	
Sufficient water resources available			√
The use of an adequate drainage system			√
The use of flowery planting			√
The use of scented planting			√
The combined use of deciduous and evergreen plants			√
BIODIVERSITY			
Features frequently included on biodiverse green roofs for shooting sessions are; varying depth and substrate compound, planting areas, stones, rope and decaying wood.		√	
WATER			
Ponds and pools should have at least 300mm depth of water to compensate for the higher evaporation rate of high, exposed buildings.			√
Wherever possible, the heaviest water elements should be located directly over support columns within the structure.			√
Minimum water depths should be used.			√

continued on following page

Table 1. Continued

DESIGN CRITERIA	POOR	AVERAGE	GOOD
A dark-colored bottom and sides of the pool, as well as agitation of the water will allow for satisfactory effects in depths as shallow as 100-400 mm (4-16 in).			√
The presence of moving water elements such as fountains and waterfalls.			√
Having extra waterproofing systems to prevent against leakage.		√	
The use of storm water management or mechanical cooling systems.	√		
Fountain heights are 90 cm	√		
Easily operable controls	√		
The use of reservoirs to gather water.	√		
Drip watering system			√
Watering conducted with automatic systems such as time setting and thermostat		√	
Adequate supply of water available in case of fire		√	
Aesthetic design of water elements			√
MAINTENANCE			
Minimal watering requirement		√	
Presence of equipment storage space		√	
Path and furniture maintenance			√
Plant maintenance			√
Regular pruning and care			√
All planting areas should receive a top dressing, about 5 mm. per year			√
Pruning and weed control			√
Regular fertilizing of planting			√
Planting installation/replacement			√
Maintenance of supporting structures			√
Waterproofing insulation			√

*Sources used in determining criteria: (Velazquez, 2005; Landschaftsentwicklung, 2008; ASTM E 2400, 2006; Council,1998; Green Roof For Healthy Cities, 2021; Tolderlund, 2010; Harris and Dines, 1998; Unite Nations, 2012; Hai, 2014; ZinCo, 2020; Borooah and Aster, 2009; Wilkinson et al., 2016)

years old (Çelikkol, 2015), which is an indication that the roof garden demonstrates a good performance in terms of flooring and structure support.

The Marmara Forum Shopping Mall roof garden was designed as a flat roof. Although roof surfaces built in many green roof projects appear flat, almost all roof surfaces must have a slope in order to provide proper drainage (Luckett, 2009). For this reason, there is no slope on the roof except to provide water flow. This allows those who use the roof garden to move around more comfortably.

As stated in Anderson (2012), shading is the most important element with roof gardens. Shading is an effective factor for the usage area of the roof garden. Thus, the roof garden is evaluated from both a sunny and shady area aspect. This roof garden allows comfortable utilization in both sunny and cloudy weather.

Access to the green roof should be considered and included in the green roof design. Moreover, the initial setup will be significantly less expensive if there is decent, secure Access (Wilkonson et al., 2016). It is crucial to determine the entrances and exits to the area while designing the roof garden. This is one of the factors that directly affect both user comfort and the choice of the roof garden. Access to the Marmara Forum AVM roof garden is provided from within the mall. There is no external access. This situation causes some problems in terms of user access. Those who only want to use the roof garden experience negative conditions such as being subject to security checks, waiting during the check and the length of the transport hub to the roof garden. However, from the standpoint of a possible terrorist attack, this situation renders the roof garden safe.

The use of electrical illumination equipment in the roof garden, the presence of roof equipment that requires electrical energy, and the efforts to meet the electrical energy needs of its users, the presence of an electrical current system, ornamental pools, irrigation systems, water systems, water discharge without any problems show the existence of a drainage system. The fact that these systems are in user service but not taken into consideration proves a successful system establishment.

No particular precautions or applications were implemented to define sustainability targets for the Marmara Forum Shopping Mall roof garden. In order to benefit from sunlight, the roof garden was positioned towards the east. Thus, maximum benefit is provided from sunrise until the afternoon hours. However, the amount of utilization during the afternoon decreases as the sun sets to the west. Gravity is not utilized in the use of watering systems. For this reason, energy is consumed and expenditures are made financially while meeting the watering requirement. The absence of photovoltaic panels in the roof garden indicates that the roof garden cannot meet its own energy needs.

Marmara Forum Mall serves many people as it is a roof garden shopping center with users of all ages and groups. The walkways in the roof garden are arranged according to an unimpeded design. There is no wheelchair area in some sections of the seating areas. Although many activities are made available in the roof garden, there is no production such as roof gardening or urban agriculture. Though interactive activities are unavailable in the Marmara Forum Mall roof garden, there is a children's playground. With the proper positioning of the seating areas in the roof garden, users can perform activities such as reading. However, the reading area was not specifically incorporated into the roof garden design. The walking paths, the right choice of playground elements and cafes show the presence of venues deemed necessary by young users. In addition, due to its location and the lack of scenery around it, the roof garden is not used as an excursion and scenery place. Because it is located in the immediate vicinity of the city's most important transportation hubs, special planting with green walls of plants around the roof has been implemented on the roof garden so as to hinder the user from sensing the noise and visual pollution caused by the nearby heavy vehicular traffic.

While there are multiple entry points where entrances and exits to the roof garden, there are no steps or stairs at the entrances. The absence of a landing and direct provide convenience to all users. The roof garden is designed with the physically challenged in mind, with no steps or stairs along the paths. The paths are cleared of obstacles for the sake of making them easier to use. Manholes are not used outside the path. Water discharges properly. The paths are of sufficient width, whereas there are no constraining elements such as fences or railings along the walkway sides.

Brick paving stones, tiles, textured wood decking (wherever local laws and weather conditions permit), and colored or exposed concrete are excellent options for roof improvements (Harris and Dines, 1998). Natural floor coverings such as stone and wood were used as well as artificial floor coverings in the children's playground section of the Marmara Forum Mall roof garden. Non-slip materials were chosen especially for the flooring. Moreover, no permeable and light materials were used. Tall plants were positioned along the outer border of the north facade of the Marmara Forum Mall roof garden, and partially used in the garden. With these plants, users are prevented from falling down, noise and visual pollution are hindered, and the impact of northerlies blowing from the north is minimized. There is no need for railings, which are deemed necessary, since there is no height difference with a slope of more than 50 cm and 50% within the garden. Care should be taken that the roof parapets are at least a meter high (Luckett, 2009). Thus, precautionary measures to keep both the users of the roof garden as well as the personnel working in the roof garden from falling have been increased. In addition, the one-meter height of the parapet wall in the roof gardens protects plants used in the garden from being harmed by powerful wind gusts. Around the roof garden, attention has been paid to the height criteria mentioned by Luckett, thus ensuring the safety of the users and protecting the plants against wind gusts. Moreover, there are no restrictive security elements such as fencing or railings over the perimeter roof parapet.

Shading is made possible thanks to the top cover element feature, which encompasses a sufficient amount of area over the roof garden and is anchored to the ground. Seating elements in the roof garden are positioned at least a meter away from the roof border. There are seating arrangements in different parts of the roof garden. The fact that the seating elements are designed in accordance with international standards is the reason wheelchair maneuvering point complies with appropriate size standards. Due to its various designs, individual and multiple seating groups can be arranged, while some elements are fixed to the floor. The presence of seating elements in both shaded and open areas provides users with different opportunities. There are no sculptured artworks in the roof garden of the Marmara Forum Mall. The roof garden reduces the amount of energy used for lighting by taking optimum advantage of the available sunlight. Elements that provide the paths and design elements adequate illumination are mounted into the floor, whereas aesthetic concerns are taken into consideration. The standby, emergency lighting and photocell lighting elements are insufficient. While the garbage bins are carefully positioned in the roof garden so as not to interrupt pedestrian flow, they are made of durable material with bolstered resistance against impacts and are mounted into the ground. There are also recycling bins for continued sustainability.

The following points should be considered for information communications and signboards that comply with standards; There should be signage that controls the flow of traffic and directs vehicles to specific points; the use of street addresses or building numbers instead of detailed, explanatory information in public spaces; minimizing the number of signboards containing high-risk structures; reducing to a minimum signage that identifies risky complexes, such as powerplants and water treatment facilities; markings to minimize accidental entry of unauthorized personnel into critical areas; signage should be hung at intervals no greater than 100 meters. Moreover, it is vitally important to hang warning signs at all entrances, in restricted, controlled and exclusion areas, bilingual (or more) signs, and used in areas where two or more languages are widely spoken (Federal Emergency Management Agency, 2007). The adequacy of the marking elements in the roof garden is quite low in accordance with the criteria determined by Federal Emergency Management Agency.

It is highly recommended to create 30 cm vegetation-free zones around a green roof, around drainage zones, around glare areas and other penetration areas (rooftop structures, skylights, playground equipment, etc.) (Tolderlund, 2010). As Tolderlund has pointed out, there are also 30 cm vegetation-free areas around the playground equipment in the study area. Considering the characteristics of plants emphasized by Johnston and Newton in their studies, attention has been paid to use perennial plants in the Marmara Forum Mall roof garden plants. A cage system was not used to cool and moisten the plants on warm days. Regarding plant selection, pains have been taken to ensure they have a low nutritional requirement, require little maintenance, are resistant to extreme hot and cold weather conditions, and are wind-resistant. In addition, while some plants grow invasive, some plants remain evergreen. Care has been taken to ensure the plants in the roof garden are not hazardous to the path surface and human health. There is a sufficient water supply and drainage system for plants grown and placed in a way that they do not interfere with promenade paths. The diversity and the choice of flowery, scented plants used in the roof garden provides a peaceful environment preferred by its users.

Sufficient depth and dark-colored bottoms were incorporated into the design of roof garden water structures. Aesthetic concerns were considered while designing ornamental pools. There is no rainwater management or use of reservoirs.

Due to the presence of different types of plants in the Marmara Forum Mall roof garden and the dense roof garden type, the amount of watering is not at a minimum value. Since it is a user-oriented place, there is inadequate equipment space. On the other hand, the path, furniture and plants are maintained on a regular basis.

When looking at the scale of Marmara Forum, it was determined that; climatic data, hard structure activities, promenade areas and designs of plant and water elements in soft structure are moderately sufficient. It has been observed there are no problems with the roof furniture design and maintenance (Table 2).

Table 2. Overall evaluation of the Marmara Forum Roof Garden design

DESIGN CRITERIA	POOR	AVERAGE	GOOD
CLIMATIC INFLUENCES		√	
HARD STRUCTURE			
ACTIVITIES		√	
PROMENADE GROUNDS		√	
ROOF FURNITURE			√
SOFT STRUCTURE			
PLANTS		√	
WATER		√	
MAINTENANCE			√

RESEARCH CONSTRAINTS

The gathering of previous studies under the same subject headings is a reason the study could not obtain reference sources. Moreover, despite dating back to ancient times, the fact the roof garden phenomenon has only started to gain the reputation it deserves today is the reason for the limited number of officials who have conducted studies in this regard. A lack of knowledge and experience, financial concerns, ignoring user needs were among the constraints of the study topic during production.

FUTURE RESEACRH DIRECTIONS

In today's world where the importance of sustainable design is gradually increasing, it is inevitable to increase the planting designs in urban environments. This study will be important from the standpoint of boosting the quality of future roof garden designs.

CONCLUSION

Climatic factors, flooring and structure support, roof slope, function and location selection, accessibility and safety, design of roof equipment use as well as structural, vegetation and maintenance parameters that may be effective in the design of roof gardens were determined in this study. The scarcity of parameters that may be considered as poor in the evaluation of the overall design in the Marmara Forum Shopping Mall sample scale is a remarkable result. As a result, this study is important in terms of creating a checklist that can be used to increase the utilization quality of roof gardens while improving user comfort.

REFERENCES

Acks, K. (2006). A framework for cost-benefit analysis of green roofs: Initial estimates. *Green roofs in the New York metropolitan region: Research report.*

AFineLyne. (2019). https://gothamtogo.com/alica-kwade-selected-to-exhibit-on-met-roof-garden-spring-2019/

Ajuntament de Barcelona. (2018). *La Fàbrica del Sol enseña su interior.* https://ajuntament.barcelona.cat/ecologiaurbana/es/noticia/la-fabrica-del-sol-ensena-su-interior_636642

Anderson, M. (2012). *Design And Development of A Roof Garden.* https://maintenance.transportation.org/Documents/10_Anderson_RoofGarden.pdf

Architecture, D. S. (2021). *Marmara Forum Commercial Complex.* http://www.dsmimarlik.com/project/Marmara-Forum-Commercial-Complex

ASTM E 2400. (2006). *Standard Guide for Selection, Installation, and Maintenance of Plants for Green Roof Systems.* ASTM International.

Austin, G. (2014). *Green infrastructure for landscape planning: integrating human and natural systems.* Routledge. doi:10.4324/9781315856780

Bass, B., & Baskaran, B. (2003). *Evaluating rooftop and vertical gardens as an adaptation strategy for urban areas.* Academic Press.

Bayhan, B. (2015). *Dünyanın En Büyük Yeşil Çatısı Tasarlandı.* https://www.arkitera.com/haber/dunyanin-en-buyuk-yesil-catisi-tasarlandi/

Borooah, A., & Aster, D. (2009). *Toronto Green Roof Construction Standard: Supplementary Guidelines.* Academic Press.

Brebbia, C. A., Longhurst, J., Marco, E., & Booth, C. (Eds.). (2017). *Sustainable development and planning IX* (Vol. 226). WIT press.

Brenneisen, S. (2003). *The Benefits of Biodiversity from Green Roofs œ Key Design Consequences* (Doctoral dissertation). Iowa State University.

Çalışkan, N. (2017). *Marmara Forum Shopping Center.* https://nilufercaliskan.info/projects/marmara-forum/

Çelikkol, U. (2015). *Alışveriş Merkezleri Değerlemesi Süreci Ve Yöntemleri, Marmara Forum Avm Değerleme Çalışması Örneği* (Doctoral dissertation). Fen Bilimleri Enstitüsü.

Costerdesign. (2021). *Foodcourt Marmara Forum Istanbul*. https://www.costerdesign.nl/post/food-court-marmara-forum-istanbul

Council, U. G. B. (1998). *US green building council*. US Green Building Council.

Davis, B. E. (2011). Rooftop hospital gardens for physical therapy: A post-occupancy evaluation. *HERD: Health Environments Research & Design Journal, 4*(3), 14–43. doi:10.1177/193758671100400303 PMID:21866502

Dorr, E., Sanyé-Mengual, E., Gabrielle, B., Grard, B. J., & Aubry, C. (2017). Proper selection of substrates and crops enhances the sustainability of Paris rooftop garden. *Agronomy for Sustainable Development, 37*(5), 1–11. doi:10.100713593-017-0459-1

Dunnett, N. (2006). *Sheffield's Green Roof Forum: a multi-stranded programme of green roof infrastructure development for the UK's greenest city*. Academic Press.

Eckert, H., & Koop, P. (2012). Roof Restoration With A Sunny Side. *ZinCo*. https://zinco.se/news/press_releases/press_release_details.php?id=76

Federal Emergency Management Agency-FEMA. (2007). *FEMA 430: Site and Urban Design for Security: GuidanceAgainstPotentialTerroristAttacks, ProvidingProtectionto People andBuildings*. Federal Emergency Management.

Fernandez-Cañero, R., Emilsson, T., Fernandez-Barba, C., & Machuca, M. Á. H. (2013). Green roof systems: A study of public attitudes and preferences in southern Spain. *Journal of Environmental Management, 128*, 106–115. doi:10.1016/j.jenvman.2013.04.052 PMID:23722180

FMIC (Factory Mutual Insurance Company). (2007). *Green Roof Systems. FM Global Property Loss Prevention Data Sheets. 2007, 6 Temmuz 2011*. http://www.ci.berkeley.ca.us/uploadedFiles/Planning_and_Development/Level_3_Energy_and_Sustainable_Development/Factory%20Mutual%20Green%20Roof%2 0System.pdf

Francis, R. A., & Lorimer, J. (2011). Urban reconciliation ecology: The potential of living roofs and walls. *Journal of Environmental Management, 92*(6), 1429–1437.

Future Green Studio. (2021). Empire Stores. *LANDEZİNE*. http://landezine.com/index.php/2021/01/empire-stores/

Gedge, D. (2003). From Rubble to Redstarts… Black Redstart Action Plan Working Group. *Proceedings from Greening Rooftops for Sustainable Communities, First North American Green Roof Infrastructure Conference*.

Getter, K. L., & Rowe, D. B. (2006). The role of extensive green roofs in sustainable development. *HortScience, 41*(5), 1276–1285. doi:10.21273/HORTSCI.41.5.1276

Green Roof For Healthy Cities. (2021). https://greenroofs.org/

Groundhog. (2021). *Keio University Roof Garden*. https://groundhog.la/projects/keio-university-roof-garden/

GVL. (2021). *Yinian Rooftop Garden for Seniors*. https://landezine-award.com/yinian-rooftop-garden-for-seniors/

Hai, C. (2014). *Building a community rooftop network: design prototypes for Taipei* (Doctoral dissertation).

Harris Charles, W., & Dines Nicholas, T. (1998). *Time-saver standards for landscape architecture: design and construction data*. Academic Press.

Herzog, T. R., Maguire, P., & Nebel, M. B. (2003). Assessing the restorative components of environments. *Journal of Environmental Psychology*, *23*(2), 159–170.

Hopper, L. J. (Ed.). (2012). *Landscape architectural graphic standards* (Vol. 27). John Wiley & Sons.

Jafari, N., Utaberta, N., Yunos, M. Y. M., Ismail, N. A., Ismail, S., Ariffin, N. F. M., ... Valikhani, M. (2015). Benefits of roof garden in order to usage of urban agriculture at roof garden in high-rise building in Malaysia. *Advances in Environmental Biology*, *9*(24), 86–92.

Kaplan, R., & Kaplan, S. (1989). *The experience of nature: A psychological perspective*. Cambridge university press.

Knaus, M., & Haase, D. (2020). Green roof effects on daytime heat in a prefabricated residential neighbourhood in Berlin, Germany. *Urban Forestry & Urban Greening*, *53*, 126738.

Köhler, M., Schmidt, M., Grimme, F. W., Laar, M., de Assunção Paiva, V. L., & Tavares, S. (2002). Green roofs in temperate climates and in the hot-humid tropics–far beyond the aesthetics. *Environmental Management and Health*.

Landschaftsentwicklung, F. (2008). *Guidelines for the planning, construction and maintenance of green roofing: Green roofing guideline*. Forschungsgesellschaft Landschaftsentwickung Landschaftsbau.

Laumann, K., Gärling, T., & Stormark, K. M. (2003). Selective attention and heart rate responses to natural and urban environments. *Journal of Environmental Psychology*, *23*(2), 125–134.

Lazzarin, R. M., Castellotti, F., & Busato, F. (2005). Experimental measurements and numerical modelling of a green roof. *Energy and Building*, *37*(12), 1260–1267.

Lee, T. (1982). *Rooftop landscape development: design implications for cool northern climates*. Academic Press.

LIGHTDESIGN. (2021). *Seıbu Ike Bukuro Roof Garden*. https://lightdesign.jp/gallery/seibu-ikebukuro-roof-garden/

Liu, K., & Baskaran, B. (2003). *Thermal performance of green roofs through field evaluation*. Academic Press.

Luckett, K. (2009). *Green roof construction and maintenance*. McGraw-Hill Education.

Mairs, J. (2017). *Selgascano Adds Roof Extension With Pools And Plants To Second Home Offices İn London*. Academic Press.

Meteoblue. (2021). *İklim Bakırköy*. https://www.meteoblue.com/tr/hava/historyclimate/climatemodelled/bak%c4%b1rk%c3%b6y_t%c3%bcrkiye_751214

National Park Board. (2017). *A handbook on developing sustainable highrise gardens, Bringing Greenery Skywards*. https://www.nparks.gov.sg/-/media/srg/files/handbook-1.pdf

National Park Service. (2021). *Green Roof Benefits*. https://www.nps.gov/tps/sustainability/new-technology/green-roofs/benefits.htm

Oberndorfer, E., Lundholm, J., Bass, B., Coffman, R. R., Doshi, H., Dunnett, N., Gaffin, S., Köhler, M., Liu, K. Y., & Rowe, B. (2007). Green Roofs as Urban Ecosystems: Ecological Structures, Functions and Services. *BioScience, 57*(10), 823-833. www.biosciencemag.org

Olson Family Garden. (2021). *St. Louıs Chıldren's Hospıtal*. https://www.greenroofs.com/projects/olson-family-garden-st-louis-childrens-hospital/

Osmundson, T. (1999). *Roof gardens: history, design, and construction*. WW Norton & Company.

Peck, S. W., Callaghan, C., Kuhn, M. E., & Bass, B. (1999). *Greenbacks from green roofs: forging a new industry in Canada*. Academic Press.

Peck, S. W., & Kuhn, M. (2003). *Design guidelines for green roofs*. Ontario Association of Architects.

Pintos, P. (2021). *Marmara Forum Cloud Playground / Carv*. https://www.archdaily.com/939901/marmara-forum-cloud-playground-carve?ad_medium=gallery

Pouya, S. (2019). Evaluation of Roof Gardens as Recreation Areas. *Türkiye Peyzaj Araştırmaları Dergisi*, *2*(1), 40–49.

Priority Zone. (2021). *Rooftop Garden Inner-City Greening & Beautification*. http://priorityzone.weebly.com/rooftop-garden.html#

Proxima (2021). Compherensive Green Roof in Mexico City (INFONAVIT). *Landezine*. https://landezine-award.com/comprehensive-green-roof-in-mexico-city-infonavit/

Sailor, D. J. (1995). Simulated urban climate response to modifications in surface albedo and vegetative cover. *Journal of Applied Meteorology and Climatology*, *34*(7), 1694–1704.

Sanyé-Mengual, E., Orsini, F., Oliver-Solà, J., Rieradevall, J., Montero, J. I., & Gianquinto, G. (2015). Techniques and crops for efficient rooftop gardens in Bologna, Italy. *Agronomy for Sustainable Development*, *35*(4), 1477–1488.

Section 504. (2021). *Building And Rooftop Acces*. https://up.codes/s/building-and-rooftop-access

Shuang, H. (2021). *Pıxeland/100architects*. Https://www.Archdaily.Com/915563/Pixeland-100architects

Snodgrass, E. C., & Snodgrass, L. L. (2006). Green roof plants: a resource and planting guide (No. 04; SB419. 5, S5.). Portland, OR: Timber Press.

Srenco. (2007). *Looking at Rooftop Garden at St. Louis Childrens Hospital in St. Louis MO 63108*. http://www.srencoaerialphoto.com/srencobuildings/Pages/12.html

Tolderlund, L. (2010). *Design guidelines and maintenance manual for green roofs in the semi-arid and arid west*. Green Roofs for Healthy Cities.

Tooke, T. R., Coops, N. C., Voogt, J. A., & Meitner, M. J. (2011). Tree structure influences on rooftop-received solar radiation. *Landscape and Urban Planning*, *102*(2), 73–81.

Ulrich, R. S. (1998). View through a window may influence recovery from surgery. *Science, 224*, 42M21.

Ulrich, R. S., Simons, R. F., Losito, B. D., Fiorito, E., Miles, M. A., & Zelson, M. (1991). Stress recovery during exposure to natural and urban environments. *Journal of Environmental Psychology*, *11*(3), 201–230.

Unite Nations. (2012). *Enable. Accessibility for the disabled-A design manual for a barrier Free environment.* https://www.un.org/esa/socdev/enable/designm/AD4-01.htm

Velazquez, S. L. (2005). *Organic Greenroof Architecture: Sustainable Design for the New Millennium; Making the most of your building's fifth façade.* Wiley Periodicals, Inc.

Wang, T., & Pryor, M. (2019). *Social Value of Urban Rooftop Farming: A Hong Kong Case Study.* Agricultural Economics-Current Issues.

Weiler, S. K., & Scholz-Barth, K. (2009). Green Roof Systems – A Guide to the Planning, Design and Construction of Landscape Over Structure. Hoboken, NJ: John Wiley & Sons, Inc.

Werthmann, C. (2007). *Green Roof-A Case Study: Michael Van Valkenburgh Associates' Design for the Headquarters of the American Society of Landscape Architects.* Princeton Architectural Press.

Wilkinson, S. J., Knott, J., Goddard, J. G., & Craft, L. (2016). *RICS Best Practice Guidance Note on Green Roofs and Green Walls.* RICS Best Practice Guidance Note on Green Roofs and Green Walls.

Willem, V. C. (2005, April). ROOFTOP GARDENING, a big step to the future. *Conference Paper, First International Summit for Aforestation Roof Gardens in China.*

Wong, N. H., Chen, Y., Ong, C. L., & Sia, A. (2003). Investigation of thermal benefits of rooftop garden in the tropical environment. *Building and Environment*, *38*(2), 261–270.

WorldPress. (2021). *Roof Garden of The Metropolitan Museum of Art.* http://wirednewyork.com/museums/met-museum/roof-garden/

Yuen, B., & Hien, W. N. (2005). Resident perceptions and expectations of rooftop gardens in Singapore. *Landscape and Urban Planning*, *73*(4), 263–276.

ZinCo. (2020). *Planning Guide Walkways and Driveways on Roofs and Decks.* https://docs.google.com/viewerng/viewer?url=https%3A%2F%2Fzinco-greenroof.com%2Fsites%2Fdefault%2Ffiles%2F2020-

Chapter 8
Ground Air Temperature Control for Heat Pump Exchange. APTAE System:
Justification of HS6 (Radon Protection)

David Palomar Aguilar
ETSAM, Spain

Carlos Miguel Iglesias Sanz
Universidad CEU San Pablo, Spain

Sofia Corsini Fuhrmann
Universidad CEU San Pablo, Spain

ABSTRACT

Heating and cooling consume a high amount of energy, which is today mainly provided by fossil fuels. To save fossil resources and simultaneously reduce pollutants and CO2, heating and cooling energy consumption should be reduced. Geothermal energy is a clean, inexhaustible source of energy that is available all year round because it does not depend on the weather. Nevertheless, the use of tempered subsoil air has been used as a traditional air conditioning strategy; however, nowadays, its use has been questioned by the discovery of the leaks of radon gas from the ground. The investigation searches a heat exchange system with the subsoil which prevents the introduction of radon gas into living spaces. The system that is exposed increases the performance of aerothermal heat pumps by means of thermal exchange with tempered air in the sanitary chamber. This exchange is more favorable than air at the outside temperature, increasing the COP of the machine. This system complies with the regulations for protection against radon, protecting the building from this radioactive gas.

DOI: 10.4018/978-1-7998-7279-5.ch008

INTRODUCTION

Heating and Cooling Consume of CO_2. Emission Reduction Strategies

The growing concern for environmental sustainability and the fragile balance in which many of the ecosystems are found has substantially increased the need to reduce the impact of energy consumption on our planet. A significant part of this contribution to energy consumption lies in the construction sector (Zeiler & Boxem, 2009). The Global Situation Report of (2018) establishes the guidelines for efficient, resilient and emission-free construction and buildings. The built environment, which is one of the main drivers of the world economy, accounted:

- 39% of total CO_2 emissions in 2017 of carbon dioxide related to energy, where 28% of global energy-related CO_2 emissions and another 11% of CO_2 emissions from the energy sector.
- 36% of global final energy; this consumed almost 125 exajoules (EJ) in 2016, or 30% of total global final energy use and building construction, including the manufacture of materials for its construction, represented an additional consumption of 26 EJ (almost 6%) in the overall estimated final energy use.

Although buildings and construction sector emissions appear to have levelled off since 2015, they still represent the largest rate of total energy-related CO_2 emissions:

"If we don't make buildings more efficient, the increase in energy use will affect us all, whether through lack of access to affordable energy services, poor air quality or higher energy bills," says Dr. Fatih Birol, Executive Director of the International Energy Agency (IEA).

Building standards must change to reflect the urgency of buildings that are more resilient to climate change, with lower energy needs or mainly near-zero energy buildings, and their progressive decarbonization or mainly carbon-neutral buildings. Thus, global dialogue is supporting progress in developing policies for sustainable buildings and countries are continuing to implement and update building energy codes and certification policies. From here arose the Net Zero Carbon Buildings Commitment officially that launched at the Global Climate Action Summit on 13th September 2018 (C40 Cities, 2018). The aim is to reach net zero carbon in operation for all assets under their direct control by 2030, and to advocate for all buildings to be net zero carbon in operation by 2050 (ADEME, 2018). Unfortunately, investment in energy efficiency in buildings has slowed in 2017, with the slowest rate of increase in recent years.

The shift towards this desirable double new situation is promoting interest in passive geothermal cooling and heating and natural ventilation techniques in order to decrease energy consumption and carbon footprint (Soltani et al., 2018). The use of the high heat capacity of earth´s soil enable us to preheat the air in winter cold days and cool it in summer hot days (Wachenfeldt & Bell 2003). Moreover, there are various passive systems that combine strategies for passive cooling, passive heating as well as heat storage, aided or not by mechanical means. Thus, with earth air heat exchangers, it´s posible to capture heat from the ground or dissipate to it, preheating the air inside the buildings in winter and cooling it in summer (Peretti et al., 2013). The use and application of such mechanical ventilation systems in search, of low-energy buildings is the main aspect for creating a desirable level of indoor air quality, IAQ (Balvers et al., 2008). Several studies collect the latest advancements with different combinations of earth air heat exchangers and their thermal performance (Kaushal, 2017), (Bordoloi, 2018).

BACKGROUND

Origins of the Use of the Thermal Inertia of the Ground

Now it´s time to go back to the beginning, the backgrounds: the origins of exploiting the thermal inertia of the ground. In Nature itself, we can see that the search for comfort is inherent in living beings. We can find examples of the use and modification of the environment in the form of nests and burrows. For example prairie dogs, rodents who live in the soil of North American plains, take shelter in burrows that are 2-3m below the Earth's surface and can reach up to 10m in length, surviving harsh climatic conditions with temperatures ranging from 38°C in the summer to -37°C in winter.

Unconsciously, they take advantage of the physical law described in Bernoulli's principle, the same law that enables ventilate people's houses. It´s about achieving a change in air pressure inside the burrows to create a movement of air in a desired direction getting optimal ventilation and better temperature.

But when these achievements come to architecture, it seems to create a naturally ventilated building requires us to also understand how pressure is created and how it can be used actively or passively. We realise that architectural space should be composed as a flowing, interconnected space as opposed to a strongly fixed subdivided space, and then air pressure should to be controlled by means of directing natural wind or manipulating air temperature actively or passively.

The basis of conditioning buildings is from the Greek and Romans. The Greeks discovered the ground heating system on the cold Anatolian plateau. They pioneered with heating using double hollow floors through whose the hot fumes of a fire were passed. It consisted, as its own word indicates, in "making a fire below", that is, the fire heats the ceiling of the lower room so that it reaches the upper room near the ceiling through the stone floor. They checked the heat rising from the floor heats up much more and better than a direct heat source from the room itself, because the hot air rises and spreads throughout the room. However, it was an inefficient and dangerous system that consumed a lot of fuel for a small space with a high fire risk.

The Romans took over the Greek heating system, keeping its name but managing to improve it by developing something substantially better (Florides et al., 2002). Its design is attributed to the Roman engineer Gaius Sergius Orata: now the hot air that was obtained was not lost, because it was channelled through the subsoil of the whole building in an empty space like an air chamber with tiles supported on hundreds of columns of refractory bricks with thermal inertia.

This singular system was called *hypocauste* (Latin for *hypocaustum*, from gr. *ὑπόκαυστον*, from *ὑπό-*, below, and *καυστόν*) (Fig. 01) It was the ground heating system, used especially in the baths of the Roman Empire. The oldest remains have been found in Olympia, dating back to the 1st century BC. In Olympia. In the following centuries the system was perfected with its use in the *caldarium* of the thermal baths and also in the richest private houses (roman villas) (Oetelaar et al., 2013).

More recently there were heating systems similar to the hypocaust that were used, or are still used, like the *Ondol* Korean traditional heating system (Fig. 02), and the so-called *Glorias* used in large areas of Castile, Spain, during the Middle Ages, from the Roman legacy (Sansone, 1999). The latter consisted in a channel system under the floor of the house, where here straw was burned as fuel, and which carried heat throughout the house floor. There have been increasingly sophisticated examples of exploiting the thermal inertia of the subsoil since then.

Figure 1. Roman ground heating system. (Oetelaar et al., 2013).

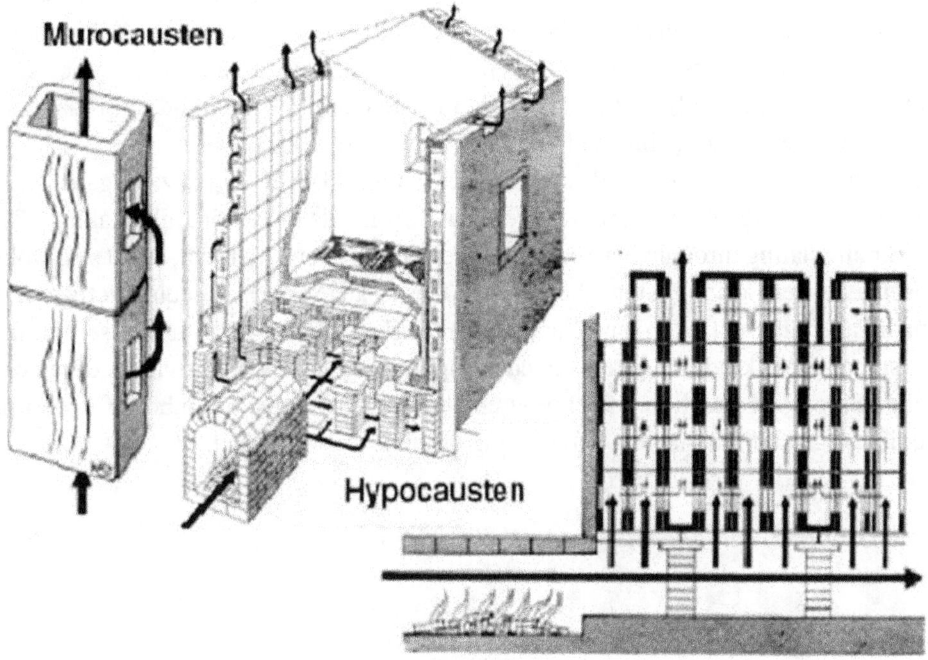

Figure 2. Korean ondol floor heating system. (Kim, 2006)

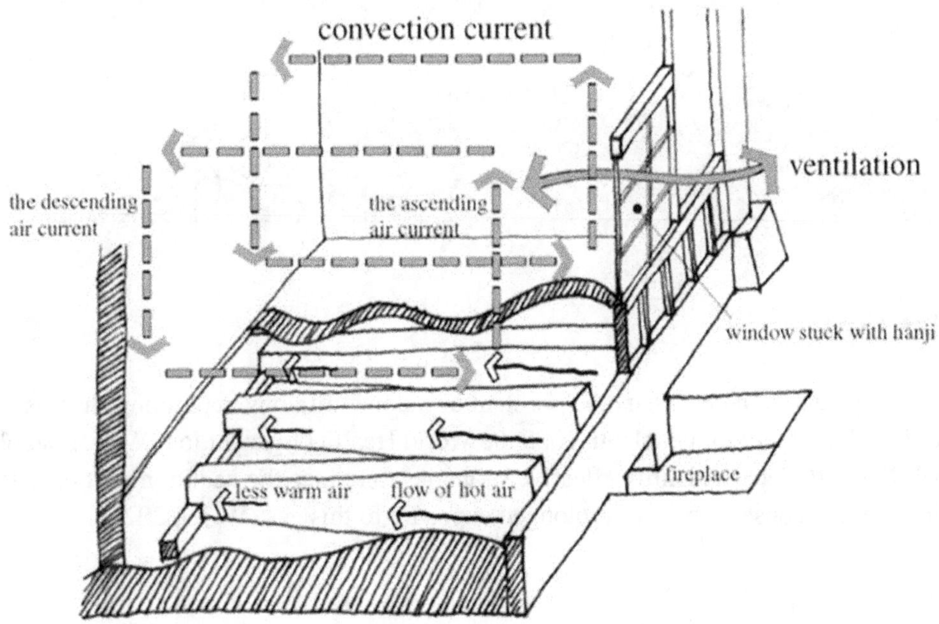

The physical principle that cold air is high pressured and warm air is low pressured was not known before the 18th century, but long before that houses were still unconsciously designed following that principle. For example, Palladio's Villa da Schio was erected in the mid-16th century and utilizes a cave to cool the interior spaces. How that works? The low pressured cool air is drawn through the villa towards the existing high pressured warm air on the outside. The thermal mass of the nearby mountain constantly cools the air in the cave, and as long as the outside air is warmer, the system will be active. Also, the greater the temperature difference between the cave and the outside, the greater the flow of air will be increasing its effectiveness. Similar case is Villa da Rotonda: the air cools in the basement and accesses of the villa through marble lattices arranged in the centre of the building. Finally, the hot air rises and exits through several openings in the dome (Panizzoni, 2001).

Another example are the Aeolian Villas in Costozza (Fig. 03) Veneto (Cazzaniga et al., 1981) are ventilated and cooled through connection with cool cave air inside the Berici hills, taking advantage of the cooling of air circulating through these caves, called "covoli" beneath them, and it still woks (Kenda, 2006). This Renaissance cooling system (Ferrucci & Peron, 2018) and subsequent others as the cave-houses of Guadix and Paterna (Spain) and Cappadocia (Turkey) (Fig. 04-05), are a useful reference and can help us to spread these kinds of systems in contemporary buildings, improving indoor comfort, and also decreasing energy consumption and carbon emissions. Currently, a number of experimental and analytical studies of geothermal heating and cooling systems are discussed.

Figure 3. Costozza Villas ventilation diagram. (Neila, 2004)

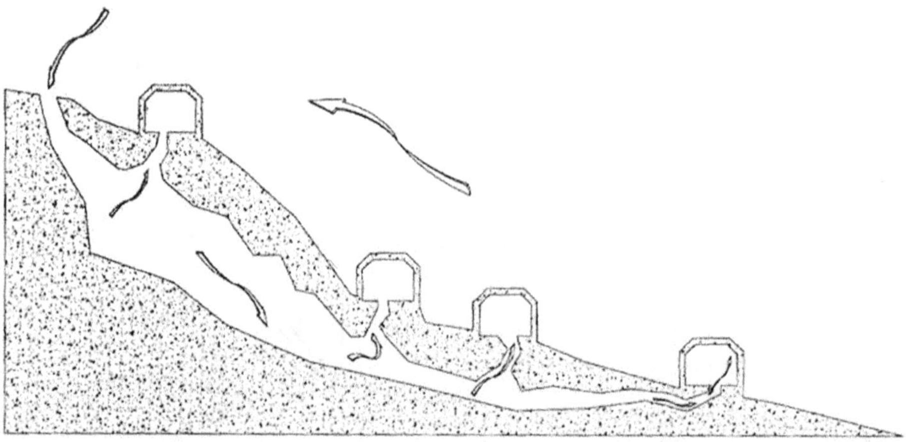

Radon Gas (Rn)

In another development, in recent years the problem of radon emissions in buildings has risen, becoming a serious health problem for people. In 2005 the World Health Organization (WHO) established the International Radon Project to identify effective strategies to reduce the health impact of radon, and to raise awareness of the consequences of prolonged exposure to this gas (WHO, 2021)

Figure 4. Derinkuyu underground city scheme in Cappadocia. (Nelila, 2004)

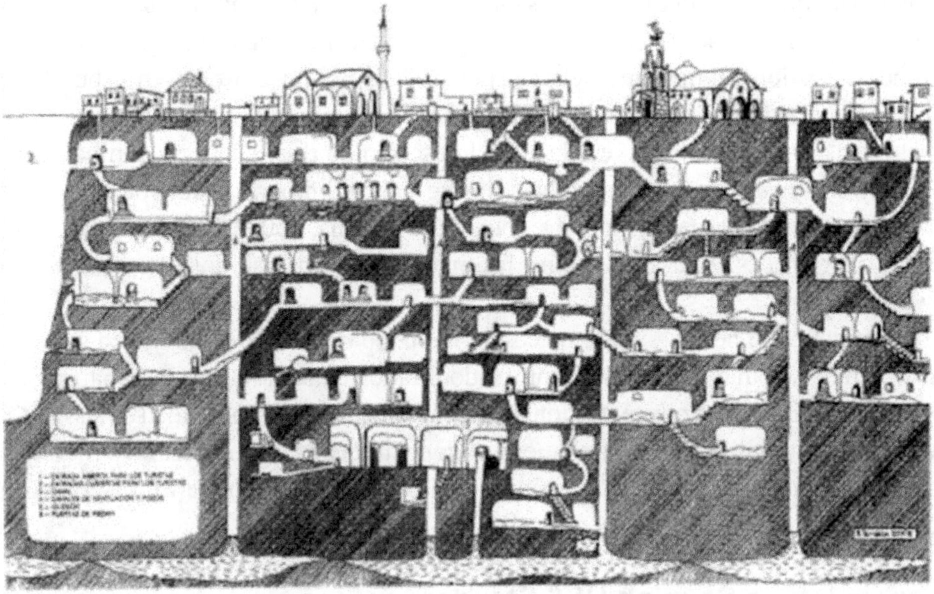

Figure 5. Göreme cave houses in Cappadocia. Own Photograph.

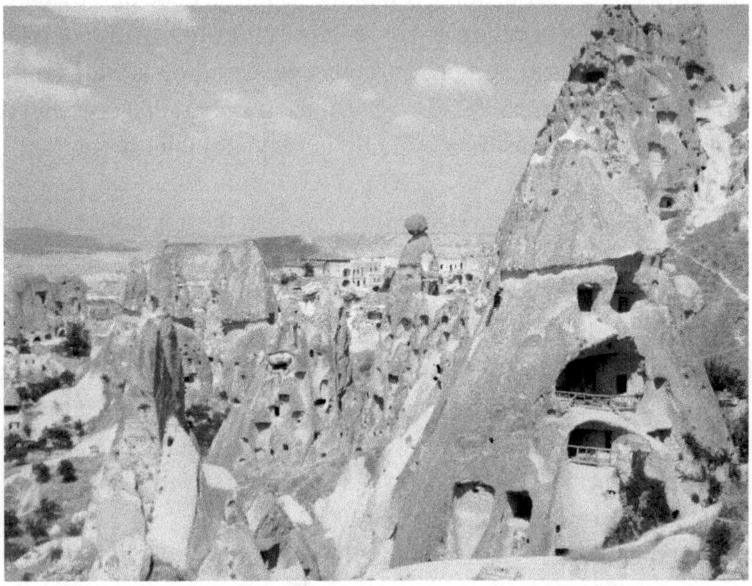

Radon gas (Rn) is a colorless, odorless, and tasteless noble gas from uranium and radium found in granitic and volcanic rocks that are often large emitters of this radioactive gas. It accumulates inside the dwelling and can be dangerous to the health of its occupants. Radon in its decay process produces radioactive particles. In France, it is considered responsible for 25% of lung cancer cases in non-smokers, and is thus recognized by the World Health Organization (WHO, 2021) (Darby et al. 2006). The natural disintegration of Rn 222 results in successive unstable isotopes and alpha radiation emissions, being Po the most dangerous. Mineral building materials may contain radon that ends up inside buildings (mainly natural stone, cement, bricks and concrete), but the highest concentration usually comes from the subsoil by diffusion and convection through the cracks and pores of the ground, as well as from building materials.

The best way to get rid of it is venting (Cavallo et al. 1991), you can ventilate the floor of the building to let it out. It is also effective to ventilate the house. To do this, windows can be opened twice a day for at least 15 minutes. To avoid losing heat during the cold months, some buildings are designed with ventilation ducts that preheat the air, (De Paepe & Janssens, 2003). But those systems leak more radon in to the living spaces. That goes against heath and latest Spanish normative, as we will explain in the following chapter.

Therefore, ventilation of non-habitable spaces between the floor and the inhabited space (e.g., ventilated sanitary chambers) can reduce significantly indoor radon concentrations by separating the interior from the soil and reducing radon concentration below inhabited space. The effectiveness of this strategy improves increasing ventilation, with passive or mechanical means. In the case of ventilation of living spaces, it is desirable that there be an exchange between indoor and outdoor air for a good general quality of indoor air.

Consequences of the Spanish HS6 Standard in the Use of Tempered Air in the Subsoil

Additionally, regulating this issue, the Section HS-6 of the technical code of the Spanish building (CTE-DB HS-6, 2019) (determines that it is necessary to limit the risk of exposure of users to inappropriate radon concentrations. The unit of measurement of radon concentration is Bq/m^3(becquerel per metre). The reference level shall be 300 Bq/m^3 as the average annual indoor radon concentration. Do not forget that the level of radon concentration inside a building is very variable throughout the year; therefore 300 Bq/m^3 is not an absolute value.

The regulation, through this new Section HS6, aims to protect the population from the harmful health effects that may result from prolonged exposure to high concentrations of radon gas inside buildings. The radon of the ground can penetrate the interior of the buildings through the cracks and joints of the building enclosure in contact with the ground (basement walls, floors, etc.), and even through the mass of porous materials that form the enclosures themselves. When radon comes from the ground, the highest concentrations in a building are located on the lower floors, such as the basements and the ground floors, since the radon density is also higher than that of the air. If radon reaches the outside environment, it is quickly diluted in the air, but when it does so to a closed and poorly ventilated space, such as the inside of basement floors, it can concentrate and be dangerous.

The current Spanish standard CTE-DB HS6 classifies municipalities into two categories (Fig. 06), depending on the presence of this radioactive natural gas. Even in *zone I* category, with the lowest concentration, it is clear that radon must be prevented from entering the inhabited areas of buildings and being inhaled by their inhabitants. This consideration complicates the use of the subsoil for the renewal air tempering techniques that have been carried out in favour of energy saving. Either the ducts are completely gas-tight or, as developed in this article, this tempered air is used for heat exchange.

Figure 6. Radon risk potential map of Spain. (ISN, 2021)

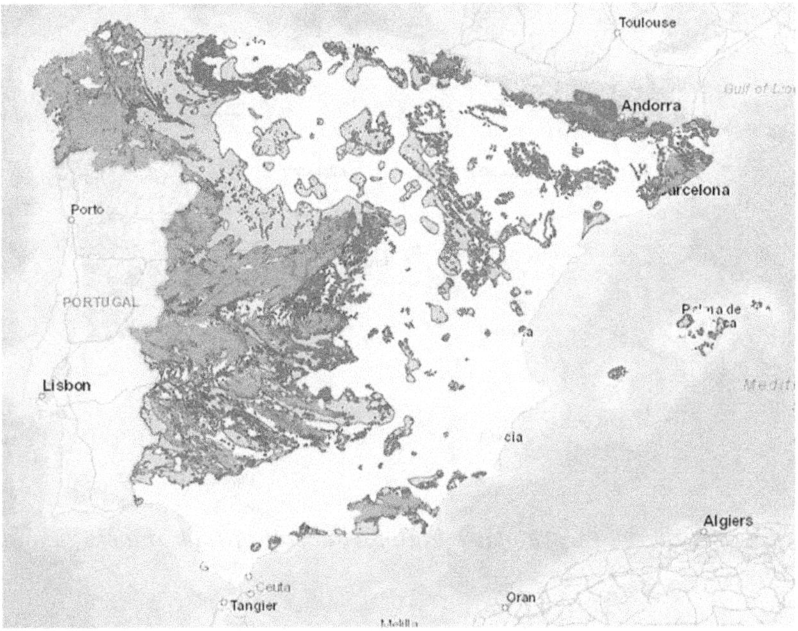

MAIN FOCUS OF THE CHAPTER

The use of tempered subsurface air has been adversely affected by the discovery of radon gas emissions through the ground. As a solution to continue using the climatic benefits of the subsoil air and, at the same, time guaranteeing the health of the space, a heat exchange system is proposed between the stable temperature air from the ground and the air from the living space, without mixing.

Thermal Properties of the Subsoil

The presence of water increases the thermal conductivity of the ground, especially in those granular or porous, susceptible to being clogged with water, improving thermal exchange, but at the same time they are more susceptible to variations of outside temperature. As the ground temperature is a function of the thermal diffusivity up to a depth of 20m (Kusuda & Achenbach, 1965), and the presence of water increases this value, the cladding and drainage that usually surround the walls to keep them dry influences the thermal gradient. Dry soils achieve thermal stability at shallower depths, as shown in the comparative graphs (Fig. 07):

A side effect of keeping the ground next to the building dry is that it increases the permeability to gases such as radon, reducing their concentration under the slab. For this reason, it is more advisable to promote drainage systems than to waterproof the surrounding soil.

Daily temperature fluctuations are no longer perceived in the subsoil from approximately 1m depth, depending on the factors mentioned (presence of water, diffusivity, among others). At greater depths, below 10 to 12m, you can take advantage of the time lag due to the inertia of the land mass, where the temperature corresponds to the average of the previous month or quarter as the depth increases, as can be seen in the diagram (Fig. 08):

Figure 7. Comparative graph of subsoil temperature (clays and silt) with different saturations. Own diagram

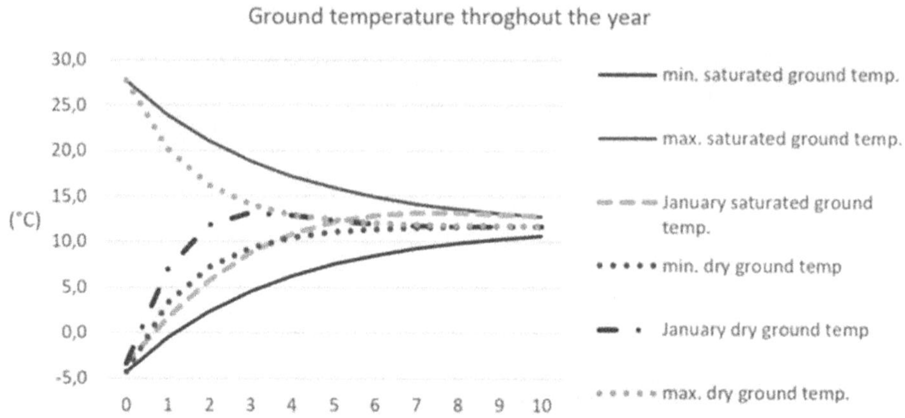

Figure 8. Evolution of the thermal wave phase lag of a subsoil of rocky blocks and clays, with depth. Own diagram

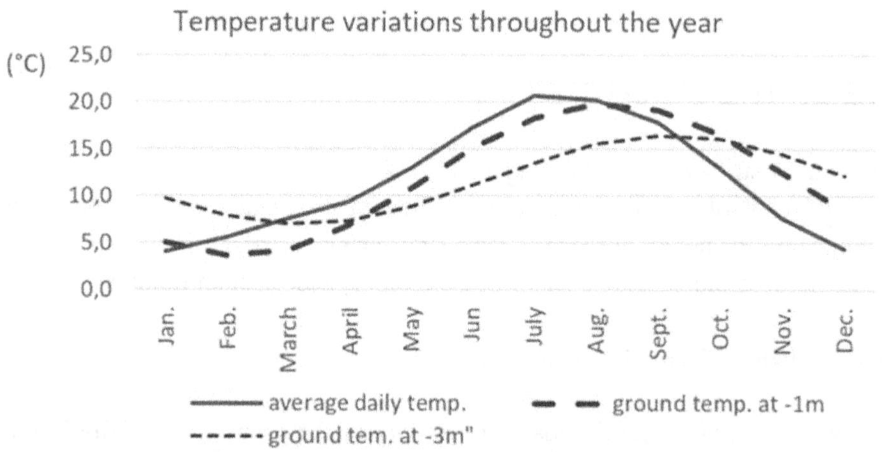

This effect is particularly desirable at depths above 3m, since the maximum temperature of the subsoil is reached after the summer, favouring a better extraction of thermal energy.

Surface and Demand

For the viability of the system, a ratio between the exchange surface and the energy demand is necessary. It becomes inefficient for tall buildings or poorly insulated, where the demands for heating and cooling have a very large proportion in relation to their contact surface with the ground. In any case, for a precise calculation the alteration of the temperature of the exchange surface due to the recirculation of air should be considered.

Hereunder are described the two demand cases:

- **Unbalanced Demand**: The worst case corresponds to very unequal heating and cooling demands. The characteristics of the building, its use and the climate, are the factors that give rise to this situation, in which the inertia of the terrain no longer influences the calculation, and the model becomes a unidirectional flow dominated by the exchange surface and the conductivity of the ground. By not reversing the energy flow seasonally, this last factor will limit the extractable power from the terrain.
- **Balanced Demand**: The most favourable situation is one in which the heating and cooling demands are similar, and their difference does not exceed the energy flow that the subsoil is capable of contributing to the exchange surface. In this situation the seasonal thermal lag comes into play, that is, the layer of the land with which energy is exchanged reaches its maximum temperature coinciding with the demand for heating and vice versa, reaching its minimum temperature in the hot season, when the building demands refrigeration.

Modification of Terrain Isotherms

A building whose construction does not have measures aimed to modifying the isotherms of the terrain, will not benefit efficiently from the stable temperature that the subsoil can provide as the depth increases. (Fig.09).

This technique consists of achieving a stable temperature of the ground at shallower depths than those that would occur in undisturbed conditions, with the aim of reducing energy losses due to conduction with the ground or, in the case proposed, favouring thermal convective exchange. Any building that is not elevated above the ground alters the temperature of the subsoil as we enter the perimeter of its floor. The perimeter thermal gradient, affected by variations in outside temperature, is called the *edge effect* and has a length of less than 5m (Neila, 2004). To reduce the edge effect there are several techniques: Isolate the perimeter of the slab, extend the insulation of the facade under the subfloor, or isolate the surface that surrounds the building. An example would be to have a thick layer of tree bark (mulch) commonly used in gardening.

Another measure, which can be complementary to the previous ones, is to increase the relative depth of the floor by means of a land slope (Fig. 10). The effect on thermal inertia is similar to that of a semi-basement. It allows access to the ground plan in a specific way, while, in general, the elevation of the land is flush with the windowsill as seen in one of the sections represented.

Figure 9. Section without extension of the insulation below the ground level (stone blocks and clays). Own diagram

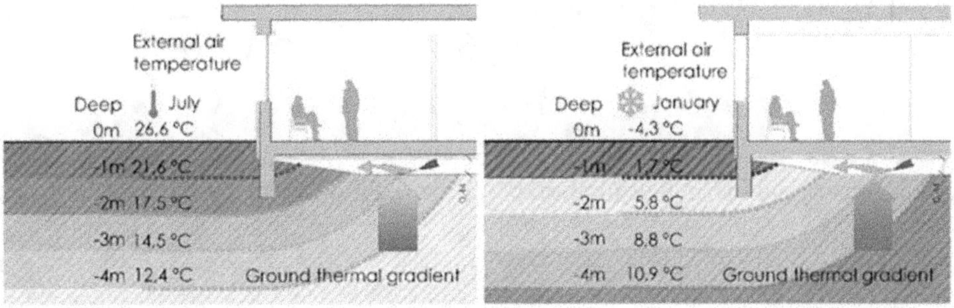

Figure 10. Section with slope and extension of the insulation under the ground (stone blocks and clays). Own diagram

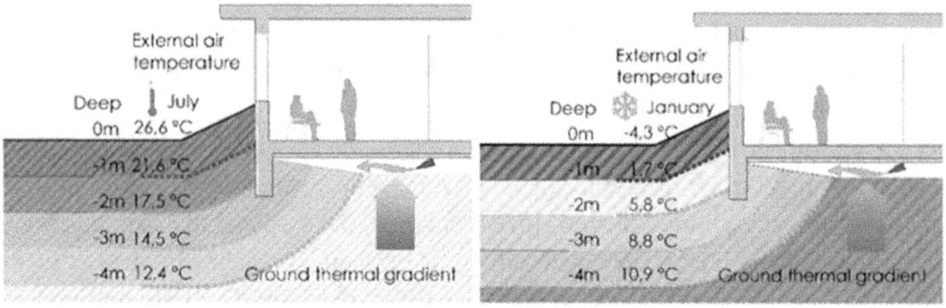

Figure 11. Section with isolated basement, (terrain of blocks, edges and clays). Own diagram

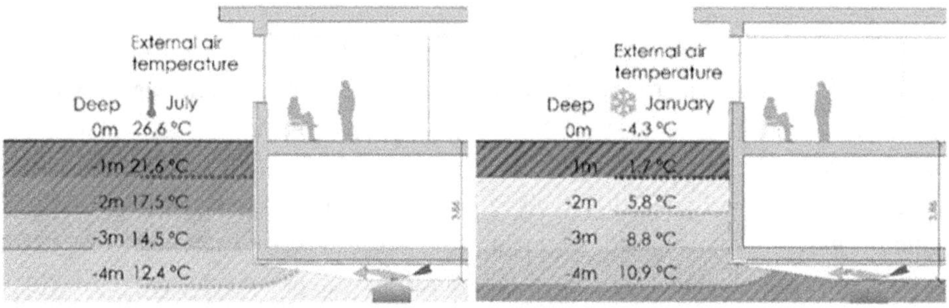

One way to reduce the edge effect in sills over a sanitary chamber is to reduce their free height at the perimeter, to limit convection. In the case of proposing recirculation of the air in the chamber, the effect could be compared to that of a river bed, where the water circulates faster on its axis than on the banks. (represented in Fig. 09-11)

Methodology

In the first place, the subsoil temperature is calculated in the first meters of the subsoil for the months of January and July, using the expression of Kusuda and Achenbach (1965), valid up to 20m depth.

$$T(z,t)=T_m - A_s e^{-z\sqrt{\frac{\pi}{365\alpha}}}\cos\left[\frac{2\pi}{365}\left(t-t_o-\frac{z}{2}\sqrt{\frac{365}{\pi\alpha}}\right)\right]$$

Where:

- *Z*: Depth (m)
- *As*: Annual superficial thermal oscillation (° C)
- *t*: Time (days)
- t_o: Lag (days)

- *α:* thermal diffusivity of the soil (m^2 / day)
- *Tm*: Average soil temperature.

From the data obtained, the graphs of the modified terrain isotherms are made for each of the three sections represented, taking into account their geometry and position of the insulation. For each of the variants, the temperatures are calculated for the summer and winter months with the highest cooling and heating demands respectively.

The ground-air exchange can be calculated as a fluid circulating on a plane assuming that the hearth is sufficiently isolated by the expression:

$$Q = h \cdot A \cdot (T^{a}a - Ts.)$$

Where:

- *Q:* Heat exchange (W)
- *h:* is the film coefficient in (W / m^2 · ° C) dependent on the speed v in (m / s). For forced convection (Blesa, 1994):

Table 1.

h values	v ≤ 5 (m/s)	V > 5(m/s)
Flat surface	5,6 + 4v	$7{,}12 * v^{0{,}78}$
Rough surface	5,8 + 4v	$7{,}14 * v^{0{,}78}$
Very rough surface	6,6 + 4v	$7{,}52 * v^{0{,}78}$

- *A*: Area of the plane (m^2)
- *T^a a*: is the air temperature (° C)
- *Ts:* Surface temperature of the plane in (° C)

Giving rise to multiple hypotheses based on:

1. Ground temperature higher or lower than that of the air flow, where vertical upward or downward thermal flow variants should be considered. If we consider that it is a forced convection we could simplify both possibilities in a single one (Blesa, 1994)
2. Roughness of the plane
3. Laminar or turbulent flow, the latter being the most desirable for greater energy exchange.

As the development of each of these variants is known and does not contribute novelty, it is assumed that the air path is long enough to reach the ground temperature at the end of its path.

The last calculation step is the estimation of the COP improvement through a progression of the performance curves stated for each technology and station (IDAE, 2008)

Location data:

Figure 12. Variation of the temperature throughout the day. Own elaboration from climatic data of the locality. (Palencia-Spain)

Hour/month:	Jan.	Feb.	Mar.	Apr.	May	Jun	July	Aug.	Sep.	Oct.	Nov	Dec.
3,00	-2,4	-0,9	1,0	2,9	6,5	10,7	14,2	13,8	11,4	6,5	1,1	-2,1
6,00	-3,9	-2,4	-0,5	1,4	5,0	9,2	12,7	12,3	9,9	5,0	-0,4	-3,6
9,00	0,1	1,6	3,5	5,4	9,0	13,2	16,7	16,3	13,9	9,0	3,6	0,4
12,00	8,1	9,6	11,5	13,4	17,0	21,2	24,7	24,3	21,9	17,0	11,6	8,4
15,00	12,1	13,6	15,5	17,4	21,0	25,2	28,7	28,3	25,9	21,0	15,6	12,4
18,00	10,6	12,1	14,0	15,9	19,5	23,7	27,2	26,8	24,4	19,5	14,1	10,9
21,00	6,6	8,1	10,0	11,9	15,5	19,7	23,2	22,8	20,4	15,5	10,1	6,9
24,00	1,6	3,1	5,0	6,9	10,5	14,7	18,2	17,8	15,4	10,5	5,1	1,9

Exchange with the Heat Pump

One of the solutions to continue using the inertia of the subsoil without increasing exposure to radon, is to use it for heat exchange with the outdoor unit (evaporator / condenser) instead of using it as fresh air.

The outside air is introduced through perimeter grilles in the sanitary chamber, driven by mechanical means. The inlet grilles are located at the far end of the facilities room, where the heat pump will be housed, maximizing the air path. The large section allows speeds low enough to take advantage of the thermal gradient of the ground and to temper the air under the sanitary slab. Additionally, you can also take advantage of the extraction air, whose temperature will be closer to comfort than outside, further reducing the consumption of air conditioning systems.

This re-circulated air travels through either the sanitary chamber or a set of buried pipes, taking with it the radon that could emerge from the ground to a non-habitable place where the heat pump is located. This machine will exchange heat with this pre-tempered air, reducing the thermal gradient that it must carry out and achieving significant savings in the energy consumed by the pump / s, (as in a mild coastal climate instead of a continental one).

It should be noted that the air with which the heat pump exchanges is subsequently expelled to the outside by a chimney on the roof and in no case is it introduced into living areas or comes into contact with the renewal air. There is only one energy exchange through the heat pump.

Estimation of the Improvement of the COP Based on a Temperature Exchange of the Outdoor Unit with an Air at the Ground Temperature under the Sanitary Chamber

COP: Coefficient of performance
EER: energy efficiency ratio

- **Cooling Mode**: For the example locality shown in the section, in the month of July, with an average outdoor air temperature of -26.6 ° C, and the chamber air was taken at 12.4 ° C, the EER corresponding to a 100% load for an invert system would go from 3.8 to 5.1, which represents a 34% improvement in efficiency.

Figure 13. Principle scheme. Own diagram

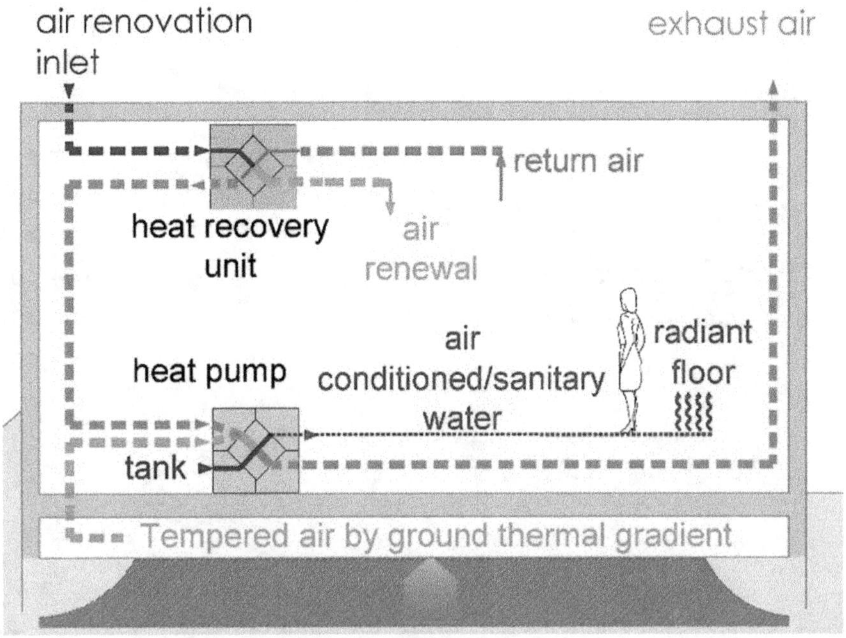

Figure 14. Influence of the energy efficiency of an Inverter type refrigeration machine, depending on the outside dry temperature (° C) and the load (%). Redrawn from (IDAE, 2008)

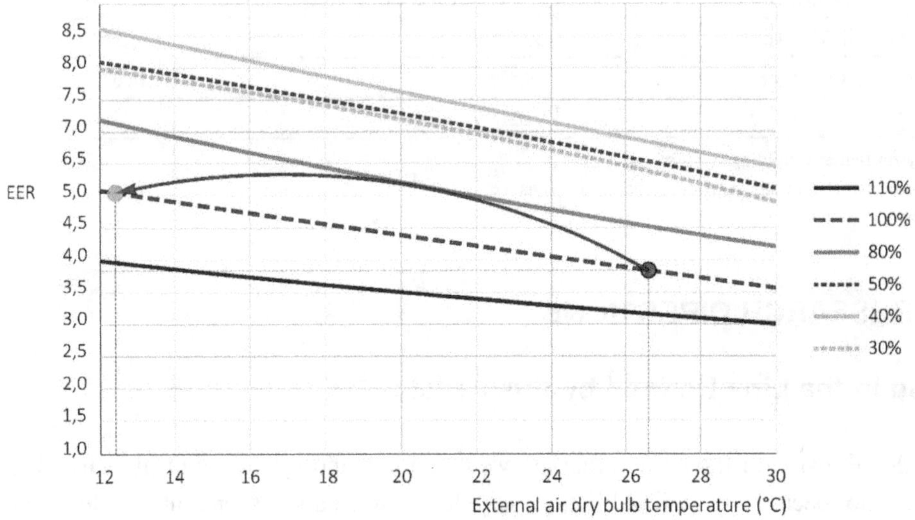

- **Heating Mode**: For the example locality shown in the section, in the month of January, with an average outdoor air temperature of -4.3 ° C, and the chamber air was taken at 10.9 ° C, the COP corresponding to a 100% load for an inverter system would go from 2.8 to 3.75, which represents a 34% improvement in efficiency.

Figure 15. COP of an inverter type refrigeration machine, operating as a heat pump, depending on the outside dry temperature (° C) and the load (%). Redrawn from (IDAE, 2008)

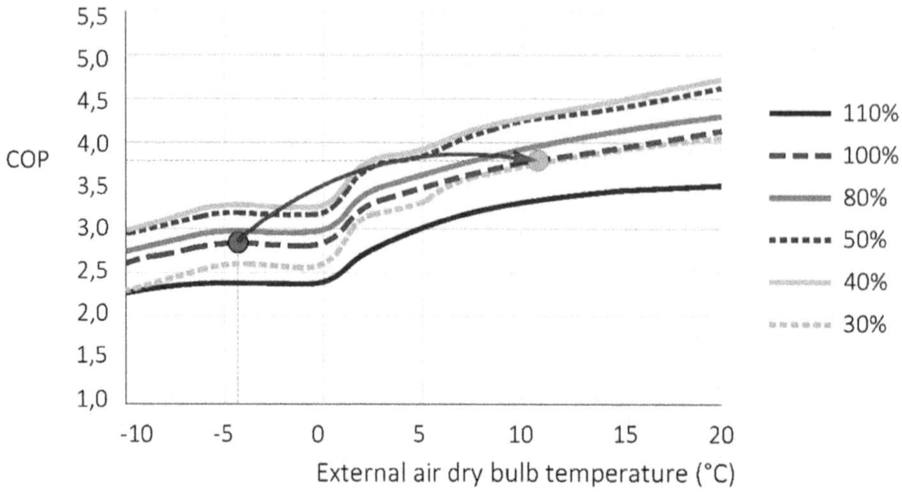

The following chart details the achievable heating savings for a high-efficiency building by adding APTAE.

Table 2.

Comparison:	NZEB with Aerothermal HP	+ APTAE	saving
Heating consumption (kWh / year)	37.588	28.917	↓30,0%
Heating emissions (kg CO_2 / year)	19.583	14.622	↓33,9%
Heating cost (€ / year)	9.021	6.736	↓33,9%

NZEB: Nearly zero-energy buildings (energy rating A)
APTAE: Aerothermal heat pump with pre-tempered air exchange
HP: Heat Pump

FUTURE RESEARCH DIRECTIONS

Deepening in the Line Defined by this Article

To allow a global vision of the system that allows its understanding, the multiple variables of thermal exchange have not been developed. Although they do not have a transcendental influence, all of them can be optimized by comparing the energy savings obtained with the necessary investment. Among these variables, those of greatest interest would be those related to the ground-air interface:

1. The movement of air through a granular matrix.
2. The effect of the different finishes that can be given to the terrain at no additional cost, such as the alternation of trenches or, on a smaller scale, the notches in the teeth of a backhoe, and their influence on heat exchange

Complementary and Combinable Topics to this Article

- **Combination with Passive Extraction Systems:** As the need for air filtration for heat pumps is much lower than that required for fresh air and is reduced to prevent the entry of animals or insects, the pressure drops of these grilles are compatible with under-pressure that it can be achieved through passive systems, such as solar chimneys or wind extraction systems. All of them result in an additional initial investment, but also in a reduction in electricity demand to be considered by those buildings that aspire to passive operation.
- **Combination with Solar Preheating:** As previously noted, the system is compatible with solar preheating with parietodynamic walls, attached greenhouses, allowing higher performance in cold seasons, as well as inertial systems using phase change materials for any time of the year. The advantage of solar systems linked to the envelope is that they increase their capture capacity in proportion to their size, solving the aforementioned shortage for buildings with high demand in proportion to their floor, as occurs in high-rise buildings.
- **Combination with Evaporative Cooling:** In climates with hot and dry seasons, such as the interior of the Iberian Peninsula, or the southwestern United States, the demand for refrigeration may be such that the described system may not reach the necessary power. In this situation, the incorporation of evaporative cooling systems is compatible.

The commercialized systems are associated with a low carbon footprint by extracting the energy from the change of state of the water and their electricity consumption is fundamentally reduced to that necessary to circulate the air (IDAE, 2007).

One of the advantages of evaporative cooling of the air for its exchange with a heat pump is the elimination of the risk of infection by Legionella pneumophila for people.

As described in this article for the tempering of air in vernacular architecture, there is an important research niche in the application of systems used by traditional architecture, either for cooling living spaces or water (Fathy, 1986). With the added advantage that these systems involve a lower risk of being vectors of contagion of the infection by not producing droplets known as aerosols. The resurgence of these traditional systems, combined with heat pumps, would allow the use of non-potable water, so that this use of water as a "fuel" for large-scale cooling does not lead to a shortage in the supply of drinking water.

The alteration of subsoil isotherms by earth-cooling would fall into the same category. This technique consists of watering the land during the hot season to obtain evaporative cooling (Givoni, 1994 and 1998) If repeated for a long time, it would alter the lower layers, being necessary to establish a new formulation to determine the temperature of the subsoil and thus calculate the ground-air heat exchange.

CONCLUSION

The use of tempered air, reusing the extraction air, or through the subsoil, through the sanitary chamber or set of buried ducts, for energy exchange reduces the thermal gradient that the heat pump must carry out and as well as the fall performance associated with defrosting, which leads to a higher performance coefficient and lower electricity consumption. The improvements evaluated in the case study (inverter type machines at 100% load) are between 30 and 34%.

The system baptized as APTAE (aerothermal pre-tempered air exchange), favours the ventilation of the subsoil under the building, reducing the possibility that radon emanations can leak into inhabited areas. It is indicated in low-rise buildings in which there is a sufficient proportion between heat exchange surface with the ground and energy demand. For taller buildings, it could be supplemented with Canadian wells, or accumulator beds (gravel, MCF spheres, etc.). Leaving aside the elimination of radon in the lower floors, it could be connected to the expulsion of the renewal air, and for prevailing heating demands, it could be combined with a preheating by means of parietodynamic walls, attached greenhouses or the like.

REFERENCES

C40 Cities. (2018). *19 Global Cities Commit to Make New Buildings "Net-Zero Carbon" by 2030.* https://www.c40.org/press_releases/global-cities-commit-to-make-new-buildings-net-zero-carbon-by-2030

ADEME. (2018). *Updated Energy-climate Scenario 2035-2050.* ADEME. https://www.ademe.fr/sites/default/files/assets/documents/energy-climate-scenario-ademe-2035-2050-010603.pdf

Balvers, J. R., Boxem, G., & de Wit, M. H. (2008). Indoor air quality in low-energy houses in the Netherlands, Does mechanical ventilation provide a healthy indoor Environment. Proceeding Indoor Air 2008.

Bordoloi, N., Sharma, A., Nautiyal, H., & Goel, V. (2018). An intense review on the latest advancements of Earth Air Heat Exchangers. *Renewable & Sustainable Energy Reviews*, *89*, 261–280. doi:10.1016/j.rser.2018.03.056

Cavallo, A., Gatsby, K., & Reddy, T. (1991). Natural basement ventilation as a radon mitigation technique. *Proceedings of the 1991 International Symposium on Radon and Radon Reduction Technology, US Environmental Protection Agency*, *2*, 1-24.

Cazzaniga, A., Furlanetto, L., & Molon, D. (1981). *Il Sistema di Raffrescamento Naturale delle Ville di Costozza* (Master's Thesis). Tesi di Laurea, Dipartimento di Architettura, Istituto Universitario di Architettura di Venezia, Venezia, Italy.

CTE-DB HE-0. (2019). *Limitación del consumo energético.* Código técnico de la edificación. Ministerio de Transportes, Movilidad y Agenda Urbana, Gobierno de España.

CTE-DB HS-6. (2019). *Protección frente a la exposición al radón.* Código técnico de la edificación. Ministerio de Transportes, Movilidad y Agenda Urbana, Gobierno de España.

Darby, S., Hill, D., Deo, H., Auvinen, A., Barros-Dios, J.M., Baysson, H., Bochicchio, F., Falk, R., Farchi, S., Figueiras, A., Hakama, M., Heid, I., Hunter, N., Kreienbrock, L., Kreuzer, M., Lagarde, F., Mäkeläinen, I., Muirhead, C., Oberaigner, W., Pershagen, G., Ruosteenoja, E., & Schaffrath, A., Rosario, Tirmarche, M., Tomásek, L., Whitley, E., Wichmann, H-E., & Doll, R. (2006). Residential radon and lung cancer: Detailed results of a collaborative analysis of individual data on 7148 subjects with lung cancer and 14208 subjects without lung cancer from 13 epidemiologic studies in Europe. *Scandinavian Journal of Work, Environment & Health*, *32*(Suppl 1), 1–83. PMID:16538937

De Paepe, M., & Janssens, A. (2003). Thermo-hydraulic design of earth-air heat exchangers. *Energy and Building*, *35*(4), 389–397. doi:10.1016/S0378-7788(02)00113-5

Espíndola, C., & Valderrama, J. O. (2012). Carbon Footprint. Part 1: Concepts, Estimation Methods and Methodological Complexities. *Información Tecnológica*, *23*(1), 163–176. doi:10.4067/S0718-07642012000100017

Fathy, H. (1986). *Natural energy and vernacular architecture. Principles and examples with reference to hot arid climates*. UNU.

Ferrucci, M., & Peron, F. (2018). Ancient Use of Natural Geothermal Resources: Analysis of Natural Cooling of 16th Century Villas in Costozza (Italy) as a Reference for Modern Buildings. *Sustainability*, *10*(12), 4340. doi:10.3390u10124340

Florides, G. A., Tassou, S. A., Kalogirou, S. A., & Wrobel, L. C. (2002). Review of solar and low energy cooling technologies for buildings. *Renewable & Sustainable Energy Reviews*, *6*(6), 557–572. doi:10.1016/S1364-0321(02)00016-3

Givoni, B. (1994). *Passive low energy Cooling of Buildings*. John Wiley & Sons, Inc.

Givoni, B. (1998). *Climate Considerations in Building and Urban Design*. John Wiley & Sons, Inc.

IDAE (Instituto para la Diversificación y Ahorro de la Energía). (2008). Procedimientos para la determinación del rendimiento energético de plantas enfriadoras y equipos autónomos de tratamiento de aire. Instituto para la Diversificación y Ahorro de la Energía.

IDAE (Instituto para la Diversificación y Ahorro de la Energía). (2007). Guía técnica, Torres de refrigeración. Ahorro y eficiencia energética en Climatización. MITC.

International Energy Agency and the United Nations Environment Programme. (2018). *Global Status Report: Towards a zero-emission, efficient and resilient buildings and construction sector.* Author.

ISN (Instituto de Seguridad Nuclear). (2021, February). *Mapa del potencial de radón de España.* https://www.arcgis.com/apps/SimpleViewer/index.html?appid=a3a435cfb6114e21ad03a5ac2961d8a8

Kaushal, M. (2017). Geothermal cooling/heating using ground heat exchanger for various experimental and analytical studies. Comprehensive review. *Energy and Building*, *139*, 634–652. doi:10.1016/j.enbuild.2017.01.024

Kenda, B. (2006). Pneumatology in Architecture: The Ideal Villa. Proceedings of Healthy Buildings in Lissabon.

Kim, D. (2006). The natural environment control system of korean traditional architecture: Comparison with korean contemporary architecture. *Building and Environment*, *41*(12), 1905–1912. doi:10.1016/j.buildenv.2005.07.007

Kusuda, T., & Achenbach, P. H. (1965). Earth temperature and thermal diffusivity at selected stations in the United States. U.S. Department of Commerce. National Bureau of Standards, NBS doi:10.21236/AD0472916

Neila, F. J. (2004). *Arquitectura Bioclimática en un entorno sostenible*. Munilla-Leira.

Oetelaar, T., Johnston, C., Wood, D., Hughes, L., & Humphrey, J. (2013). A computational investigation of a room heated by subcutaneous convection – A case study of a replica Roman bath. *Energy and Building*, *63*, 59–66.

Panizzoni, L. (2001). La Villa che Respira. Technical Report. Istituto Regionale delle Ville Venete.

Peretti, C., Zarrella, A., Carli, M. D., & Zecchin, R. (2013). The design and environmental evaluation of earth-to-air heat exchangers (EAHE). A literature review. *Renewable & Sustainable Energy Reviews*, *28*, 107–116. doi:10.1016/j.rser.2013.07.057

Sansone, C. (1999). Traditional Bio-Climate Building Techniques. *Proceedings Sharing Knowledge on Sustainable Buildings, Mediterranean Conference.*

Soltani, M., Kashkooli, F., Sanij, A. D., Kazemi, A., Bordbar, N., Farschini, M., Elmi, M., Gharali, K., & Dusseault, M. (2018). A comprehensive study of geothermal heating and cooling systems. *Sustainable Cities and Society.*

Wachenfeldt, B.J., & Bell, D. (2003). *Building Integrated Energy Systems in Smart Energy Efficient Buildings – A State-of-the-art.* SINTEL Project report, STF22 A04503.

WHO. (2021). *More countries act against exposure to radon and associated cancer risks*. https://www.who.int/news/item/04-02-2021-more-countries-act-against-exposure-to-radon-and-associated-cancer-risks

Zeiler, W., & Boxem, G. (2009). Geothermal Active Building Concept. In R. J. Howlett, L. C. Jain, & S. H. Lee (Eds.), *Sustainability in Energy and Buildings*. Springer. doi:10.1007/978-3-642-03454-1_32

KEY TERMS AND DEFINITIONS

Aerothermal Heat Pump: The heat pump is a thermal machine capable of pumping heat from a cold source to a hot one. In the case of aerothermal heat pumps, they extract natural environment (air) through the evaporator and transfer it to the interior of a building through the condenser.

APTAE System: Pre-tempered aerothermal air exchange system between the living space and the subsoil without mixing. This system benefits from taking advantage of the constant temperature that the ground has at shallow depth, while avoiding radon gas leaks inside, favouring its ventilation to the outside.

Carbon Footprint: The Carbon Footprint, defined in a very general way, represents the amount of greenhouse gases (GHG) emitted into the atmosphere derived from the activities of production or consumption of goods and services, and is considered one of the most important tools to quantify the emissions of these gases. GHGs, defined in the Kyoto protocol in 1997, form a permanent layer in the middle part of the atmosphere that prevents all solar radiation that is returned by the earth from leaving, thereby causing the temperature under the layer to increase (Espíndola & Valderrama, 2012).

Parietodynamic Wall: Enclosure that takes advantage of solar energy to preheat the external ventilation air. Generally, it is made up of a factory inner sheet, an air chamber and a glazed or metallic outer sheet that absorbs solar radiation. Air circulation can be natural (thermosyphon) or forced (CTE-DB-HE0, 2019).

Passive Air Conditioning System: Passive air conditioning systems take advantage of the building's constituent elements such as windows, walls, or floors to obtain thermal energy and use it to heat or cool the building. The general objective of these design strategies is to take advantage of the climatic conditions to minimize the use of active air conditioning systems and thus reduce energy consumption and CO_2 emissions.

Chapter 9
Health and Well-Being:
Considerations in the Design of Indoor Environments for the Elderly

Nerea García Cortés
Universidad de Sevilla, Spain

Samuel Dominguez-Amarillo
https://orcid.org/0000-0002-9177-8736
Universidad de Sevilla, Spain

Jesica Fernandez-Agüera
Universidad de Sevilla, Spain

ABSTRACT

The older segments of the adult population in cities experience problems conditioned by the climate of each place. Since the 2003 heat wave which caused 70,000 heat deaths, the dramatic consequences of climate change and rising temperatures in Europe have led to the elderly being most at risk. Insufficient adaptability and economic resources among them also lead to repercussions on architecture, causing energy poverty issues as a result of a real consumption needed which is very different from the actual consumption. The demands of these people are determined by environmental stress, which differ greatly throughout the year. In addition, illnesses influence the daily health and the decrease in sensory capacity of the elderly, making them more vulnerable to constant changes. Faced with this problem, the main aim of this research is to analyse the degree of comfort and well-being of the elderly due to the environmental changes that occur in Andalusian rural homes in order to include some considerations in the design of indoor environments.

DOI: 10.4018/978-1-7998-7279-5.ch009

INTRODUCTION

Today's society is subject to constant transformation, altering its way of life and its way of thinking about architecture and the spaces which make it up. Currently, anywhere in the world changes are always promoted by self-interest, something which can be manipulated and directed by society. Although nature cannot be directed by the action of humans, it is influenced by their actions. Climate change continues to be one of the main axes influencing our lives, a process which cannot be modified by humans. Resilient architecture can be understood as the ability to recover from changes caused by environmental agents.

In parallel, another concept that will determine how architecture is thought about is the way in which users understand life. The degree of comfort of an individual will depend on the situation at a given point in time, their way of life, their customs, their needs, etc. It will always be personal and unique to each user.

Given the current population context in Europe, where an aging population has resulted in a significant inversion of the population pyramid, the study of this older sector of the population is of interest. At this stage in their lives, people have assimilated certain customs imposed by the culture in which they live, and certain aspects of how they use their home bring about a unique purpose in rural architecture (Figure 1).

Figure 1. Population pyramid of Spain
Source: Instituto Nacional de Estadística, Spain,2020

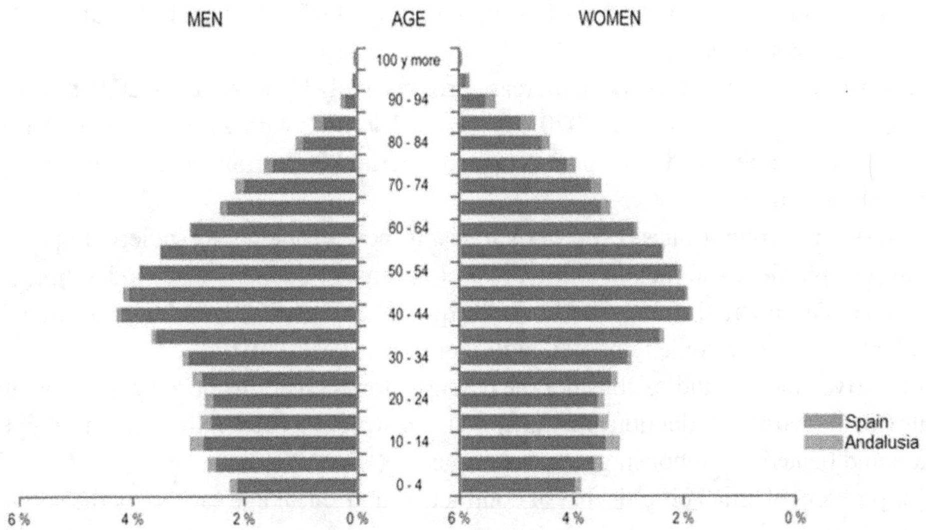

At present, the elderly make up a vital influential part of society in the development of a resilient architecture. The numerous energy poverty issues stemming from a lack of adaptability and economic resources in turn have a serious impact on the architecture. Demand is determined by environmental stress, with the situation changing drastically for them from one season to the next. In addition, the damage caused by disease to daily health and the reduced sensory capacity of the elderly makes them vulnerable to continuous change. At this stage, people are more fragile, with a more reduced adaptive capacity. A case study in Aznalcóllar, a town in Andalusia has been set up to study the comfort and well-being of users and their homes.

The main objective of this research is to analyse the degree of comfort and well-being of the elderly due to the environmental changes that occur in rural homes.

This case study aims to answer two main questions:

- Does rural architecture have the sufficient capacity to act as a climatic shelter for an aging population today?
- Will rural architecture adapt to climate change?

BACKGROUND

The conflicts and convergences that occur between climate change and the aging of society is a current reality, one to be experienced for many years. People's age and required energy demand are directly linked. The current aging population is also affected by falling fertility and mortality. This is expected to have an impact on global health and financial stability, while also constituting a greater burden on the environment. (Harper, 2006).

The city of the future will be affected by a rise in temperatures and a higher concentration of older people. Flexibility proposals are made for the city, including sustainable infrastructure and changes to urban environments. The constant increase in temperature expected until 2100 and changes in precipitation patterns have prompted consideration of an architecture which can adapt to its surroundings, where homes can act as climatic shelters

In the Mediterranean temperatures will increase progressively by + 2/4 ºC. In 2035 they will increase between + 4/6ºC; in 2050 by + 8ºC; in 2070 between + 10/12ºC; with an increase of around 15ºC expected in 2100. On the other hand, precipitation change in the Mediterranean is expected to fall by 0.05 to 0.10 metres (Peek, 2016).

This will result in drought phases for years, causing new problems to society. Population ageing causes a change in physical and mental ability, reducing sensory capacity and moderating decreases in temperature and environmental stress. Another consequence expected is that of migrations, which empty the industrial city and create some temporal agglomerations (Peek, 2016).

The constructive systems studies consider the potential for adaptation and easy functionality of housing materials (manufacture, production and transport), construction (depending on house type and user), and operation and behaviour of housing to suit user needs (Hirst, 2013).

The major problem of small cities is that of contraction and shrinkage caused by the suburbanization and deindustrialization processes, although there are also issues stemming from modern lifestyles and globalization. The strategies studied focus on a viable search for urban regeneration to be implemented in each of the city typologies which have led to the loss of population (Panagopoulos et al., 2013).

The scope of research in the older sectors of society is guided by their resilience in light of the global situation, especially as this group is considered to be the most vulnerable. The possibility or impossibility of adaptation might be questioned when establishing an approach to architecture and in order to understand the present and future situation. These problems are dynamic and in constant change but the focus should remain mostly on the individuals and their comfort conditions.

Comfort can be understood in different ways, always with the user as the focus, and with certain influential aspects linked to satisfaction and convenience. Each individual can define their level of comfort, which can lead to a variety of situations, depending on place, time of year, characteristics of the building, the building loads or user age (Roaf et al., 2013, 2015; Roberts & Henwood, 2019; Wells et al., 2015). Climate, housing typology and construction house, and temporary situation are also included. The seasonal guides characterize each place, as detailed by (Ministerio de Fomento del Gobierno de España, 2017).

The adaptation or resilient inability of the current housing system is due to user instability. Housing should answer user needs and offer protection from external change, improving their health. The economic resources of these people depend on the general population. However, the fact that energy poverty continues to exist among the elderly in society should be a widespread concern (Jenkins, 2010; Sanchez-Guevara et al., 2019; Santamouris et al., 2013; Wilkinson et al., 2007).

It is necessary to discuss between the terms capacity of adaptation and resilience in the houses to satisfy the user:

1. Ability to adapt, can occur in the long or short term, and the objective should be to increase the power of adaptation in the face of any adversity.
2. Resilience,
    - It is the ability of a living being to adapt to a disturbing agent or an adverse state of affairs.
    - Capacity of a material, mechanism or system to recover its initial state when the disturbance to which it had been subjected has ceased.

In this case, the objective is to strengthen this capacity and give the dwellings diversity, self-organization, self-sufficiency and learning capacity, always complementary to the needs, attitudes and behaviors of the users.

Susan Roaf, stablished a three-step diagram in the Workshop held at the School of Architecture of Seville about design (Roaf, 2018):

1. Base Note. Architectural elements of the building that cannot be modified.
2. Heart Note. Adaptive opportunities.
3. Top Note. All about the mind: Sensations, feelings, Perceptions, Impressions…

Susan Roaf proposes guidelines for a comfortable home:

1. Make it run thermally safe.
2. Integrate adaptability opportunities.
3. Design for thermal pleasure including "Top Notes".

This study gives the guidelines that will guide the investigation and the possibility of understanding a society with some problems. In addition to a possibility of proposal before a field of social housing formed by an elderly society.

OBJECTIVE

Today, housing stock does not respond in the same way it did in the past or what is expected to happen in the future. Equally, in housing in southern Europe, there is no correlation between energy demand

and the real use of energy due to the energy poverty (Domínguez-Amarillo, Fernández-Agüera, Sendra, et al., 2019; Domínguez Amarillo, 2015).

A rejection of comfort and living in conditions of energy poverty lead to an individual's behaviour and attitude towards housing and (active and passive) systems. This creates insecurity among users, who feel this will disrupt their comfort state, creating a problem which will become permanent in their life. (Domínguez-Amarillo et al., 2018; Domínguez-Amarillo, Fernández-Agüera, Peacock, et al., 2019; Roaf et al., 2013).

In order to truly understand the degree of comfort that a person may or may not feel, user patterns that include technical and social aspects should be studied. It is also necessary to collect quantitative data about housing.

Some publications compile essential aspects to respond to the treatment of all the parameters of interest in this research (Fernández-Agüera et al., 2019). Indoor comfort and environmental quality in housing are studied from a holistic perspective, including aspects such as in situ environmental measurements, energy consumption measurements and user patterns. The difficulty of responding to the needs of elderly people today may pose a problem in the future if there is an inability to cope with a climate change. In a few years, elderly population will increase and people over 65 will account for 22% of the world's population (2050) (Organización Mundial de la Salud, 2015).

In this case, the exposure and vulnerability of ageing populations should be addressed, considering their seasonal health and resilience (Haq, 2016). Concern for these generations has led to careful examination of their current way of life, the construction and current operation of their housing, and how it can be adapted for the future. This architecture must be designed for users who are changing over time and who require very different resources depending on their stage in life.

CASE STUDY

This research includes a case study of housing in the town of Aznalcóllar in Seville.

Interest in this case study is prompted by the population's unique nature and lifestyle. The town is inhabited by working class people who have practically devoted their entire lives to industry (working in the mines of Aznalcóllar). Those who worked in this sector were used to working in all climatic conditions, from extreme temperatures to intense rains. In this region, the unique nature and features of housing as climate refuge makes it an attraction. Most of the local dwellings are over 30 years old, and made up of many rooms and a large central space, usually occupied by large traditional working class families. The construction of housing using local materials that are easy to treat and obtain is commonplace in these areas.

Residential built stock is analysed and characterized based on a classification of the constructive elements and morphological aspects of thermal envelopes. These areas should respond to several hypotheses defined by the time period:

- Hypothesis 1: Climate action (current and future). These changes are constantly taking place and require a constructive adaptation capacity of the current social housing.
- Hypothesis 2: Lifestyle (past, current and future). Society with customs and way of understanding well-being and life are very different at each stage. Elderly people have experienced certain

Figure 2. Factors that influence comfort and well-being in homes
Source: Author, 2020

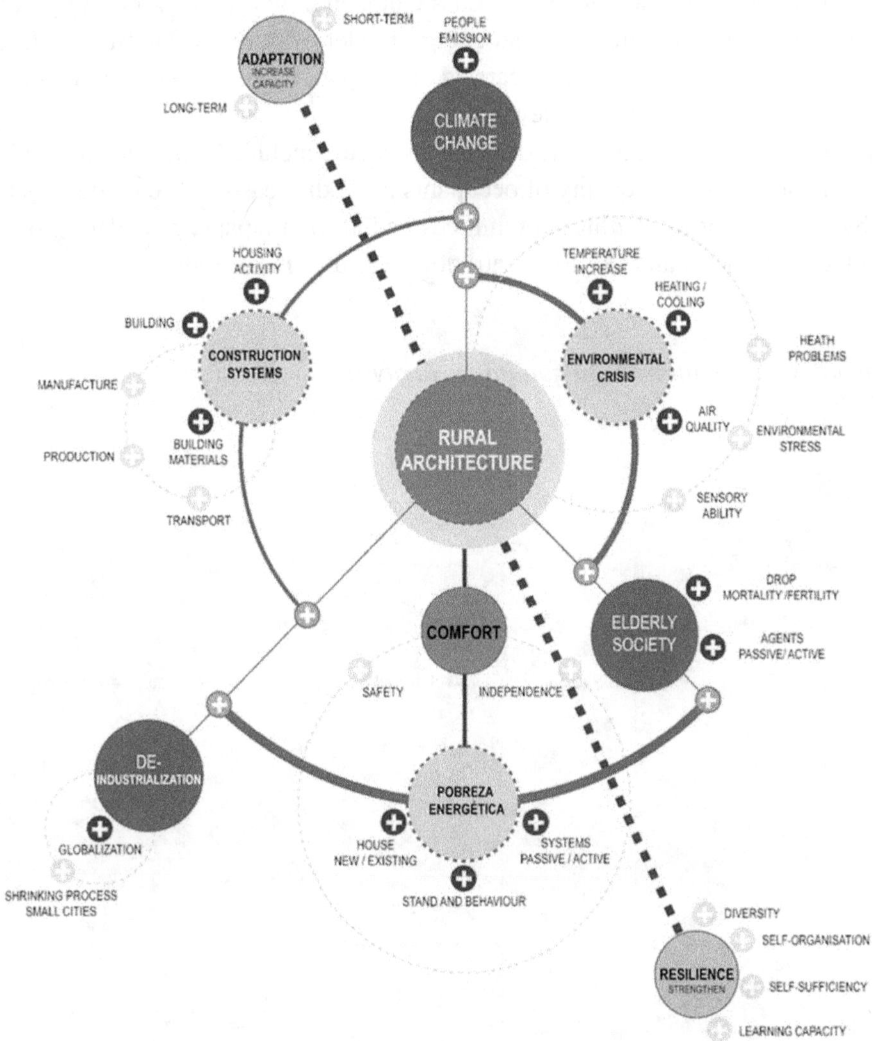

situations which have shaped their current housing, although it does not function in the same way today.

- Hypothesis 3: Location and characterization of social housing. Analysis of the usual thermal conditions in social housing and the capacities of the residential stock.

METHOD

The investigation methodology consists in the qualitative and quantitative study of dwellings, users and their needs. An initial overview was carried out on the housing: morphology, buildings and materials. Secondly, DesignBuilder was used to create an energy model to study evolution of indoor conditions within the dwelling. In parallel, surveys were carried out on patterns of use, behaviour and user comfort in order to analyse how these adjust to the level of comfort.

An in situ survey among residents of the dwellings selected included questions on habits of ventilation, comfort, symptoms and sleep quality of occupants in all the seasons throughout a year. The study was approved by the relevant local ethics committees and all participants provided informed consent. Temperature, relative humidity and CO_2 concentration were also measured.

Figure 3. Methodology: quantitative and qualitative analysis
Source: Author, 2020

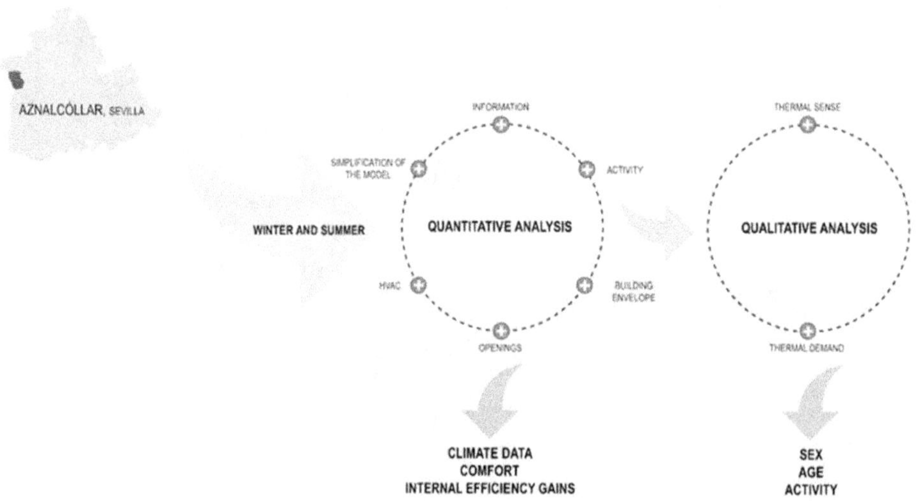

Location and Climate

The factors "location and climate" of an element is the first characteristic factor that is thought for a retrofitting, project or any activity. The Mediterranean climate is characterized by two very distinct seasons: mild rainy winters and warm dry summers. There is an intermediate variable period, between winter and summer, depending on the year. In these areas, for the most part the temperature does not display major changes.

The focus of this investigation, the town of Aznalcóllar, is located to the north-west of Seville (Figure 4). Aznalcóllar and its surrounding areas are characterized by an extensive area with a complex topography bordering the Sierra Norte mountain range.

- Surface area (2015): 199.20 m^2.

Figure 4. Location
Source: Author, 2021

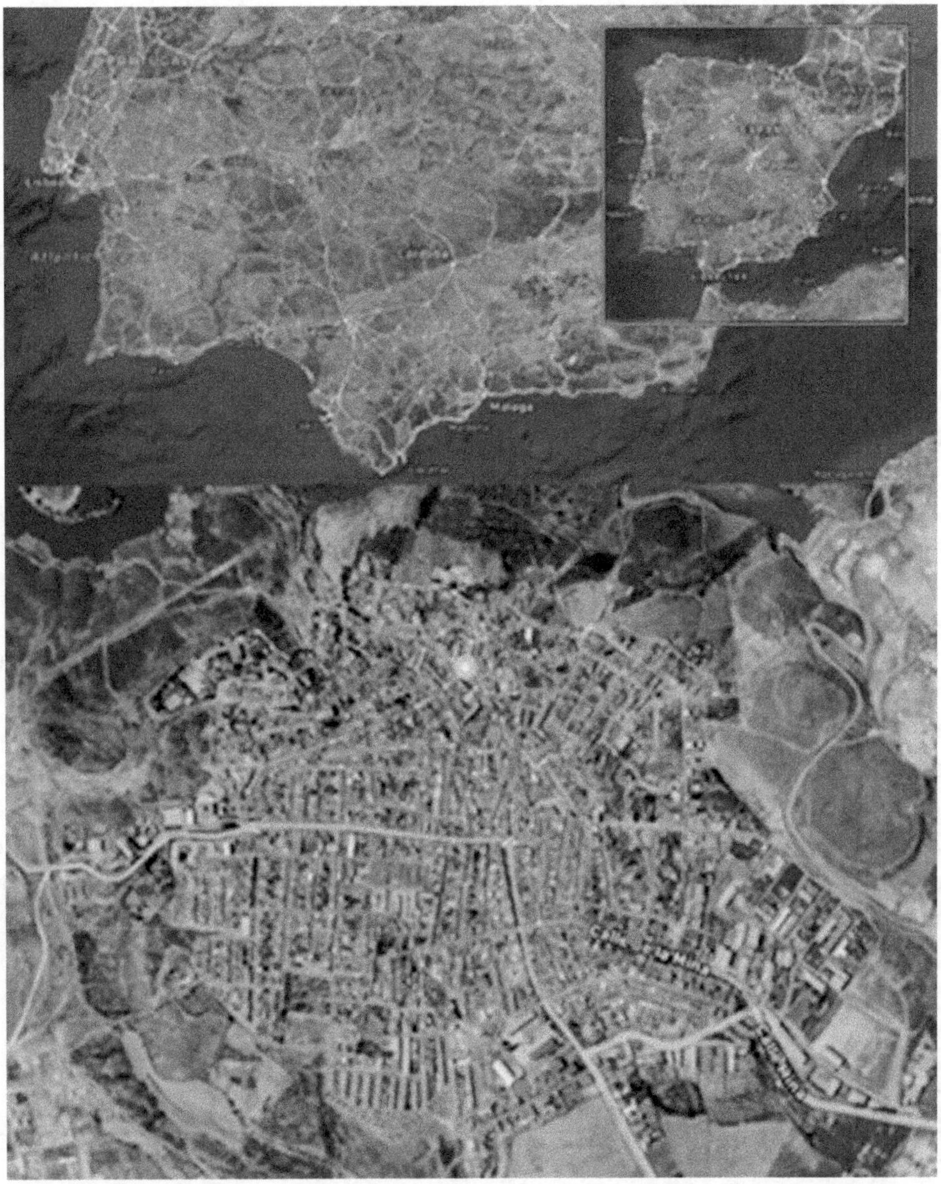

- Perimeter (2015): 68,420.10 m^2.
- Elevation above sea level (2015): 136 m.

Population.

- Total population (2017): 6,116 inhab. (51.2% male; 48.8% female).
- Population under 20 years old (2017): 1,354 inhab. (22.14%).
- Population over 65 years old (2017): 918 inhab. (15.01%).

Definition and Identification of the Target Population

Mining was traditionally the main industry in Aznalcóllar while still in production, along with agriculture and livestock farming. Throughout history these trades have shaped the local lifestyle throughout history, leaving their mark on the lives of local inhabitants. This has also conditioned the forms of construction and design used. Dwellings were for large working-class families and were often self-built following an unregulated "do-it-yourself" philosophy.

Among the population of Aznalcóllar there are families in which the man has generally spent his entire working life devoted to the mining industry, from a very young age until the collapse of the sector. As a result of this, different circumstances are encountered: the homes of many elderly people who always worked at the mine remain unchanged; middle-aged people who worked in the mine for part of their lives aim to improve their dwelling and quality of life; and a smaller number of young people and children, who have been educated in today's society.

Although research is limited to elderly users, it is necessary to acknowledge the rest of the population in order to have a broad visual field for the future. The elderly population is the main focus of this study. It is a large group compared to the rest of the population and it encounters certain difficulties in adapting to today's society. Their lifestyle is adjusted to a minimum, which plays a part in the energy poverty situation due to the inefficiency of their homes and exclusion in modern life.

The users of these case studies are:

Case study 1. Family made up of: 54-year-old male (1); 52-year-old female (2); 23-year-old female (3); 19-year-old male (4); 16-year-old male (5).

These users display an ease in adapting to any sort of circumstance. The dwelling is set up for a future situation in which adults 1 and 2 will have different requirements.

Case study 2. Family made up of: 83-year-old male (1); 78-year-old male (2).

These users are accustomed to living in this house, and making any modifications or additions to the house would require some effort. Users 1 and 2 are accustomed to living a life with the benefits which this housing has provided since living in it.

Table 1. Summary table of study samples

Sample 1: V01- A	Sample 12: S04- D
Sample 2: V01- B	Sample 13: S06- A
Sample 3: V01- C	Sample 14: S07- A
Sample 4: V01- D	Sample 15: S07- B
Sample 5: S03- A	Sample 16: S08- A
Sample 6: S04- A	Sample 17: S08- B
Sample 7: S05- A	Sample 18: S08- C
Sample 8: S05- B	Sample 19: S09- A
Sample 9: V02- A	Sample 20: S09- B
Sample 10: S04- B	Sample 21: V02- B
Sample 11: S04- C	

Source: Author, 2020

Analysis carried out provides general data on the population in which the research is located and twenty-one samples were taken in nine different houses.

Table 1 shows the sample number and table 2 the characterization of the sample.

Sample Definition

Two representative houses were sampled. The occupants had to agree to the surveys of individual dwellings and the surveys also required residents' collaboration. The characterization of each individual dwelling and the profiles of samples studied are shown in Table 2 (grey), while the case studies are in Figures 2 and 3. As none of these dwellings has ventilation systems, air renewal depends on the manual opening of windows by the users.

A progressive timeline will help to understand both the needs and benefits, as well as the operation, construction and way of thinking about architecture. A distinction must be made between:

Table 2. Characterization samples in Aznalcóllar

Samples	Code	Type of dwelling	Construction year	Retrofitting	Age	Sex	Nº of users	Outdoor activity
1	V01- A	Single-family housing	2017	-	49	F	5	No
2	V01- B		2017	-	53	M	5	Yes
3	V01- C		2017	-	16	M	5	No
4	V01- D		2017	-	19	M	5	No
5	S03- A		1988	Yes	26	M	3	No
6	S04- A		1994	Yes	22	F	4	No
7	S05- A		1988	-	27	M	5	Yes
8	S05- B		1988	-	51	F	5	No
9	V02- A		1900	Yes	78	F	2	Yes
10	S04- B		1994	Yes	51	M	4	Yes
11	S04- C		1994	Yes	50	F	4	Yes
12	S04- D		1994	Yes	27	M	4	Yes
13	S06- A		2008	-	31	F	5	Yes
14	S07- A		1975	-	65	M	2	Yes
15	S07- B		1975	-	65	F	2	Yes
16	S08- A		1990	Yes	23	F	4	No
17	S08- B		1990	Yes	54	M	4	Yes
18	S08- C		1990	Yes	54	F	4	No
19	S09- A		1998	Yes	42	M	4	Yes
20	S09- B		1998	Yes	45	F	4	Yes
21	V02- B		1900	Yes	83	M	2	Yes

Source: Author, 2020

1. Past period. Construction of the homes of the elderly today. Today's older people at this time had a very different adaptability and easy routine modification than today. In addition, their demand and consumption were conditioning variables of their life, very different from the present. It influences case 2 and may have left samples of customs in case 1.
2. Present period. Adults of the past are older people of the present (case 2), they are vulnerable to changes. And today's adults will be older people of the future (case 1), foresee future situations to increase an adaptation capacity and strengthen the individual's resilience capacity.
3. Future period. The elderly of the future will have the same requirements as the elderly of the present, but different conditions will be presented, which are the ones that must be taken into account when thinking about architecture.

The case studies analysed are:

- Case study 1 (Figure 5 and 7). The development chosen for the quantitative tests is located in a recently built area in Aznalcóllar. The dwelling was built in 2017, representative of traditional Mediterranean architecture for large family. The case study chosen has five users. The house had been kept up routinely, but not retrofitted and a split AC unit was used to cool and heat the living room.
- Case study 2 (Figure 6 and 7). The development chosen for the quantitative tests is located in the old town of Aznalcóllar. The dwelling, built in 1900, is representative of rural Mediterranean architecture with elderly users. The users in this case were an elderly couple. The house had undergone basic upkeep, with a retrofitting of external enclosures. It was fitted with two split AC units for cooling and heating, one in the bedroom and one in the living room.

Indoor Air Quality Measurements

The monitoring was carried out while the housing was occupied, so that the influence of inhabitants' behaviour on variations in the environmental parameters could be considered. For indoor temperature data, an infrared thermometer was used to measure the indoor ambient temperature and the temperature at different points in the room or space where the user is. These temperatures are recorded in ºC. A lux meter was used to obtain lighting data and the lux in the respondent's position. Outside conditions were obtained from AEMET, examining hours in Aznalcóllar. Table 3 shows the quantitative characterization of case studies.

Figures 8 and 9 show the users' positions and measuring points.

Occupant Behaviour and Perception

Personal surveys were drawn up for the qualitative analysis of the case studies and general population. A specific type of survey was created for each sample and individual user, who completed them personally.

The survey can be adapted to any person, and there are no previous requirements to prevent popular participation. While this research is specific to Aznalcóllar, where the case studies are located, it can be adapted to any other location. The surveys include questions about the previous winter but were completed during summer.

Figure 5. Case study 1
Source: Author, 2020

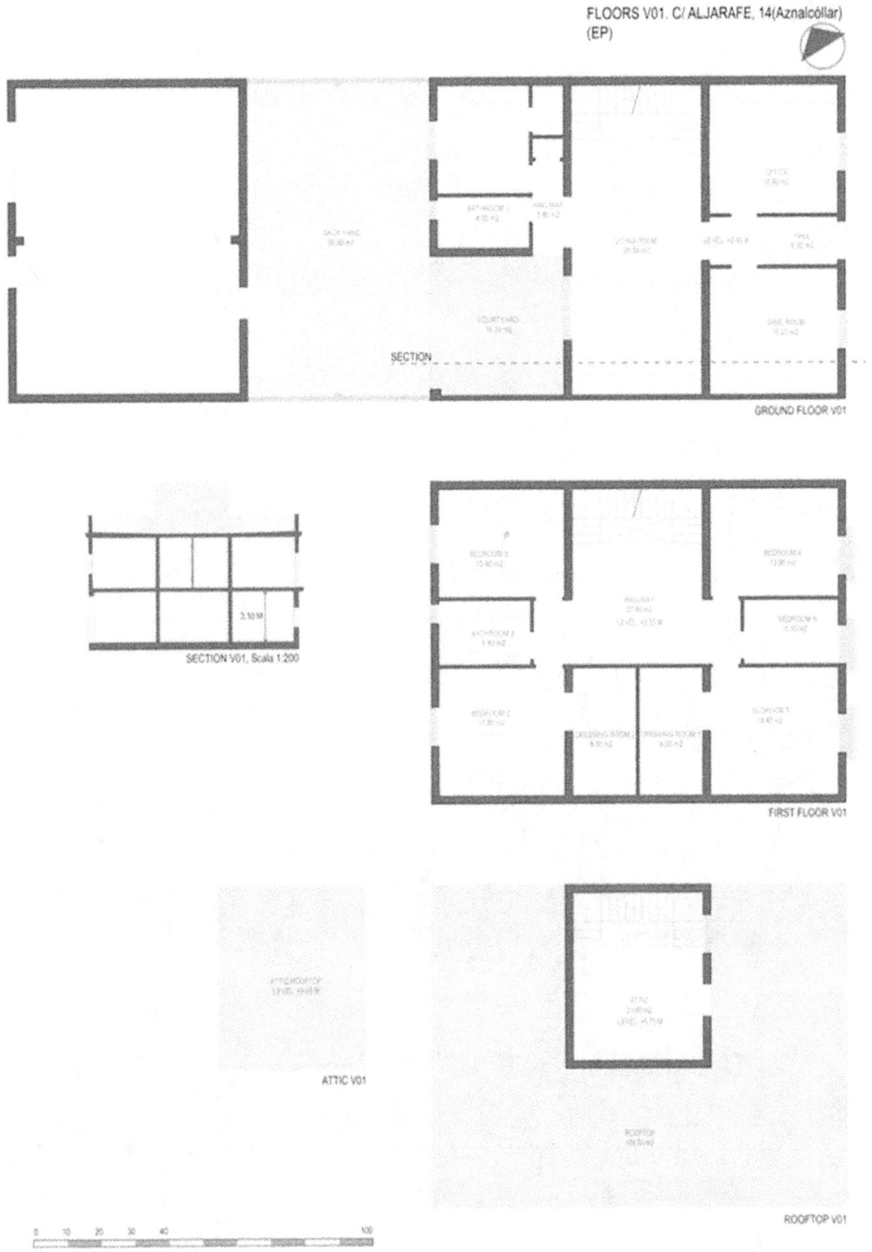

Data collection was carried out through individual, personal and anonymous surveys on paper. In this case, two parts could be distinguished, depending on whether the researcher or user collected the data:

Data provided by researcher, including variable or fixed data and determining or informative data:

- Initial data.
- General data, including: City or town; Survey date; Survey time.

- Dwelling data, including: Housing year of construction; Housing retrofitting and date; Housing typology and characterization; User position. This also includes indoor temperature, measuring points and illumination.

Figure 6. Case study 2
Source: Author, 2020

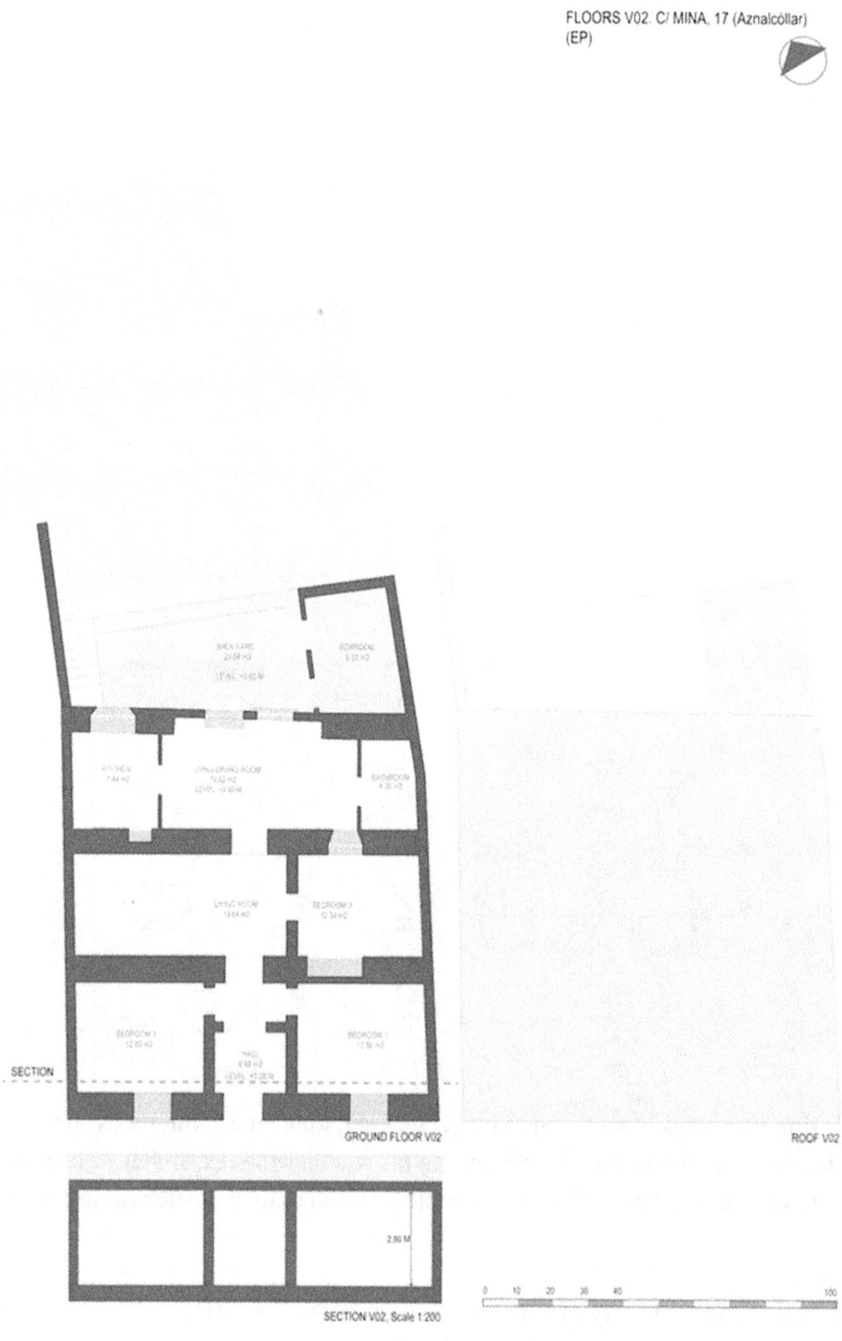

- Weather conditions, including: Outdoor temperature; Humidity; Other general information. The source must be included.
- Other data relevant to researcher, such as outdoor activity (or lack thereof) by the user during the day.

Data provided by users, provided answers on:

- Previous information data.
- Personal sensation.
- Personal demand.

Figure 7. Case studies
Source: Author, 2021

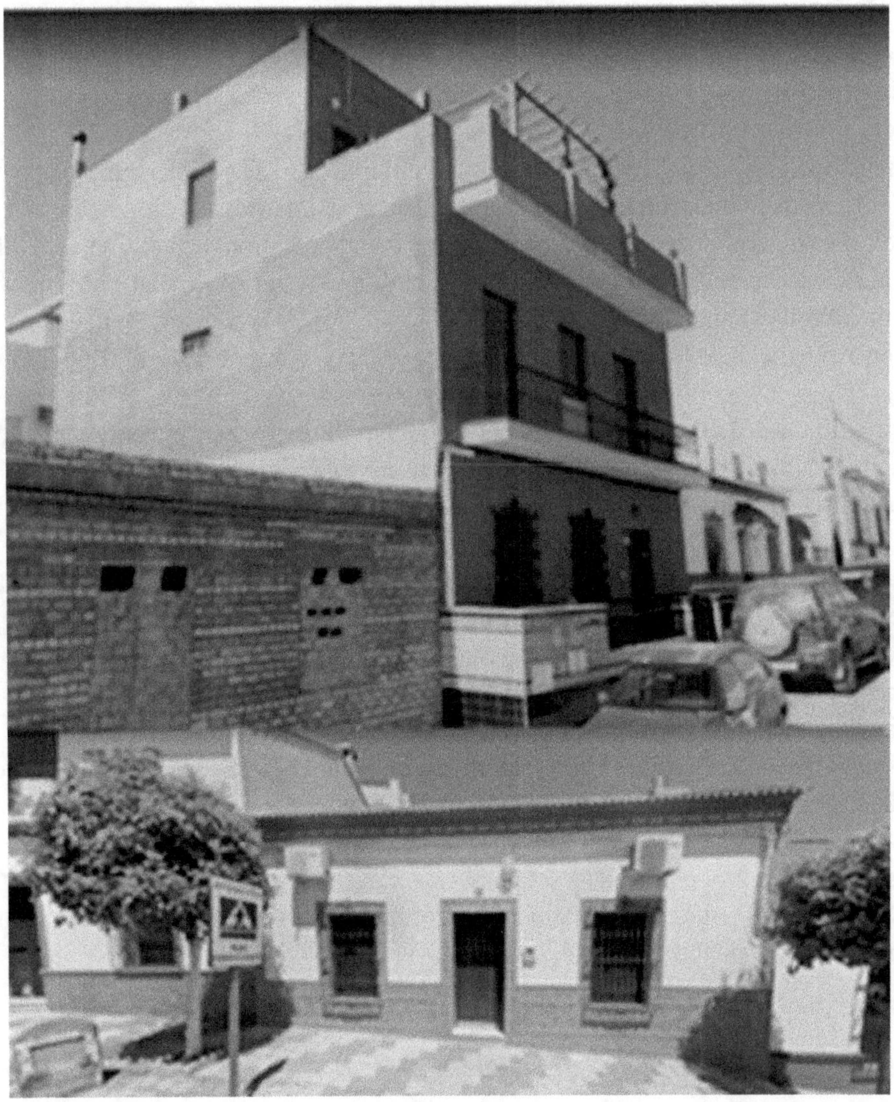

Table 3. Quantitative characterization of case studies

Samples	Code	Date	Time	Indoor temperature (°C)	Ilumination (lux)	Outdoor temperature (°C)	Mean relative humidity (%)
CASE STUDY 1							
1	V01- A	17/06/2018	18:30h.	26.7 °C	134.1 lux	36 °C	26%
2	V01- B	17/06/2018	18:30h.	26.7 °C	106.7 lux	36 °C	26%
3	V01- C	20/06/2018	19:15h.	27.3 °C	100.1 lux	31 °C	32%
4	V01- D	20/06/2018	19:15h.	27.3 °C	99.8 lux	31 °C	32%
CASE STUDY 2							
9	V02- A	21/06/2018	22:00h.	29.1 °C *(courtyard)*	-	24 °C	50%
21	V02- B	24/06/2018	22:00h.	27.9 °C *(courtyard)*	-	24 °C	61%

Source: Author, 2020

Energy Simulation

Virtual building models were generated from the study sample (selected through analysis of the housing stock) in order to recreate their fundamental characteristics: geometric, morphological and typological characteristics; construction systems; urban environment; and operational conditions. In order to assess the thermal performance and energy demand of the buildings, energy simulation tools were used to generate synthetic and dynamic models with sufficient accuracy, including urban boundary conditions.

Building energy simulation tool EnergyPlus and energy analysis package DesignBuilder were selected for this phase.

The construction and definition of the model of the buildings for subsequent simulation has been carried out under the methodology directives detailed in ANSI/ASHRAE/IES Standard 90.1-2013. Operational protocols were established based on Spanish official energy labelling procedures, which were subsequently adapted for a more realistic approach.

A calibration procedure contrasted with an actual model was developed to check the validity of the energy modelling of the buildings. The adjustment and calibration process was conducted in accordance with the specifications of ASHRAE 14-2002 (Ashrae, 2002).

The real people density has been established in each of the study cases and the usual timetable. There are 2 different situations: one in winter and other in summer.

Different clothing conditions have been established in summer (0.22 clo) and winter (1 clo).

The demand for hot water has been established at 281 / day per person.

There is an electric stove for heating. It was simulated like on or off.

There is a single split for cooling. The set point was 23°C.

Household internal gains have been established according to the actual operation of existing electronic equipment and kitchen appliances.

Figure 8. User position and measuring point, case study 1
Source: Author, 2020

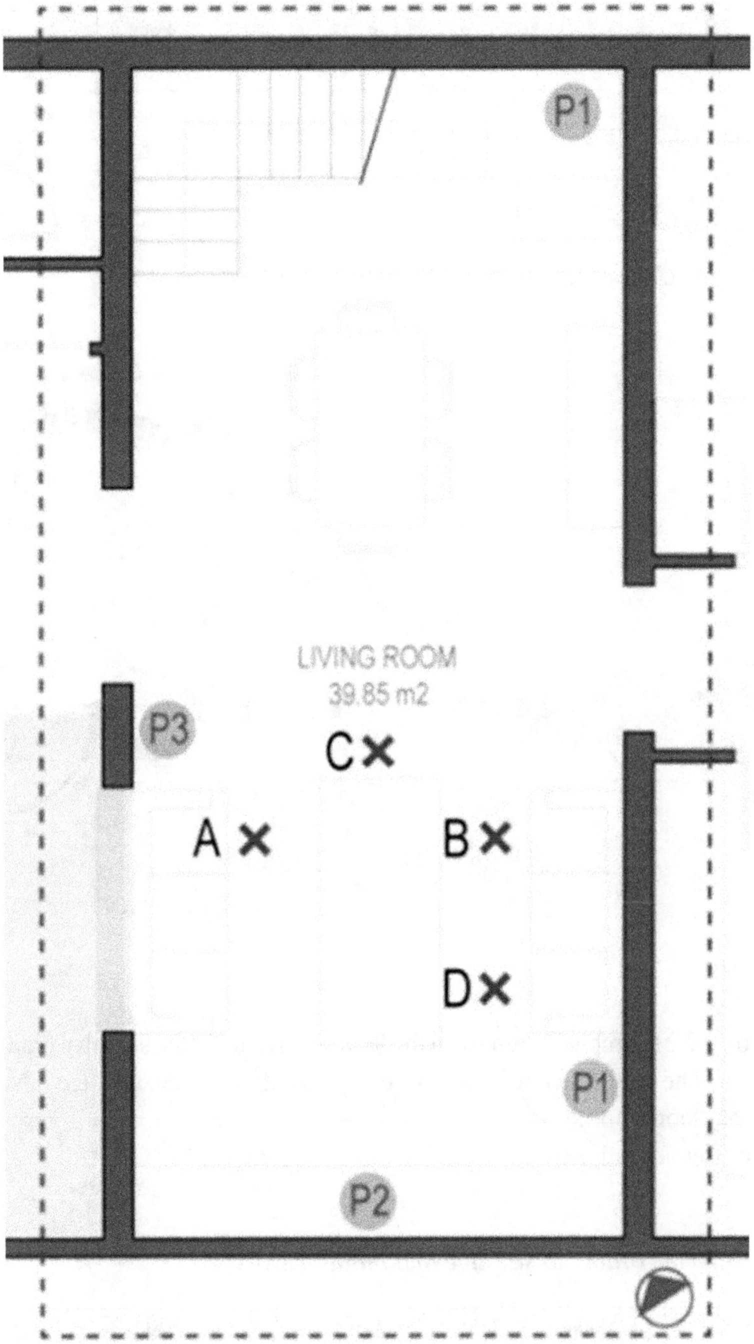

Table 4. Indoor temperature according to point, case study 1

Samples	Code	Indoor temperature (°C)	P1 (°C)	P2 (°C)	P3 (°C)	P4 (°C)
1	V01- A	26.7 °C	27.4 °C	27.9 °C	28.6 °C	26.5 °C
2	V01- B	26.7 °C	27.4 °C	27.9 °C	28.6 °C	26.5 °C
3	V01- C	27.3 °C	28.7 °C	29.3 °C	29.9 °C	27.8 °C
4	V01- D	27.3 °C	28.7 °C	29.3 °C	29.9 °C	27.8 °C

Source: Author, 2020

Figure 9. Users position, Case Study 2
Source: Author, 2020

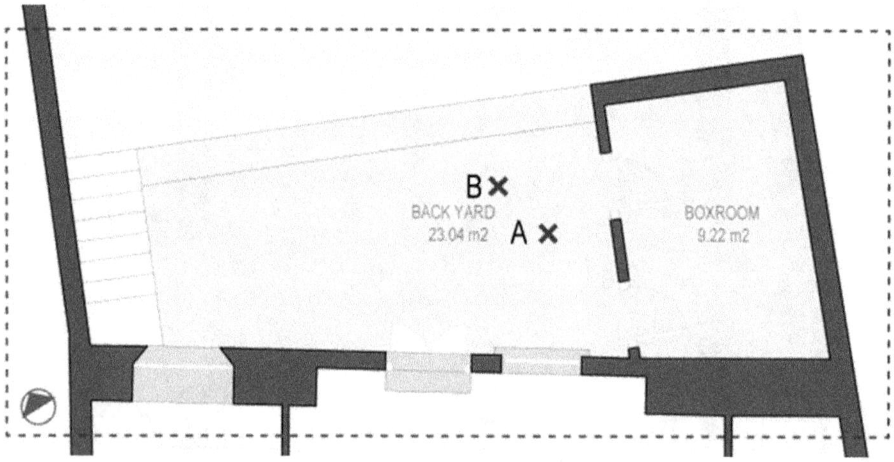

RESULTS

Qualitative Results

The results depend on the 21 samples taken from the 9 different study cases, with a data collection process carried out in summer. The qualitative results have been classified by sex and age of sample participants and whether or not outdoor work .

Results linked to user sensations.

Table 5. Data collection according to sex, age and outdoor work

SAMPLE DATA	Young	Adult	Elderly	Outdoor work
Male	2	6	2	8
Female	2	7	2	5

Source: Author, 2020

Analysis of issues relating to climate, weather and health in winter, by sex:

- *How did the winter climate of 2018 feel?*
- *How did the winter weather of 2018 feel?*
- *What has the predominant thermal sensation been in the dwelling during winter?*
- *How often did you experience health problems during winter 2018? What where these linked to?*

The overall population trend has been:

- Winter climate, 2018: Wet (45%, male; 40% female).
- Winter weather, 2018: Rainy (45%, male; 50% female).

Male participants felt winter 2018 with less intensity than female participants. These results are linked to the outdoor work of male participants. In contrast, female participants spend more time indoors. A range of health problems of between 45% (male) and 80% (female) has also been established.

Analysis of issues relating to thermal sensations and immediate needs, according to age:

- *What is your thermal sensation in this room right now?*
- *What thermal sensation would you like to have right now?*

Participants perceived a heat sensation as this research was carried out in summer.

Young and elderly participants reported a similar thermal sensation (75% warm) and needs (50% more cool). However, adult participants reported a normal sensation (48% normal) with no needs (48% well) at that specific moment. The results of adult participants are influenced by outdoor activity being carried out.

Analysis of issues relating to thermal comfort and needs, according to sex:

- *Which is the most comfortable part of your house? Why?*
- *Which is the least comfortable part of your house? Why?*

Social culture in rural society leads to certain parts of a dwelling being used more than others depending on whether the users are male or female. The overall population trend observed has been:

- Most comfortable area: Living room.
- Least comfortable area: Attic or other unspecified area.

In addition, based on the consequences analysed, users have identified the reasons for the comfort or lack of comfort in their homes. Overall trends are:

Comfortable area due to:

- Natural illumination: Male (36%); Female (70%).
- Air-conditioning systems: Male (36%); Female (60%).
- Room features: Male (45%); Female (40%).

Areas that are not comfortable are due to:

- Air-conditioning systems: Male (54%); Female (70%).

Results relating to user demands.

Analysis of issues relating to personal sensations and thermal comfort, according to sex:

- *Which room of the house is most frequently used in winter? What measures are taken?*
- *Which room of the house is most frequently used in summer? What measures are taken?*

The most comfortable area for users in both winter and summer is the living room. Reasons mentioned include comfort, habit, good climate control, good ventilation and good lighting. The overall population trend is:

- Cold stages: Comfort (81% Male; 100% Female); Good climate control (54% Male; 60% Female).
- Warm stages: Comfort (45% Male; 90% Female); Good climate control (72% Male; 90% Female).

It should be pointed out that female participants reported a preference for active measures over passive measures in cold stages. In the warmer stages both male and female participants would take passive measures.

Analysis of issues relating to personal sensations and thermal comfort, according to samples:

- *What elements are necessary to ensure a good state of comfort at home?*
- *What would you include in the house to reduce the cold in winter?*
- *What would you include in the house to reduce the warmth in summer?*

The results of activities have been analysed in order to establish the implications of the term "comfort". According to users good comfort conditions are due to aspects such as Furniture; Air-conditioning systems; Building systems ; Light; Open space.

Participants have identified their needs:

- Cold stages: stove; fireplace; shelter; furniture.
- Warm stages: Air conditioning; furniture; taking a shower; removing clothing.

These issues have been considered of interest in their classification as a reflection of the main interests and concerns of participants.

Quantitative Results

Case Study 1. Analysis of issues relating to the most and least comfortable area, according to the dwelling occupants. A comparison has been carried out for the results of energy simulation and the information from users in these areas during summer. According to the survey of V01 users the most comfortable area is the living room. This area, located on the ground floor, has a north-west orientation with no direct solar incidence. Figure 10 shows the results of the most comfortable room in case study 1.

Figure 10. The most comfortable room (living room), case study 1
Source: Author, 2020

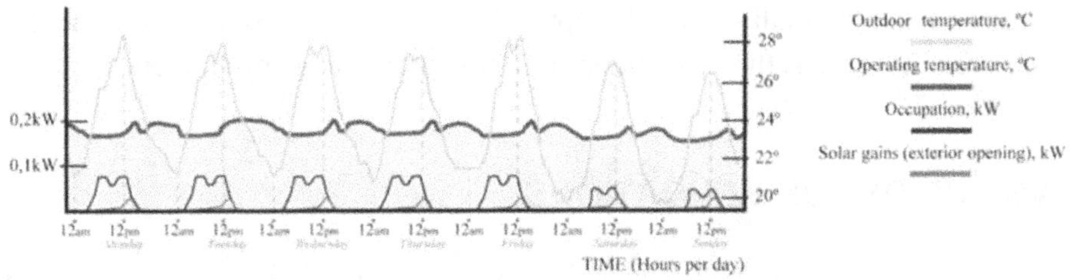

In contrast, according to the survey of V01 users the least comfortable area is the attic. This area is located on the rooftop and receives direct solar incidence from all sides. Figure 11 shows the results of the least comfortable room in case study 1.

Figure 11. The least comfortable room (attic), case study 1
Source: Author, 2020

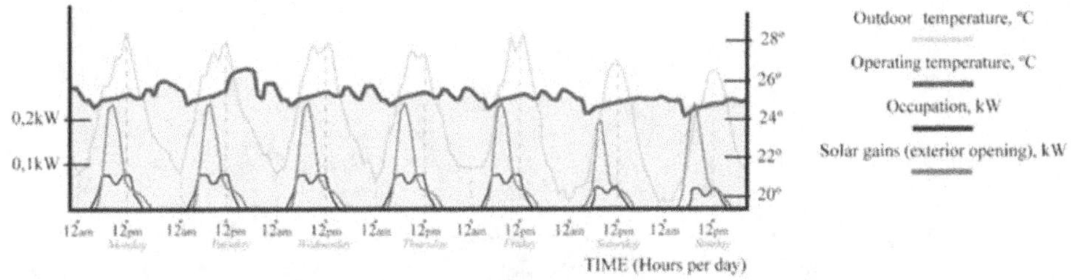

Case Study 2. Analysis of issues relating to the most and least comfortable area, according to the dwelling users.

A comparison has been carried out for the results of energy simulation and the information from users in these areas during summer. According to the survey of V02 users the most comfortable area is the living room, located on the ground floor with a north-west orientation. In this case, the living room receives direct solar incidence. Figure 12 shows the results of the most comfortable room in case study 2.

Figure 12. The most comfortable room (living room), case study 2
Source: Author,2020

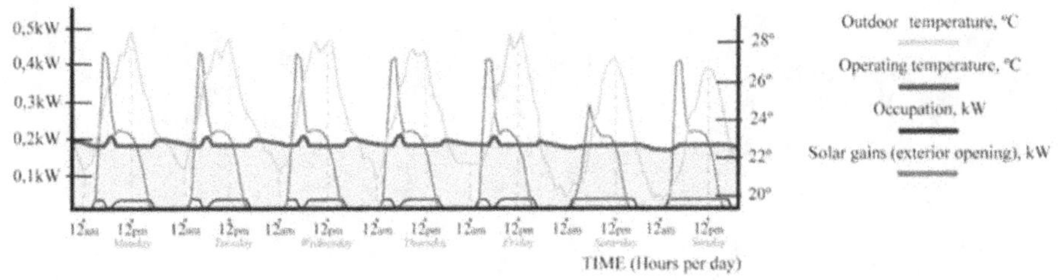

In contrast, both users of the dwelling have highlighted that there is no uncomfortable area. All areas of the house meet their needs and comforts. This is important to note as older people are usually set in their ways and this could potentially cause disruptions to their life. These users do not require elements to improve their comfort state as they find their current situation comfortable enough.

SOLUTIONS AND RECOMMENDATIONS

Opportunities, strengths and weaknesses are proposed when seeking to adapt housing as climate shelter in rural architecture.

The main opportunity is the possibility of adaptation as a climate shelter, according to the needs and potential housing of the user. These dwellings also have many advantages relating to the user lifestyle and their architecture, including local customs and traditions, the use of energy gains or construction systems, the natural ventilation of the dwelling and use of the back yard.

Figure 13. Climate shelter approach
Source: Author, 2020

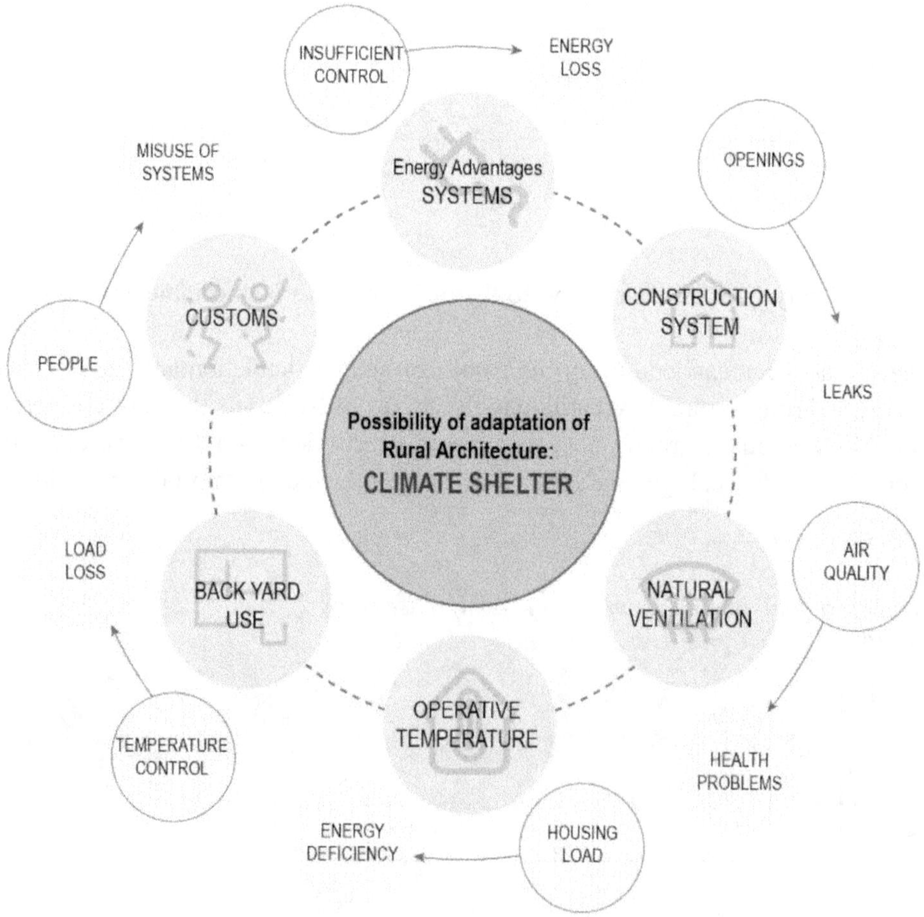

Weaknesses in these key points can lead to problems and threats for the future housing adaptation. These points include misuse of the system on the part of the user; energy loss due to poor control of systems and housing loads; continuous leaks caused by dwelling openings; health problems due to low air quality; and finally, continuous load loss caused by inefficient temperature control (Figure 13).

FUTURE RESEARCH DIRECTIONS

This methodology is proposed to raise awareness among the local population and construction professionals, as well as the retrofitting of social housing in cases specific to elderly users. Future research scopes proposed are:

- An increase in the study samples.
- Study of lighting in case studies, observing its effect on user comfort.
- Analysis of natural ventilation, identified by users as a key aspect in their dwellings.

CONCLUSION

The conclusions met the initial requirements established thanks to energy simulation and surveys among specific sectors of the population, depending on the winter and summer stages, thermal sensation and thermal demand.

Thermal sensation.

- The real characteristics of winter 2018 do not match the participants' perception of a wet and rainy winter. The perception and recollections of most users differed greatly from reality. The thermal response of the dwelling should be suited to user needs and external agents (climate, weather).
- The overall user trend has been characterized by the way of life, culture and customs of rural architecture in the dwellings. Users generally prefer the living room and back yard. The different usage habits of spaces are different for young people, adults and more elderly people. Currently, the spaces in constant use display better thermal behaviour in rural architecture. In both cases, this space is the north-facing living room.
- There is a tendency to associate the most/least comfortable areas with the most/least used areas due to the features and customs of the population. In this case, it can be stated that:
  The most comfortable area is the living room, where families spend most time.
  The spaces on the upper floors are considered the least comfortable areas.
- The most/least comfortable areas vary depending on whether the users are male or female, with men and women preferring different areas.

Thermal demand.

The main issue faced by this society at present is the lack of autonomy experienced by elderly occupants in their homes. Energy performance benefits users in their dwellings because it offers better comfort condition. However, the energy produced does not fit the needs of these elderly occupants. It becomes necessary to consider areas with different levels of thermal control. Thermal comfort depends on the sensations and demands of individuals at each specific moment.

ACKNOWLEDGMENT

Access Contract for the VI Research Plan of the University of Seville (Contrato de Acceso del VI Plan Propio de Investigación de la Universidad de Sevilla).

REFERENCES

Domínguez Amarillo, S. (2015). *Building envelopes and social housing in southern Europe energy assessment of the residential social stock of the city of Seville under the climate change scenario*. Academic Press.

Domínguez-Amarillo, S., Fernández-Agüera, J., Peacock, A., & Acosta, I. (2019). Energy related practices in Mediterranean low-income housing. *Building Research and Information*. Advance online publication. doi:10.1080/09613218.2019.1661764

Domínguez-Amarillo, S., Fernández-Agüera, J., Sendra, J. J., & Roaf, S. (2018). Rethinking User Behaviour Comfort Patterns in the South of Spain—What Users Really Do. *Sustainability*, *10*(12), 4448. doi:10.3390u10124448

Domínguez-Amarillo, S., Fernández-Agüera, J., Sendra, J. J., & Roaf, S. (2019). The performance of Mediterranean low-income housing in scenarios involving climate change. *Energy and Building*, *202*, 109374. doi:10.1016/j.enbuild.2019.109374

Fernández-Agüera, J., Domínguez-Amarillo, S., Alonso, C., & Martín-Consuegra, F. (2019). Thermal comfort and indoor air quality in low-income housing in Spain: The influence of airtightness and occupant behaviour. *Energy and Building*, *199*, 102–114. doi:10.1016/j.enbuild.2019.06.052

Haq, G. (2016). *Win-win strategies to help older people face climate change*. https://www.sei.org/perspectives/older-people-climate-change/

Harper, S. (2006). *Climate Change and the Ageing Population – Oxford Programme for the Future of Cities*. Oxford Institute of Ageing, University of Oxford. http://www.futureofcities.ox.ac.uk/research/climate-change-and-the-ageing-population/

Hirst, N. (2013). Buildings and climate change. In Design and Management of Sustainable Built Environments. doi:10.1007/978-1-4471-4781-7_2

Jenkins, D. P. (2010). The value of retrofitting carbon-saving measures into fuel poor social housing. *Energy Policy*, *38*(2), 832–839. Advance online publication. doi:10.1016/j.enpol.2009.10.030

Ministerio de Fomento del Gobierno de España. (2017). Código técnico de la Edificación (CTE). Author.

Organización Mundial de la Salud. (2015). *OMS | Datos interesantes acerca del envejecimiento*. WHO. https://www.who.int/ageing/about/facts/es/

Panagopoulos, T., Guimaraes, M., Barreira, A. P., & Pana, R. (2013). *aging population and climate change induced migration as causes of urban decline in Portugal*. Academic Press.

Peek, K. (2016). How to Survive in a Warmer World. *Scientific American*. https://www.scientificamerican.com/article/how-to-survive-in-a-warmer-world-interactive/

Roaf, S., Nicol, F., & De Dear, R. (2013). The wicked problem of designing for comfort in a rapidly changing world. *Architectural Science Review*, *56*(1), 1–3. Advance online publication. doi:10.1080/00038628.2012.753783

Roaf, S., Nicol, F., & Rijal, H. (2015). Designing for comfort at high temperatures. *Architectural Science Review*, *58*(1), 35–38. doi:10.1080/00038628.2014.972069

Roberts, E., & Henwood, K. (2019). "It's an Old House and That's How It Works": Living Sufficiently Well in Inefficient Homes. *Housing Theory and Society*, *36*(4), 1–20. doi:10.1080/14036096.2019.1568296

Sanchez-Guevara, C., Núñez Peiró, M., Taylor, J., Mavrogianni, A., & Neila González, J. (2019). Assessing population vulnerability towards summer energy poverty: Case studies of Madrid and London. *Energy and Building*, *190*, 132–143. doi:10.1016/j.enbuild.2019.02.024

Santamouris, M., Paravantis, J. A., Founda, D., Kolokotsa, D., Michalakakou, P., Papadopoulos, A. M., Kontoulis, N., Tzavali, A., Stigka, E. K., Ioannidis, Z., Mehilli, A., Matthiessen, A., & Servou, E. (2013). Financial crisis and energy consumption: A household survey in Greece. *Energy and Building*, *65*, 477–487. doi:10.1016/j.enbuild.2013.06.024

Wells, E. M., Berges, M., Metcalf, M., Kinsella, A., Foreman, K., Dearborn, D. G., & Greenberg, S. (2015). Indoor air quality and occupant comfort in homes with deep versus conventional energy efficiency renovations. *Building and Environment*, *93*(P2), 331–338. doi:10.1016/j.buildenv.2015.06.021

Wilkinson, P., Smith, K. R., Joffe, M., & Haines, A. (2007). A global perspective on energy: health effects and injustices. Lancet. doi:10.1016/S0140-6736(07)61252-5

ADDITIONAL READING

Attia, S., Eleftheriou, P., Xeni, F., Morlot, R., Ménézo, C., Kostopoulos, V., & Hidalgo-Betanzos, J. M. (2017). Overview and future challenges of nearly zero energy buildings (nZEB) design in Southern Europe. *Energy and Building*, *155*, 439–458. doi:10.1016/j.enbuild.2017.09.043

Brambilla, A., Bonvin, J., Flourentzou, F., & Jusselme, T. (2018). Life cycle efficiency ratio: A new performance indicator for a life cycle driven approach to evaluate the potential of ventilative cooling and thermal inertia. *Energy and Building*, *163*, 22–33. doi:10.1016/j.enbuild.2017.12.010

Campblell-Dollaghan, K. (2014). Storm-Proofing NYC Will Cost At Least $11 Billion, But It's Worth It. Retrieved from https://gizmodo.com/storm-proofing-nyc-will-cost-at-least-11-billion-but-1570873371

Frumkin, H., Fried, L., & Moody, R. (2012). Aging, climate change, and legacy thinking. *American Journal of Public Health*, *102*(8), 1434–1438. doi:10.2105/AJPH.2012.300663 PMID:22698047

Jacobs, S. (2016). The human population is aging. Can our cities handle it? | Grist. Retrieved June 24, 2018, from https://grist.org/cities/the-human-population-is-aging-can-our-cities-handle-it/

Laros, M., Birch, S., Clover, J., & ICLEI-Africa. (2013). Ecosystem-based approaches to building resilience in urban areas: towards a framework for decision-making criteria. *Workshop Background Paper*. Retrieved from http://durbanadaptationcharter.org/wp-content/uploads/2015/06/Urban-EBA-Background-Literature-Review-2013.pdf

OECD. (2015). Ageing in Cities. *Ageing in Cities*, 161–168. doi:10.1787/9789264231160-en

Oree, V., & Anatah, H. K. (2017). Investigating the feasibility of positive energy residential buildings in tropical climates. *Energy Efficiency*, *10*(2), 383–404. doi:10.100712053-016-9462-7

Simone, G. De, Janeiro, R. De, Toronto, T. D., Jack, D., York, N., Toronto, J. P., & Rahman, M. (2011). Climate change and human health in cities Coordinating Lead Authors : Lead Authors : *Cities And Climate Change - First Assessment Report of the Urban Climate Change Research Network.*

Sorokanich, B. (2014). Report: Climate Change Will Be Our Aging Cities' Biggest Problem. Retrieved June 24, 2018, from https://gizmodo.com/report-climate-change-will-be-our-aging-cities-biggest-1572403936

Survey, A. (1981). Lecture Notes in Computer Science. *Lecture Notes in Computer Science*.

Susan Roaf, L. B. and N. F. (2017). Design to thrive. Legacy Document. In *Legacy Document of 33rd PLEA International Conference* (pp. 5–64).

Yach, D. (2013). The link between ageing and climate change | World Economic Forum. Retrieved June 24, 2018, from https://www.weforum.org/agenda/2015/02/the-link-between-ageing-and-climate-change/

Zainudin, H., Haron, N. A., Bachek, S. H., & Jusoh, A. (2016). Utilization of building information modeling (BIM) in planning an adaptive reuse project of a Traditional Malay House (TMH). *Proceedings of the 2016 International Conference on Virtual Systems and Multimedia, VSMM 2016*. 10.1109/VSMM.2016.7863193

Zheng, D. L., Yu, L. J., & Tan, H. W. (2017). Design and optimization of zero-energy-consumption based solar energy residential building systems. *IOP Conference Series. Earth and Environmental Science*, *93*(1), 012055. Advance online publication. doi:10.1088/1755-1315/93/1/012055

KEY TERMS AND DEFINITIONS

Adaptive Capacity: Its aim is to increase the power of adaptation to any adversity either in the long or short term.

Comfortable Area: Areas which have characteristics that make users feel better.

Resilience: Adaptive capacity of a living being or thing against an external agent which alters its common state.

Thermal Demand: This is the demand required by each user and the features offered by each dwelling. It is the user's response.

Thermal Sensation: This refers to the sensations, impressions, feelings, and satisfaction produced at the time of the specific research.

Uncomfortable Area: Areas which display characteristics that users consider unsatisfactory.

Chapter 10
Integration of Tellurism and Sacred Geometry in Professional Training:
Innovation, Healthy Architecture, and Landscape

Guadalupe Cantarero-García
Universidad CEU San Pablo, Spain

ABSTRACT

At present, the implementation of the concepts of tellurism and sacred geometry in the schools of architecture is neither obvious nor simple. It starts with the historical heritage of patterns that are shaped and molded according to professorships that have worked independently in territories at different scales within building and urbanism. Moreover, they share the same premise of the occupation of space and creation. In this study, the authors focus on the intrinsic value of the land, its energy, and how this affects not only the overall design of the building, but also the interior of a healthy dwelling. The psychological, psychosomatic, and symptomatic effects on the human being are related to the intrinsic use of a dwelling, as well as to the building's placement on the land. The work method in this investigation has implemented a comparative case study carried out in El Pardo and Carabanchel.

INTRODUCTION

It is unusual to talk about *Tellurism* in Schools of Architecture, even more so in relation to the design of interior space in a dwelling. However, the location and surrounding landscape of a dwelling are key in order to achieve the ideal home.

Although, for the architect the foundation is the building's base, he or she has not always taken into consideration whether the foundation has been built on land contaminated by energy that will impact

DOI: 10.4018/978-1-7998-7279-5.ch010

the inhabitant's health. In architecture, tectonics is the great forgotten, as is archaeology, which provides the basis to work utilizing the perspective of history and ways of living.

At present, the implementation of the concepts of *Tellurism* and *Sacred Geometry* in the Schools of Architecture is neither obvious nor simple. It starts with the historical heritage of patterns that are shaped and molded according to professorships that have worked independently in territories at different scales within building and urbanism. Moreover, they share the same premise of the occupation of space and creation. However, town planning addresses the external context and architecture deals with the interior and the exterior according to what is most precious to the architect such as the facade, the building's appearance and its expression in the city. On the other hand, interior architects have established a career almost devoid of any appreciation of exterior spaces.

This study focuses on the intrinsic value of the land, its energy and how this affects, not only the overall design of the building, but the healthy interior of a dwelling as well. The research also includes a case study that investigates the concept of *Sacred Geometry* and how it can transform a house into a home as well as its possible effect on health and its relationship with the landscape. It is illogical to address the interior without taking into account the exterior too. Luminary and chromatic perception, as well as identifying the horizon line of urban or natural landscape, have a direct effect on the inhabitant's feelings.

Reflecting on the need to call a house a home is a starting point for this study. There are times when a person likes a house but cannot explain why. That house surely contains noble materials, such as the wood used in its carpentry, its latticework, the coffering, the floors and finishes, but what is clear is that it constitutes a home, which, in turn, implies warmth like the hearth as a place to gather in order to keep warm. Without wood there is no fire, without wood there is no hearth or home. Water, fire and air are vital elements in a home, as is the geometry applied to house them. Oriental feng shui works on the understanding of plans and the distribution of space inside the house in order to optimize well-being. It is, however, unthinkable to contemplate this concept in the West.

The purpose of this study is to highlight the need to publicize the concepts of tellurism and Sacred Geometry in an architect's training and thus raise the designer's awareness of the positive consequences of the inhabitants' health. Presenting guidelines on concepts unknown in the West, such as feng shui, may even appear to be obvious for design optimization. A secondary objective proposes architecture as a service to the people and must include empathy when dealing with inhabitants. The psychological, psychosomatic and symptomatic effects on the human being are related to the intrinsic use of a dwelling, as well as to the building's placement on the land. Developing a living space is very different in an apartment than in a house with a garden. Looking through a window at an urban landscape has more limitations than looking out of a balcony and seeing a natural landscape. The location of the horizon line plays an important role in visuospatial optometry.

The work method of this study has implemented a comparative case study carried out in El Pardo and Carabanchel. Both are located in the outskirts of Madrid and have a strong historical background, though their distinctive characteristics have led them in very different directions. This analysis first shows how the artesian wells built on the Royal Site have also conditioned the configuration of the area and its houses. Secondly, it shows how the water table and the vegetation have made Monte de El Pardo a protected natural area and its relation to the stretch of the Manzanares River in lower Carabanchel. Therefore, the perception from inside the homes of the inhabitants of El Pardo is very different from the inhabitants of Carabanchel. (this case study is part of the funded project PID2019-110693RB-I00 published in the BOE (June 11, 2020) and the provisional resolution of the "Research Projects Oriented for the Challenges of Society in the Federal Plan for RD&I", and our project "The Peri-urban Landscape of Madrid: Visions from Memory Towards the New City", which is proposed for funding with a start date of June 1, 2020)

Finally, the pandemic caused by COVID-19 has been crucial in awakening the people's appreciation of their home as part of who they are. Staying longer than necessary inside the house has meant a radical conceptual change of the spatial relationship between the interior and the exterior. This awareness of space has led to a greater financial investment in items for the home, thus demanding more interior refurbishments. There has also been a rise in the real estate sector with people relocating to the outskirts of the city.

One of the conclusions derived from this study is that the landscape is a determining element in the way a person lives within the interior space of their home and it has direct repercussions on a person's health. It is necessary to reflect on how technologies have led to changes in work habits such as working from home, as well as reflecting on the warmth that the land acquires when building on it and considering the dwelling's appearance and how it opens up to the exterior.

Optometrist scientific researchers, doctors, psychologists, *Tellurism* experts, topographers and architects have worked with a multidisciplinary approach and have taken an active part in this study and have contributed with new conclusions to the status and knowledge of the issue. Students with intellectual disabilities from the TP Consultant in Universal Accessibility1 as well as educational psychologists from the University of Monterrey have also participated.

BACKGROUND: HISTORICAL REFERENCES

In Plato's Timaeus, he sets forth an arrangement of the physical universe based on five, regular polyhedrons. The tetrahedron, the hexahedron, the octahedron and the icosahedron. They "are the four basic elements and the dodecahedron allows for the proportional composition of the universe," narrates Rafael Leoz, architect and creator of the HELE module, in the treatise where Luis Moya describes contemporary artists (Moya 1978).

Since prehistoric times, man has been aware that geometry is a system for making order out of the ''whole.''[2] Rivaud said that there must be permanent or, as he called it, perennial proportions within the disorder of appearances (A. Rivaud in Associacion Guillaume Budé, 1949). As Aristotle stated, "The Universe is a continuous 'whole', a sphere rounded with such precision that it cannot be compared to any human work of art."[3]

Kepler's laws were the first "laws of nature" in the modern sense. "These laws divorced astronomy from theology and united it with physics. Finally, they put an end to the nightmare that had been the obsession of cosmology for the last two millennia: the obsession of spheres revolving around spheres." (Alvarez Garcia, Marquina and Ridaura Sanz 1993).

Geometry demarcates the symbolism of the circle as being the first form that the human being understood. An example being the wheel and the movement of kinematic physics that it implies. The circle is the shape that protects us when we are inside it. Dwellings were built within that pure morphology. In the beginning, that graphic representation on the ground symbolically demarcated access points, which later became a moat. The first settlements could be described as proto-urban with a large number of inhabitants within a powerful fortification system. Humans of the Stone Age already made drawings by carving the first geometrical forms of triangles and parallel lines. These patterns were reproduced in textiles as well. As well as Neolithic human works, without knowledge of geometry as such, used

Figure 1. Image a: Late Chalcolithic settlement (late 2600-2200 BC).
Image b: Idols. Barbacena (Elvas, Portugal). Temporary exhibition piece of the Regional Archaeological Museum of the Community of Madrid.
Image c: Wool and linen cushion from the Coptic period c. IV-V BC. Akhim.

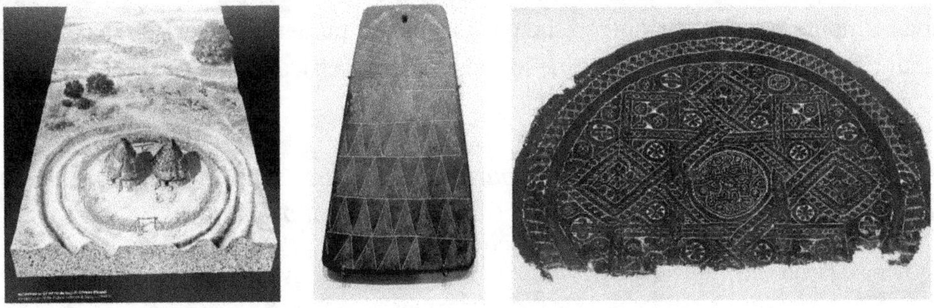

concepts of repetition of forms and pure symmetry that is generated both in clay designs, clothing and household items such as cushions (Fig.1).

The construction of the Sumerian ziggurat is highlighted when regarding cultures and the people that lived in the Near East between the 4th and 1st millennium BC. They are made of adobe with linteled and exceptionally vaulted forms (half-barrel and close walls). They were built between 2,700 BC to 2100 BC.

Following a thorough site selection, these structures were placed in strategic locations and were built with design lines regulated by pure geometry (Fig. 2).

Figure 2. Image a: Sumerian ziggurat 2500 B.C. Source: contenidos.educarest.es Image b: Sargon II palace at Khorsabad (717-705 BC) Source: https://archeologie.culture.fr/khorsabad/en

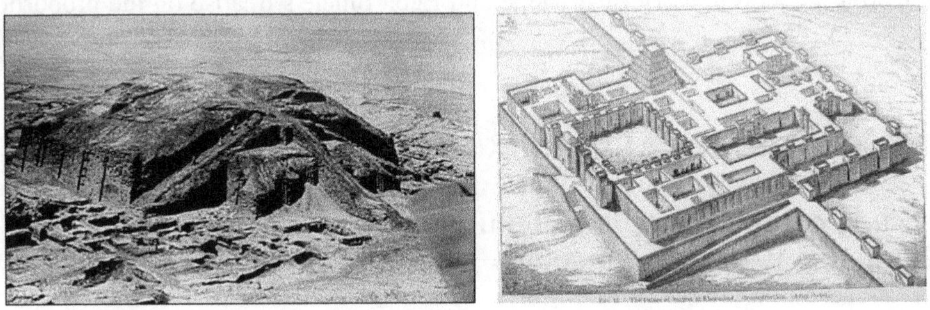

Geometry is inherent and intrinsic to nature and its application in design and construction is essential. Geometry as a science constitutes a collection of practical knowledge in relation to length, area and volume. Herodotus, Strabo and Euclid (in the 2nd century B.C.) configured geometry in an axiomatic and constructive way. Later, Descartes developed analytical geometry, which was used by Gauss and Euler to establish new topographical measurement systems thanks to differential geometry. The 19th century is a key period as far as topography is concerned. The military engineering corps developed more accurate surveying methods that allowed for understanding the terrain with exact coordinates and contour lines. However, it was not until 1950 that educators in mathematics began to link mathematics with geometry. This was a turning point for Schools of Architecture and Engineering.

In design, proportion and scale are linked to geometry. Whether it is an object or an architectural construction, there is proportion and its analysis has characterized the classical orders of Greek architecture and the Roman Empire. Dr. Caskey studied the proportions of numerous Greek vases on display in the Boston Museum, which led him to draw some interesting geometrical conclusions[4] (Fig. 3).

Figure 3. Image a: From the Villard d'Honnecourt album. Source: Bibliothèque Nationale de Paris (plate 39). Image b: Kylix or Greek vase and Dr. Caskey's study of proportions.
Image c: Projection of a grouping of Kelvin's polyhedra (plate 28).
Images b and c Source: Published in Matila C. Ghyka's plates 1983.

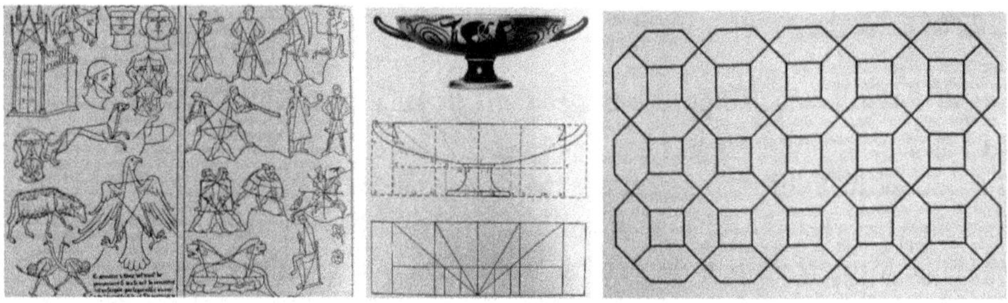

Arabesques also give clues as to how rhythm, music, poetry and mathematics took shape with this graphic language. Interlaced surface ornamental and decorative elements used in friezes, plinths and borders are generally based on complex geometric designs devised by Arab artists. (Fig. 4).

Finally, while discussing proportions in architecture, inevitably one must talk about Leonardo, Palladio and le Corbusier, as well as Herman Helle and Egon Shiele's treatise on the proportions of the human body (Fig.5).

OBJECTIVE, CASE STUDY AND WORK METHOD

In-Depth Study of the Concepts of Tellurism and Sacred Geometry as a Work Objective

Proportion theories vary just as the size of the men, women and children from the different hemispheres and continents vary. Specific proportions cannot be applied to human beings as such, but rather the use of an average proportion helps scale the space of homes, public spaces and, ultimately, architecture and urban planning. Ergonomics also plays an important role in industrial design. In fact, the constant search for the adaptation of models to the human being is endless. The search for the ideal and comfortable interior space must be adapted to personal and family needs, but also to the space-time we live in, that is to say, to permanent and temporary needs.

Given the awareness of the importance of geometry throughout history and of its study for the knowledge of architecture, why has it not been considered in current housing design? Is it really mere symbolism

Figure 4. Fine architectural detail at the Alhambra Palace in Southern Spain. Ataurique. Published in Arabesco Source: Yves, Remedios in: https://ceramica.fandom.com/wiki/Arabesco?file=Atauriques.jpg

Figure 5. Figure a. Heller, Hermann y Schiele, Egon (1913) Proportionstafeln der menschlichen gestalt: für kunstwerkstätten und fachschulen. Source: Ghyka, M. La estética de las proporciones en la naturaleza y en las artes. Figure b. The Modulor: A Set of Harmonious Dimensions on the Human Scale, Universally Applicable in Architecture and Mechanics. Le Corbusier. Source: (Boesiger, 1992, p.88-89)

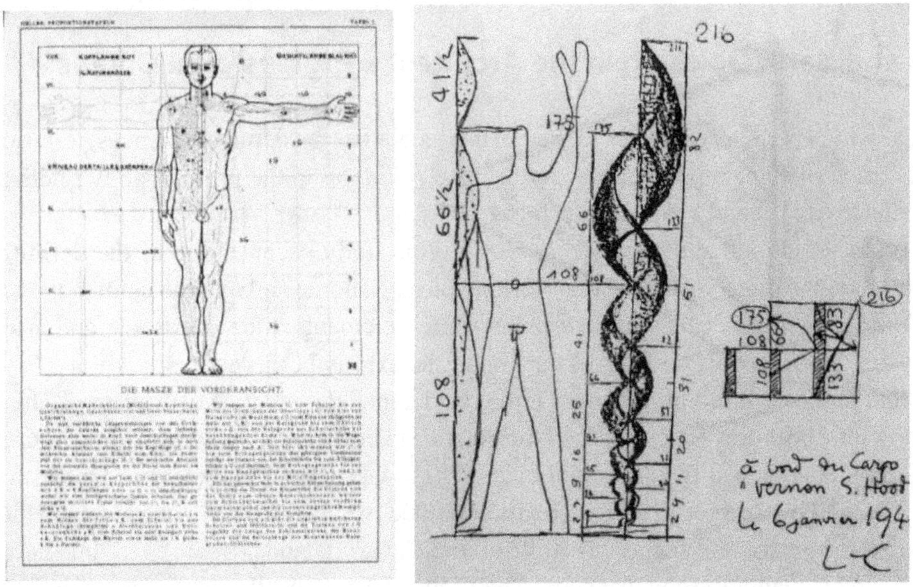

that does not have a beneficial effect on the dweller?. This study focuses on the importance of learning about the concepts of tellurism and Sacred Geometry within the study of architecture. These concepts and their implementation in the professional career are also important for the architect's academic training. Many architects do not know about tellurism and know even less about Sacred Geometry. Should these concepts be known to architects? Would architects be open to including them in their projects? Furthermore, if residents of the same city were familiar with these concepts and they were asked to evaluate the quality of life in their homes, would they be able to identify, according to these two concepts, the key points that optimize their homes and make them more comfortable and therefore healthier?

Case Study at El Pardo and Carabanchel: Work Method

The case study completes the research presented here. The investigation focuses on two very different points that share a common element, the Manzanares River. There are different ways of living on the banks of the same river and in the same city of Madrid, however, there are significant differences such as landscape and types of housing. The work method is carried out through two surveys taken with forms on a digital application. Architects and citizens from the Royal Site of El Pardo and the neighborhood of Carabanchel were surveyed.

First, the architects survey examines whether the architect is familiar with both concepts. Should the answer be positive, they are asked if they would integrate the concepts as part of the curriculum in the degree and if they would apply them to their work or if they do not consider the concepts to be pertinent enough to apply them. Additionally, the survey asks the architects what their daily life has been like during the lockdown and whether they feel it has affected either their psychological or physical health, both of them or neither one.

In the citizen survey, the questions are the same, but we go further by asking about the comfort of their dwelling place and whether they would choose another place or neighborhood to live in.

INTRODUCTION TO TELLURISM AND SACRED GEOMETRY IN ARCHITECTURE

Tellurism and Earth Dowsing in the Architect's Professional Career

Telluric is that which pertains or relates to the Earth as a planet. In chemical sciences, telluric also refers to the qualification of an acid produced by tellurium.[5] *Tellurism* in the present study refers to the earth and how it behaves above and below the surface.

It is important to introduce the term *Tellurism* in this study because one of the definitions of this concept is based on the direct influence that the land has on a home and a home contributes to the health of the dwellers.[6] The study deals with two underground elements, the water table and artesian wells, because they are considered essential in determining the external character.

It seems that in the 18th century, Father Feijóo condemned the practice of dowsing.[7] The Inquisition persecuted dowsers[8] because they considered the practice to be sorcery.[9] However, the dowsing technique was not officially condemned by the Catholic Church, in fact, the first Society of Friends of Dowsing was founded in 1890 by the French abbot Alexis-Timothée Bouly, who was a priest from Hardelot. This practice favored the creation of numerous wells on the Canary Islands (Spain) and thus helped provide irrigation for banana plantations on drylands. The French term radiesthesia first appeared in English in

1930. Numerous scientific studies throughout the 20th century, mostly in Germany, have not yielded positive results to reinforce dowsing as a reliable practice.

In the late 20th century, architects knowledgeable in the field used radiesthesia on very few occasions. In the Schools of Architecture there is no mention of the practice of these methods, not even for project site location on a plot of land. Just as alternative medicine such as acupuncture has been imported to Europe to complete treatments that allopathic medicine was not able to heal, oriental techniques such as Feng Shui, I Ching and tellurism intervene to identify pathogenic geological points such as groundwater flow, faults or diaclases, Hartman nets or Curry grids. The Bovis Biometer is a device that measures the energy of an outdoor or indoor location. 6500 Bovis is considered to be the optimal vital average. Thus, places with a lower vibration would be devitalizing and those with an energy between 7000 and 9000 Bovis would be optimal for balance and health.

The study of telluric disturbances is subject to external conditions such as the earth's magnetism. Magnetic storms also indicate if the earth's magnetic field are unstable, which can have considerable variations. According to Einstein, matter is a particular form of energy and, therefore, material objects also emit radiation.

The divining rods contain a ring ideally designed with a 3 mm brass rod to make them reactive and receptive. These rods, with their crossover movement, favor the detection of networks, waves and locations considered to have a high ionic charge.

Water Table and Artesian Wells

In 1904, Alfonso XIII encouraged agriculture and livestock usage within the Royal Site of El Pardo. As a result, the Royal Palace cultivated large plots in the woodlands with around five hundred hectares of non-irrigated land. A wire fence was built around it to protect the crops from both large and small game. Numerous wells were dug on several plots (Fig. 6) that reached about one hundred and ten meters in depth. These wells, near Queen Victoria's Bridge, yielded about eight hundred liters of water per minute and could shoot out of the ground more than twenty meters high.

There were also four electrohydraulic pump installations. Two of the most powerful of these pumps could draw out 3,300 and 6,000 L. of water per minute, respectively. With these installations, it was expected that the total extension of irrigated land would reach 187 hectares. Grains, legumes and vegetables such as wheat, barley, oats, rye, grass peas, beans, chickpeas, carob, potatoes, alfalfa, corn, turnips, beets and other foods that are currently consumed were harvested in these farmlands. Crops from non-irrigated gardens were worked using modern, agricultural technology of the time such as moldboard plows, rollers, harrows, seeders, cultivators, mowers as well as powerful steam powered threshers. Manure and chemicals were used as fertilizer.

This agriculture data for El Pardo was found in the Espasa Encyclopedia, where Janini is introduced as the creator of the agricultural expansion of the Royal Site.

It also makes reference to his book (Espasa Calpe, 1920): "Due to the kindness of D. Rafael Janini Janini, agricultural engineer of the Royal Household and Heritage, who had the pleasure to carry out the initiatives of Alfonso XIII. [...] Also, author Janini, who wrote the remarkable publication entitled Irrigation with Artesian Groundwater, compiled a mass of data about the great importance of cultivating the land. It is a work of true patriotism and is extremely useful, not only for the Royal Palace but for all farmers. [...]"

Figure 6. Artesian well in El Pardo (1913) Source: in Archive [BCM]

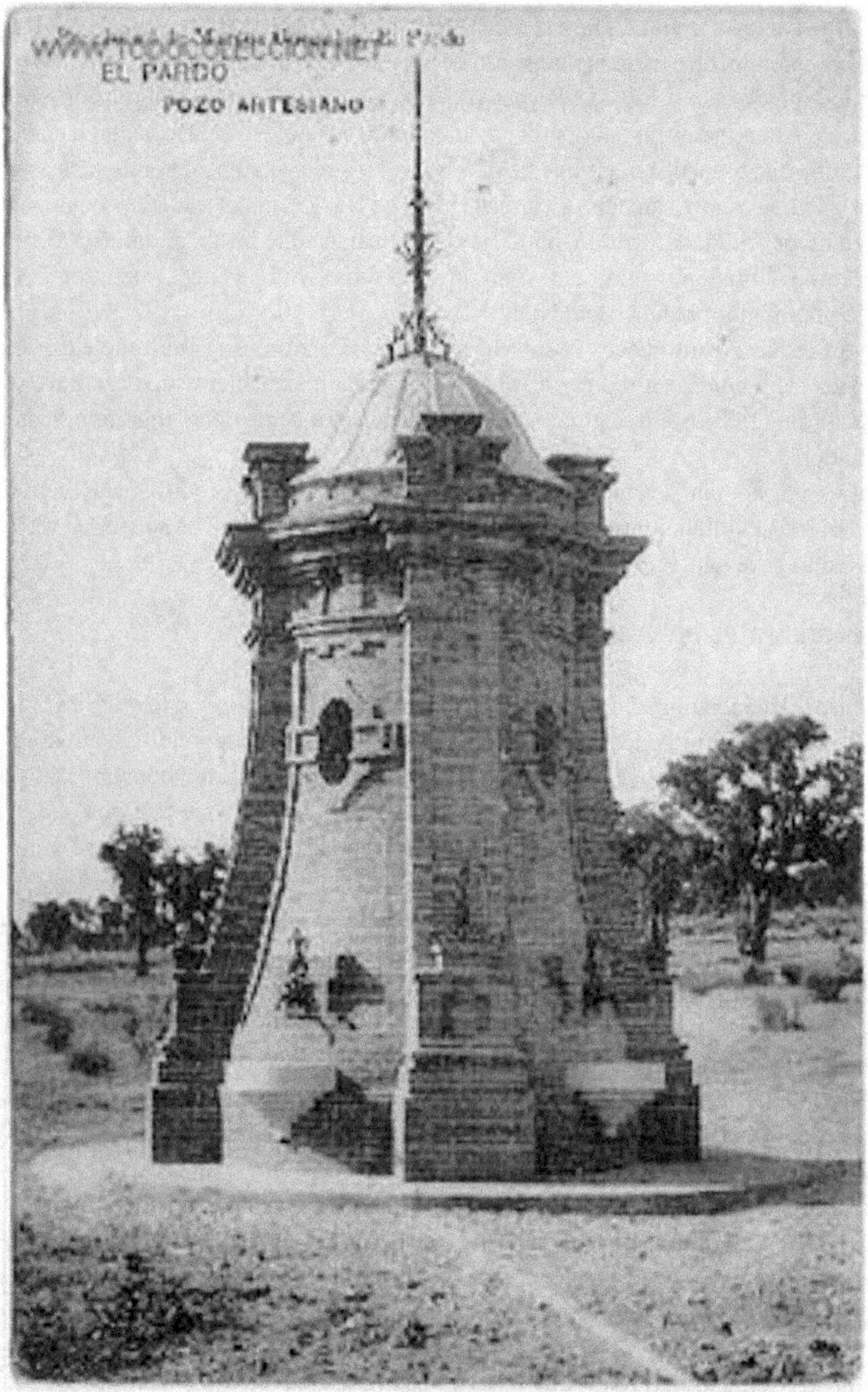

Alfonso XIII also commissioned Janini to study and promote the agricultural exploitation of the fertile plains of Manzanares. The area of study stretched from the San Fernando Bridge to the town of El Pardo. This stretch of land was considered alluvial terrain with several water tables. In 1908, Janini planned to transform the site into what he called an "urban settlement" or a true town with sanitation, culture and areas of recreation such as pavilions, hotels and villas surrounded by gardens. Many of these building projects were never developed, however, agriculture was greatly favored thanks to the artesian wells and irrigation systems that were implemented, which undoubtedly promoted the self-sufficiency of the town.

Impact on Landscape as a Result of Topographic Interventions

The El Pardo Woodlands (Fig. 7), a protected natural area, was first a hunting ground used by the Spanish monarchy. Later, the Palace was located within the reserve and the area was deemed a Royal Site. These woodlands were declared a Special Protection Area for Birds in 1987 (ZEPA)[10]

Figure 7. "Proyecto del Camino Real de El Pardo", "Royal Road Project" (1741)
Source: Sebastián de Rodolphe, in Archive: [A.G.P.]

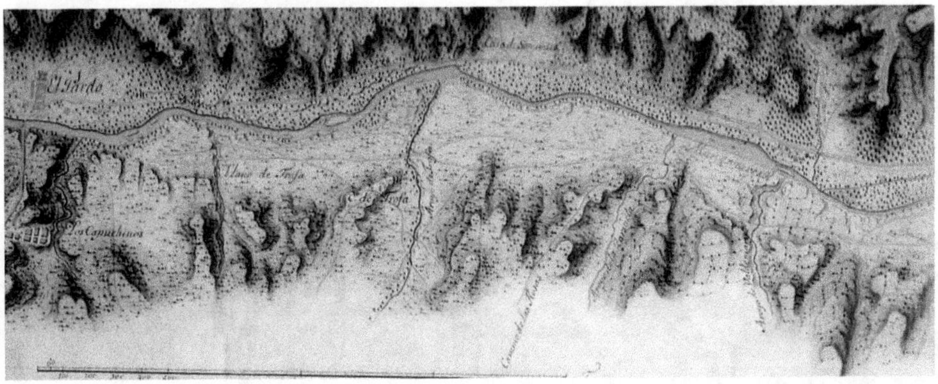

Historical underground interventions in the area, including the artesian wells and trenches presented in this research, are now undetectable. Although these elements have not yet been considered in previous scientific investigations, artesian wells and trenches are important factors in landscaping that has been conditioned by the soil and its treatment throughout history.

Several publications from the late nineteenth and early twentieth centuries were found and analysis of these bibliographical sources reveals interests other than political, economic or artistic expansion in El Pardo. These sources are published in travel guides, route maps and landscape photography, which invite travelers to better understand the natural environment of the area.

In terms of recreation, landscaping changes have been made with the creation of hiking and biking trails. Hence, surveyors and engineers write articles, essays and books, which are sometimes accompanied by cartography based on planimetry as well as cuts or profiles. Intrinsic values of the El Pardo Woodlands are recorded in a descriptive, practical and visual style, almost to lure in visitors and outdoor recreationists, many of whom are foreigners.

Sacred Geometry

Sacred Geometry has determined, throughout history, the definitive location of constructions. It has been said that the synchronicity of the universe is determined by certain mathematical constants, which express themselves in the form of 'patterns' and 'cycles' in nature. The word geometry comes from the Greek words "geos" meaning "earth" and "metron" meaning "to measure", which together literally translate as the "measuring of the earth" or "earthly measurements", an art which was traditionally restricted to the priesthood. It is often mistakenly said that geometry began with the Greeks, but before them were the Minoans, the Egyptians, Sumerians, Indus valley, Chinese, Phoenicians and, of course, the builders of the western European megaliths, all of whom left clear geometric fingerprints in their greatest constructions. The Greeks may well have been the first to offer geometry to the public at large, but they were by no means the first to make use of it.

Sacred Geometry[11] ascribes symbolic and sacred meanings to certain geometric shapes and proportions.

Figure 8. 2D and 3D open grids and closed models.
Source: www.plm.com.ar

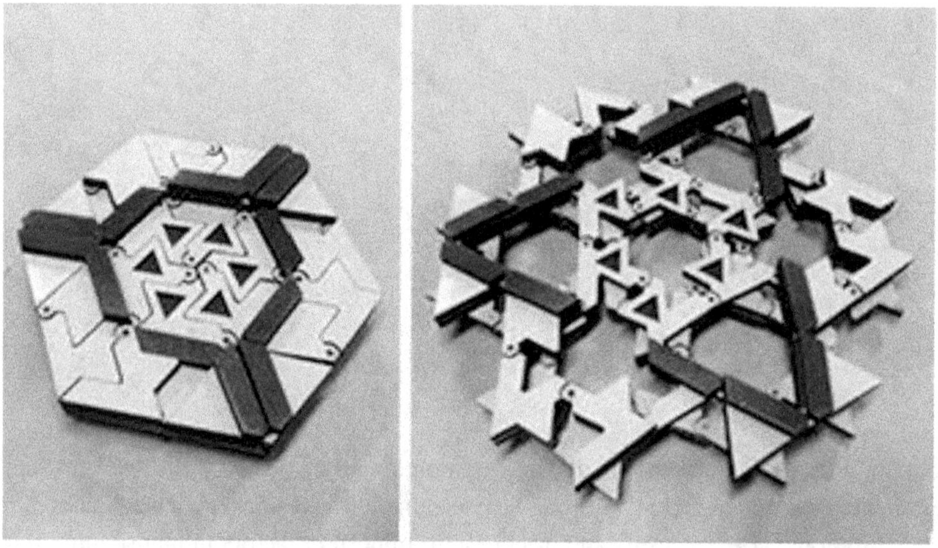

Basic Regulatory Layouts and Management Systems. Geometry, Design and Structure

The *Vesica Piscis* depicts the commitment of marriage understood as the union of one unit to another unit in which the number two creates duality (1+1=2). It is the sacred union of two identical and exact geometrical forms, such as two circles that have the same radius and, therefore, have equal diameters. Like two rings that form an oval (not an ellipse) at their intersection. This oval is the union, but it is not random. It is strategically placed where the centers of the radius touch.

The *Vesica Piscis*, also known as the Pisces symbol (Fig. 9), translates literally from Latin and its meaning refers to the fish, specifically to the fish bladder.

"This symbol is a prominent piece in the history of Pythagoras and is considered to be a sacred figure because it was believed that the ratio of its width to its height, 165:153 or 1.73203, was a sacred number. It should be noted that the number 153 is written in the Gospel of John as the number of fish that Jesus miraculously caught." (www.mownageometriasagrada.com)

"Almost every ancient civilization has considered the circle to be a symbol of the infinite or the perfect because it has no vertex, no beginning and no end. The circle is also related to the sun, the source of life, as well as to many deities. As a result, it is only logical that two circles joined in an intersection are found in a variety of cultural settings. Even without formal knowledge of geometry, the most natural choice of intersection for two circumferences is to join the centers with the perimeters. So, it is not uncommon to come across the vesica piscis construction in artefacts from many different cultures.

Since there are no extensive studies in classic mathematics concerning the vesica piscis, it is unclear whether there are subtypes, which might include the intersection of circumferences with different radii or centers that do not coincide exactly with the perimeters. Such cases may be referred to as "circle–to-circle intersections", but this study uses the term vesica piscis in a more general form, including intersections among ellipses or other curves" (Barrallo, J., González-Quintial, F. & Sánchez-Beitia, 2015).

Figure 9.

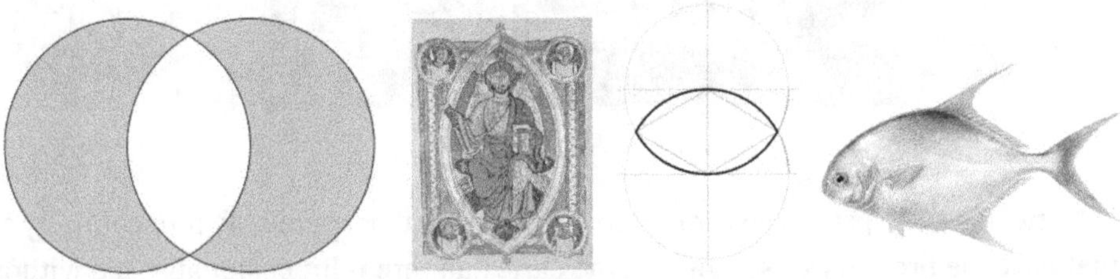

Vesica Piscis / Christ pantocrator or Jesus within a vesica piscis shape. It is usually framed in an oval border known as a mandorla (from the Italian mandorla, 'almond') which coincides with the shape of the vesica piscis / geometry of the vesica piscis is called this because of the fish-like shape that stands out. Source: (es.wikipedia.org). Pacific Pompano. Marine fish with regularly ossified skeleton. Dorsal

Figure 10. Zygote in the first weeks of development. Image b: Geometric figures: outcome of Vesica Piscis repetition and generation of new patterns: seed of life and flower of life.

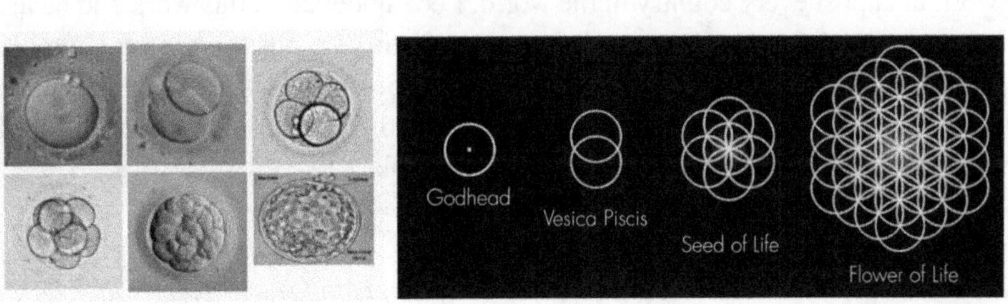

side silvery blue grey, ventrally paler. Large adults golden orange, especially snout and ventral half of body. Dorsal snout profile very steep and broadly rounded. Source:_conxemar.com

The *Vesica Piscis* is found in nature in its purest perfection. During development, the zygote multiplies repeatedly, creating this geometric form. As a result, the repetition of the geometrical shape took on the sexual reproductive concept as the "seed of life" and later as the "flower of life" (Fig.10).

In order to discuss geometry applied to architecture in the sixties, it is necessary to mention the HELE module created by Leoz[12] and Hervás, which was presented in 1961 at the Sao Paulo Biennial (Fig.11). This approach opened up other perspectives that, together with the prefabricated industry, would favor housing modulation and urban planning, not only in terms of construction. Leoz's theories were welcomed by the great architects and theorists of the time, such as Jean Prouvé, Le Corbusier and Jean Prouvé.

Figure 11. Rafael Leoz and the HELE module (Hervás and Leoz)

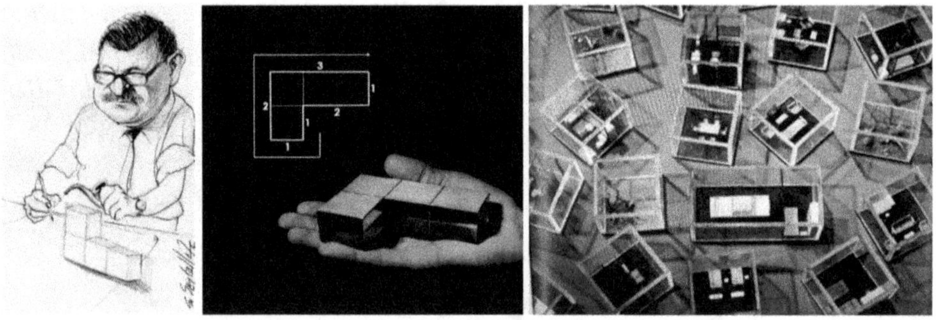

In his book, Networks and Spatial Rhythms, Leoz clarifies that there are only four centrally symmetric polyhedrons that have the property of solidifying the cartesian three-dimensional space without leaving any gaps. All four are subject to being embedded and circumscribed in a sphere. The four polyhedrons are the cube, the regular hexahedron, the right prism with a regular hexagonal base, the rhombic dodecahedron and the heptaparallelohedron or Lord Kelvin polyhedron (Fig.12). With them, four fundamental reticules, which are not limited to these four reticules, are obtained to fill the three-dimensional space.

The purpose of the work, Networks and Spatial Rhythms, is to present the unique personality of the architect Rafael Leoz. His complete dedication to the task of research compels one to address his life and his professional work in terms of that research, which was the axis of everything he did as a man and as an architect. Everything he did revolved around it and its stated purpose was to solve the problem of social housing. In this respect he was no different from many others who have dedicated themselves to the same work in almost every country in the world. Leoz understood this work and he also knew its partial achievements, its defects and, in short, its unsatisfactory results. Solving this problem was for him an ethical imperative, but a self-preserving intuition helped him understand that the standard path, the one followed by many, was based on a positivist pragmatism that could not go very far because of its attachment to circumstances that are limited in time and place.

"Since the six faces of a cube are identical regular polygons (squares) with the same angle between one face and another, the probability of any side (from one to six) is the same. That is the characteristic of

Figure 12. Image a: Cover of the book by the author Luis Moya Blanco (1978) Title: Artistas españoles contemporáneo. Rafael Leoz Collection: Contemporary Spanish Artists, n°151 Published by: Centro de Publicaciones. Ministry of Education and Science. Image b: Estructuración hiperpoliédrica del espacio, by Rafael Leoz. The work is a cube that houses a Kelvin polyhedron within its interior, formed by six squares and eight hexagons, which in turn has in its interior a regular octahedron. This sequence is repeated two more times. It is made of stainless steel. Image c: Metatron Cube: Metatron's Cube starts with the fruit of life shape and connects all 13 circles with straight lines. Metatron's Cube includes all 5 platonic solids hidden inside, symbolizing the underlying geometric patterns found throughout our universe.

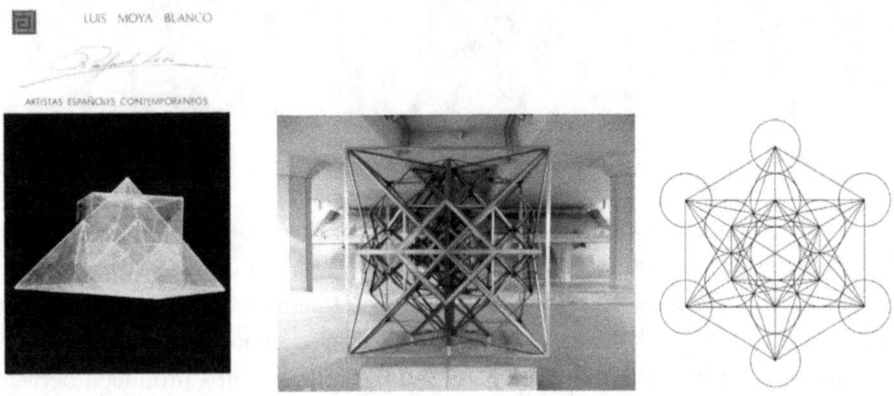

good dice. However, just as researcher Javer Sampedro points out, Frabetti also reminds us that the cube is not the only solution. He said, "There are four other polyhedrons that meet the same conditions and their faces are identical regular polygons that form the same angle. They are the tetrahedron (four equilateral triangles), the octahedron (eight equilateral triangles), the icosahedron (20 equilateral triangles) and the dodecahedron (12 regular pentagons). Together with the cube (six squares) they constitute the five platonic solids and the five perfect dice. There are no others and Euclid demonstrated this in his Elements. Plato was so fascinated with those five polyhedrons that he identified them with the elements that form the world," (Javier Sampedro in: June 2018: elpais.com)

It took two thousand years for the family of regular polyhedrons to grow and include four new members, which are the small stellated dodecahedron, the large stellated dodecahedron, the large dodecahedron and the large icosahedron non-convex regular polyhedron. The earliest known representation of the small stellated dodecahedron (Fig 13) is a mosaic by Paolo Ucello in St. Mark's Basilica, Venice, dated 1430. The four non-convex regular polyhedrons were rediscovered and studied by Kepler in the 16th century and then again by Louis Poinsot in the early 19th century, so they are called Kepler-Poinsot solids.

Leoz followed some of the geometric patterns and devised others that were undoubtedly exemplary for architects who came after him. Twenty years before the HELE module, Mies opened up an important avenue on housing and health. The premise was that housing should have the capacity to influence the overall environment of the landscape. It is, therefore, relevant to present in this investigation the architect's project called, *50x50* (Fig. 14) where, in his previous study, Avila Caro indicates that *"the transparency*

Figure 13. Image a: Moya. Image b: Moya. Image 3: Small stellated dodecahedron by Paolo Ucello in St. Mark's Basilica in Venice Source: Carlo Frabetti in: https://elpais.com/elpais/2018/06/28/ciencia/1530172242_068672.html

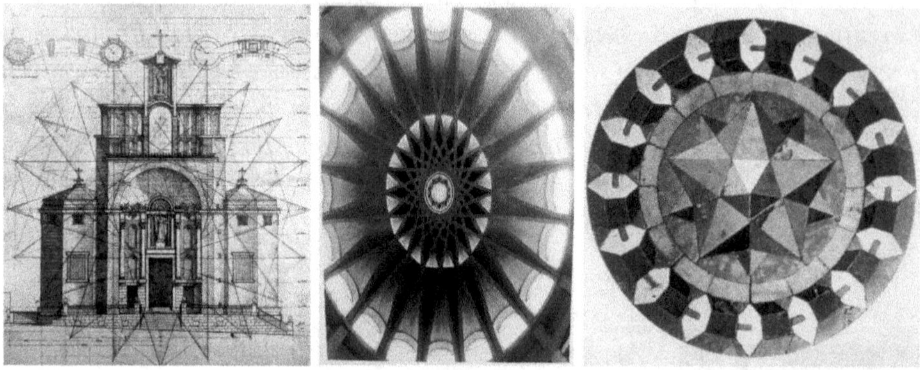

he uses in this project, as in many of his other buildings, works not only from the inside out, but from the outside in. The building is then incorporated into the site" (Avila Caro 2010).

In order to return to the concept of the "whole", it is important to also mention the work of Van Eyck (Fig.15), as Mayoral points out, "all are located in the same universe of values, where the choral and the cyclical replace the single thought; where the part, and the relationships produced between them, are as important as the whole .... a proposal of architectural thought, which from the tiny to the enormous, claims the multiple and the fragmentary .... In this project, the architect designs the exhibition strategy and the containing space, returning to some previously discussed concepts of intermediate space, the inside-outside relationship and the interaction between work, space and visitor as being integral parts of the same narrative. The proposed space investigates the concept of threshold, understood as a meeting place, through a series of longitudinal walls arranged in parallel and building a filter. A passing through place, emphasized by the interruption of the walls by cylindrical elements. Again the circle as a space of integration, a place to stop" (Mayoral 2014 p. 74.).

The figure of Van Eyck has been a reference in today's architecture causing one to reflect on the foundations of vernacular architecture. "Van Eyck aims to enter into direct contact with those primitive societies that still survive today. It is done in such a way that, beyond archaeological studies, it is possible to learn from the testimony and observation of these peoples' ways of life" (Fernández 2013).

Educational Innovation Applied to Healthy Interior Architecture in Relation to the Landscape

Comfort in the Interior Living Space According to its Geometry

The international pandemic caused by Covid-19 has been crucial in *awakening* people's appreciation of their home. As stated in the introduction, staying longer than necessary inside the house has meant a radical conceptual change of the interior spatial relationship with the exterior.

Also, in the introduction the term *home* instead of house was introduced as a starting point to establish some reflections. The term *home* in Spanish is *hogar* and its Latin root is *fogar,* which in Spanish is *fuego*

Figure 14. 50x50 Mies Van der Rohe House. Source: cavicaplace.blogspot.com

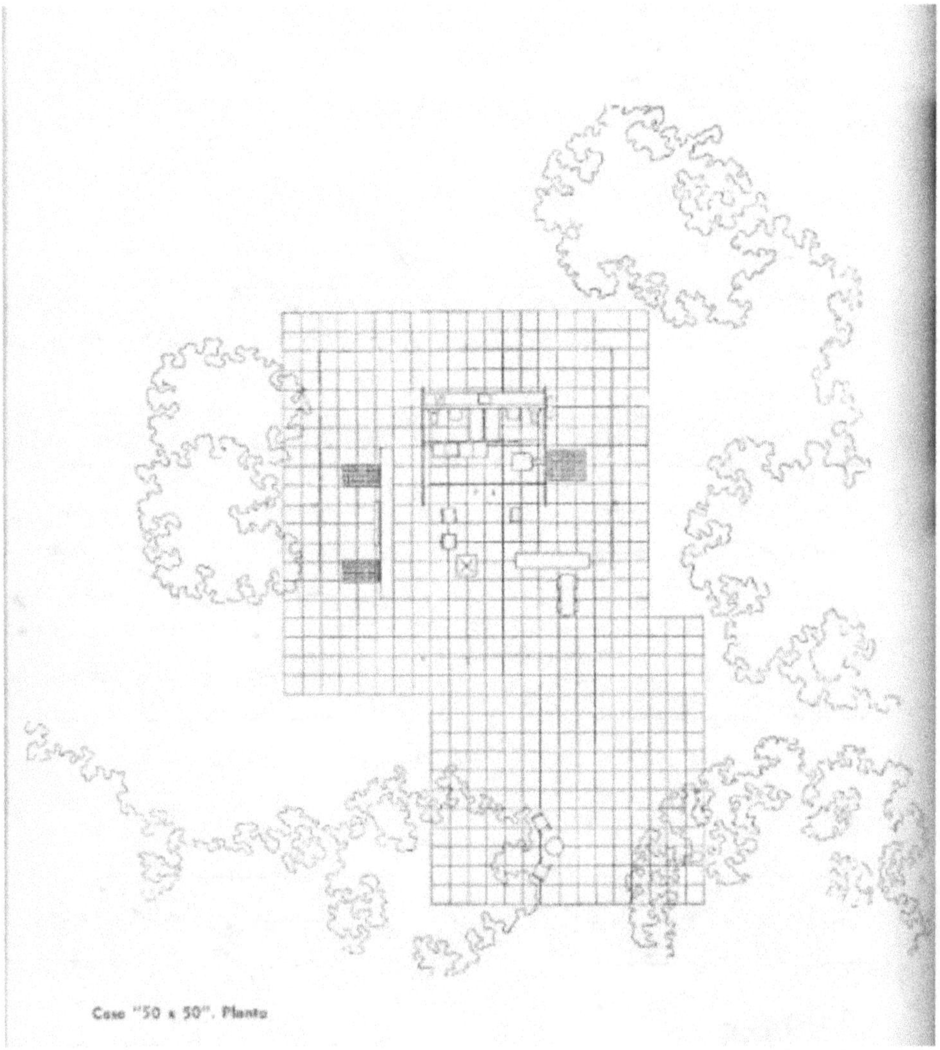

(in English *fire*), implies warmth given to the *hearth,* around which people gather to keep warm. Water, fire and air are vital elements in a home, as is the geometry applied to house them. Oriental feng shui works on the understanding of plans and the distribution of space inside the house in order to optimize well-being. It is, however, unthinkable to contemplate this concept in the West.

The awareness of space has led to a greater financial investment in items for the home, thus demanding more interior refurbishments.

Parallel to the concept of ergonomics is the concept of Universal Accessibility when it is integrated in the learning of the responsibilities acquired by an architect insofar as the interior or exterior space is to be designed as accessible to all. The motto *Design for All*[13] is a holistic and innovative approach, which constitutes an ethical and creative challenge for all designers, entrepreneurs, administrators and political leaders to optimize accessible and comfortable spaces.

Figure 15. Temporary pavillion. Sonsbeek by Van Eyck in Arnhem. Source: archiveofspace.tumblr.com

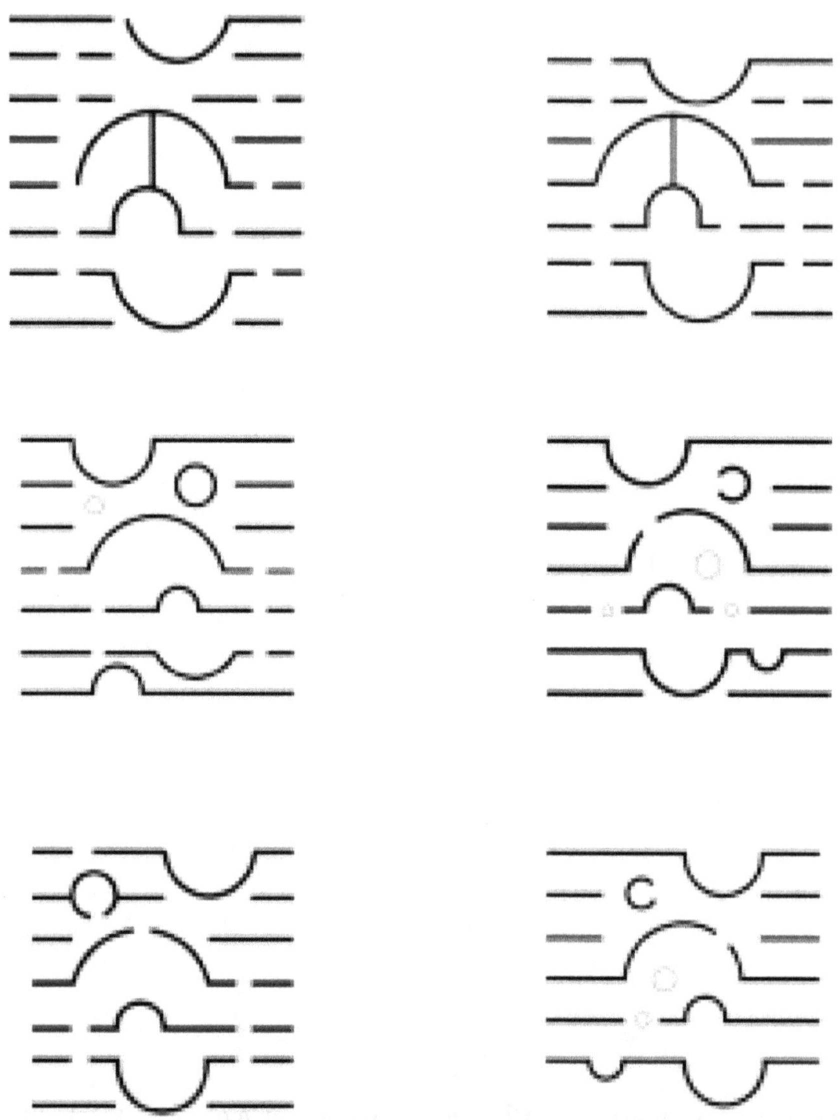

At present, students of the School of Architecture,[14] along with students with intellectual disabilities from the TP Consultant in Universal Accessibility[15] and educational psychologists from the University of Monterey, have worked together in a special evaluation of the interior of their own house. Although this activity has been part of an educational innovation experience, it was also inspired by the international lockdown.[16]

Relationship Between Interior Comfort and Exterior Perception. Landscape and Horizon Line

Since 2005, the concept of smart cities has burst into architecture and engineering schools in Spain. Researchers on the subject try to implement some theories about the intelligence of a city within the study of each specific case. In Madrid, a great change has taken place in the first twenty years of the twenty-first century: *"Madrid is a complex, historical city in terms of topography and orography as well as landscape and urban aspects. The architecture of Madrid, as in other cities with a concentration of historical heritage, is rich in language and culture and therefore its diversity makes this city a complicated area in which to intervene.*

Madrid's population has been growing in the outskirts of the city as well as upwards, as shown in the example of the Four Towers. This trend is changing northern Madrid's skyline. Urban planners of the nineteenth century already considered the scale of vegetation, the sun and shadows produced by surrounding plants in relation to their height and angle of projection on the buildings and the street" (Cantarero 2019) (Fig. 16).

Figure 16. Madrid skyline. The Four Towers built.
Source: https://www.expansion.com/empresas/inmobiliario

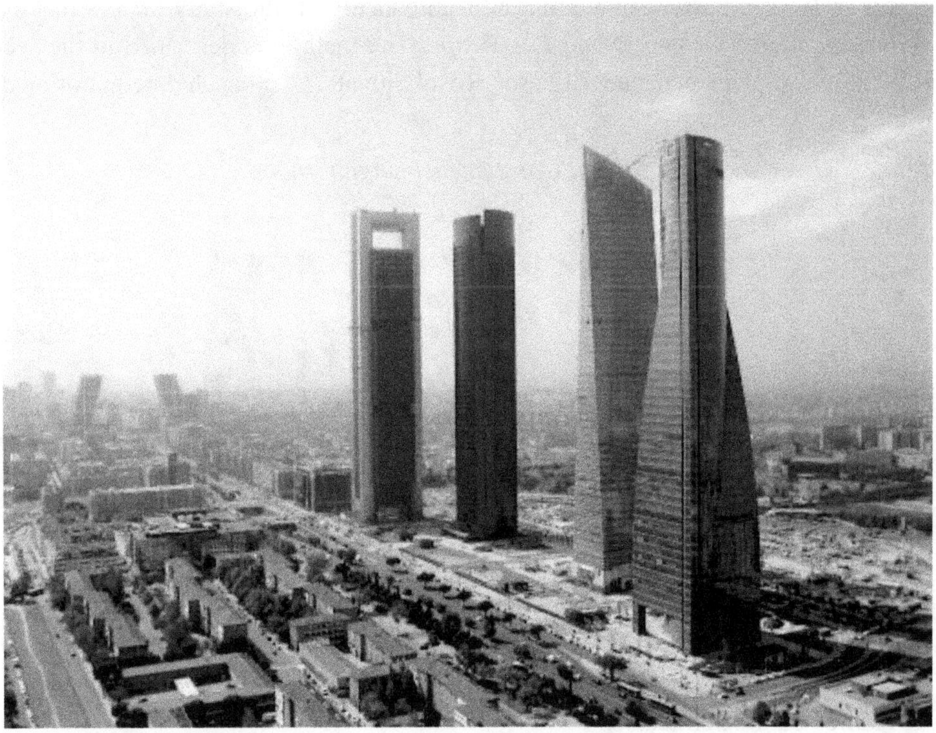

There is a common interest in offering citizens climatic as well as perceptive comfort. The city of Madrid is one of the most well-kept cities in terms of landscape and environment. The green belt defined by the countryside areas surrounding the capital protects the urban core from pollution. Projects in the southwest, such as the *Pasillo Verde Ferroviario* and *Madrid Rio*, have given the city a complete 180º change and, in the west, the *Casa de Campo* and *Monte de El Pardo* preserve the city's growth and its origins as the capital of Spain. Researchers from architecture and engineering schools are beginning to look more deeply into landscape and how it is essential to the citizen. The intelligence of a city is transmitted by the intelligence of its citizens. The concept of the "smart citizen"[17] as the main agent and deviser of the smart city is beginning to emerge rather than the other way around.

COVID -19 has undoubtedly led to reflections on the suitability of housing in the city, such as housing scale in relation to the number of dwellers and how basic, essential resources reach the people when they are unable to leave their homes. Following the lockdown experienced in Spain in 2020, Madrid was drastically affected by a snowstorm, which produced declared, catastrophic areas. Surprisingly, the flexible and adaptable nature of human beings demonstrated that their response to this new lockdown was better assumed because of the previous experience due to the pandemic. Also, the pandemic caused by COVID -19 has affected the real estate sector in terms of people relocating to the outskirts of the city.

The case study, which is presented below, analyzes a parallel comparison about tellurism, sacred geometry and health between two places in Madrid on the banks of the Manzanares river.

Case Study in Madrid: Royal Site of El Pardo and Carabanchel Neighborhood

In order to demonstrate a specific case of interior well-being in relation to the landscape, two different exterior contexts in Madrid have been studied in accordance with the study factors of this research, which are *Tellurism*, *Sacred Geometry* and *Landscape*. The method is described in the section titled *Work Method*. These two placements are El Pardo Royal Site and Carabanchel neighborhood (Fig.17).

Figure 17. Mar Océana Park El Pardo and Carabanchel neighborhood
Source: author's pictures

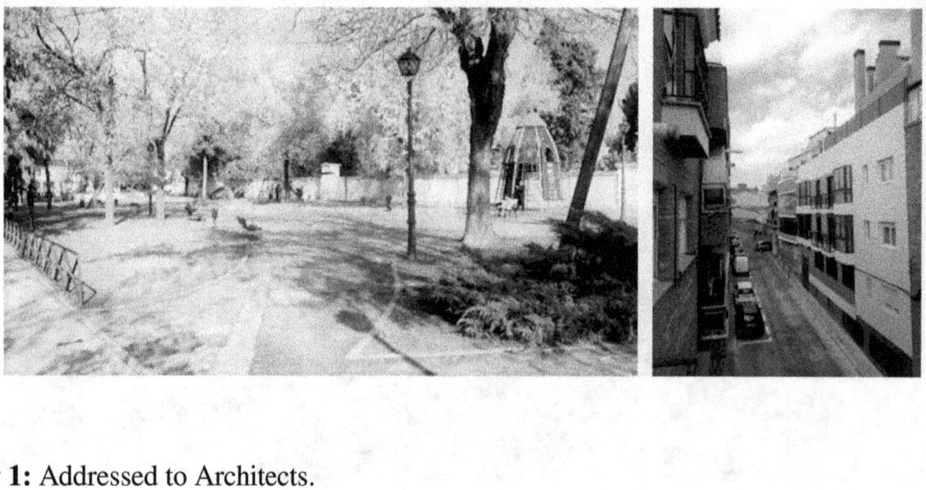

Survey 1: Addressed to Architects.
Survey 2: Addressed to citizens of El Pardo and citizens of the Carabanchel neighborhood.
Both surveys (1 and 2) include the following questions:

1. Gender: male / female/ prefer not to say

2. Age: 18-40/ 40-60/ more than 60
3. Do you know the term *Tellurism*? Yes/ no
4. Do you know the concept of *Sacred Geometry*? Yes/ no
5. Tellurism is "The influence of the soil and landscape of a region on its inhabitants' and Sacred Geometry refers to the geometric shapes that are present in the design of certain sites that are considered sacred. Do you think they should be taught in architecture degree programs? Yes/no
6. Why? It is not applicable/ it is not relevant/ it would be interesting.
7. Do you think it would be important to apply knowledge of these subjects in real projects? Yes/no/ maybe.
8. Do you think that the soil where your home is located affects your health? Yes/no/maybe.
9. In which sense? Subway or underground activity/ wells activity or water underground/ electric network/ earth ionization/ all previous answers/ none of them.
10. Do you think the Geometry or shape of your house affects your health? Yes/no/maybe.
11. Do you think that the height at which your home is located affects your health? Yes/no/maybe.
12. Do you think that the lack of natural light and vegetation affect your health? Yes/no/maybe.
13. Do you think that the sleep quality could depend on whether you have a water or electricity network close to your headboard? Yes/no/maybe.
14. Select the space-room in which you feel more comfortable at home. Living room/ bathroom/ bedroom/garden or terrace/ kitchen/another one.
15. During the COVID-19 quarantine, in which space/room of your home did you stay the longest? Living room/ bathroom/ bedroom/garden or terrace/ kitchen/another one.
16. Do you think the COVID-19 quarantine affected your health? Yes/no/maybe.
17. Evaluate how the quarantine could have affected to your health. Psychological health/ physical health/none of them/ both of them.
    a. SURVEY 2 include also these following questions:
18. Where do you prefer to live? El Pardo/ Carabanchel/ None of them/both of them
19. Do you feel happy living in your home? Yes/no/maybe

Surveys Results Analysis

- -In total a number of 87 people participated in these surveys.
- -Question Q1: shows the gender participation: 54% are women, 42% are men and 3,47% preferred not to say.
- -*Question Q2:* shows the average of age of people participating. 16% (18-40 years old), 62% (40-60 years old) and 22% (more than 60 years old).
- -Questions Q3 - Q19: Below is shown the results in terms of relevant percentages (table 1) according to questions 3 to 17 (SURVEYS 1 and 2) and questions 18 to 19 (SURVEY 1)
- Q3. 63% of architects, 35% in El Pardo and 62,50% in Carabanchel, know the term *Tellurism.*
- Q4. 45,45% of architects, 22,81% in El Pardo and 37,50% in Carabanchel, know the concept of *Sacred Geometry*
- Q5. 81,82% of architects, 100% in El Pardo and 87,50% in Carabanchel, think that these concepts should be taught in architecture degree programs
- Q6. 68,18% of architects, 71,93% in El Pardo and 62,50% in Carabanchel, think that it would be interesting.

Table 1. Results

	people interviewed	Question 3	Question 4	Question 5	Question 6	Question 7
Architects	22	63,64	45,45	81,82	68,18	59,09
El Pardo	57	35,09	22,81	100,00	71,93	82,46
Carabanchel	8	62,50	37,50	87,50	62,50	75,00

	people interviewed	Question 8	Question 9	Question 10	Question 11	Question 12	Question 13	Question 14	
Architects	22	68,18	72,73	68,18	59,09	95,45	50,00	31,82	living room/garden or terrace
El Pardo	57	78,95	52,63	54,39	68,42	91,23	52,63	56,14	
Carabanchel	8	62,50	62,50	75,00	62,50	100,00	37,50	62,50	

empate con maybe

	people interviewed	Question 15	Question 16	Question 17	
Architects	22	50,00	59,09	36,36	both
El Pardo	57	57,89	68,42	42,11	psychological health
Carabanchel	8	62,50	62,50	62,50	physical health

	people interviewed	Question 18	Question 19
El Pardo	57	96,49	85,96
Carabanchel	8	50,00	100,00

% percentage

- Q7. 59,09% of architects, 82,46% in El Pardo and 75% in Carabanchel, think that it would be important to apply knowledge of these subjects in real projects.
- Q8. 68,18% of architects, 78,95% in El Pardo and 62,50% in Carabanchel, think that the soil where their home is located affects their health and according to the next question:
- Q9. 72,73% of architects, 52,63% in El Pardo and 62,50% in Carabanchel, think that all previous answers (Subway or underground activity, wells activity or water underground, electric network and earth ionization) affects their health.
- Q10. 68,18% of architects, 54,39% in El Pardo and 75% in Carabanchel, think the Geometry or shape of their house affects their health.
- Q11. 59,09% of architects, 68,42% in El Pardo and 62,50% in Carabanchel, think that the height at which their home is located affects their health.
- Q12. 95,45% of architects, 91,23% in El Pardo and 100% in Carabanchel, think that the lack of natural light and vegetation affect their health.
- Q13. 50% of architects, 52,63% in El Pardo and 37,50% in Carabanchel, think that the sleep quality could depend on whether there is a water or electricity network close to their headboard.
- Q14. 31,82% of architects, 56,14% in El Pardo and 62,50% in Carabanchel, selected the living room as the space-room in which they feel more comfortable at home. It is remarkable that as well another 31,82% of architects selected the garden or terrace.
- Q15. 50% of architects, 57,89% in El Pardo and 62,50% in Carabanchel, selected the living room as the space/room in which they stay the longest during the COVID-19 quarantine.
- Q16. 59,09% of architects, 68,42% in El Pardo and 62,50% in Carabanchel think the COVID-19 quarantine affected their health.
- Q17. According to the evaluation about how the quarantine affected to their health, we could conclude that this last question is the one in which the results have been more varied:

36,36% of architects think that their psychological and physical health were affected, 42,11% in El Pardo the citizens think that their psychological health was affected and 62,50% in Carabanchel the citizens think that their physical health was affected.

SURVEY 2 include also these following questions:

Q18. 96,49% of El Pardo citizens prefer living in El Pardo and not in Carabanchel and 50% of Carabanchel citizens prefer living in Carabanchel.

Q19. 85,96% of El Pardo citizens and 100% of Carabanchel citizens feel happy living in their own homes.

DIRECTION OF FUTURE RESEARCH

The pandemic due to COVID-19 has generated an emotional shock in the citizen. The home has been taken as a refuge and we have seen ourselves investing a long time inside the house. New ways of living would imply new behaviors and therefore a new social and collective intelligence. It is then possible to speak of changing human ways of living and citizen intelligences.

As a result, lines of research that open up are:

- Creation of practical, multidisciplinary teams at the university level to combine health and architecture from scratch in the project
- Study of applied emotional understanding and the psychology of the citizen for architects
- Deepen the concepts of “architectural barriers” and “Universal Accessibility”

CONCLUSION

The introduction showed that one of the conclusions derived from this study is that the landscape is a determining element in the way a person lives within the interior space and it has direct repercussions on a person’s health.

To conclude, and according to the analysis of the surveys’ results, we may highlight the following appraisals:

Not every architects know about the concept of Tellurism (63%) and those who do not know what is it about do not think is relevant to include it in the Degree of Architecture studies but those who have heard about it find it very interesting to introduce it not just in the Degree courses (81,82%) but also in real projects. (59,09%). The concept of Sacred Geometry is even less known in general (architects and citizens)

More than an 87,50% of citizens think that these concepts should be taught in Architecture Degree programs.

More than a 62% of people think that the soil where their home is located affects their health and, according to this question, more than a 52% of people think that all these factors affect to their health: ‘The subway or underground activity, the wells activity or water underground, the electric network and the earth ionization’. As well, this same percentage of people think that the height at which their home is located affects their health. Less than a 45% of citizens think the sleep quality could depend on whether there is a water or electricity network close to their headboard, although architects are are more receptive to this affection.

Which is remarkable is that more than a 54% of people (architects and/ or citizens) are concerned about the Geometry or shape of their house and believe that it affects their health.

As well we point up in these research that the highest punctuation is for the light and natural landscape. More than a 90% of people support that a lack of natural light and vegetation affect their health. In general terms, this study asserts that citizens feel happy living in their own homes and this has been demonstrated by the resulted average (over the 90%), although the 50% of Carabanchel citizens would like to live in other places (due overall to environmental and acoustic contamination).

According to the quarantine due to COVID-19 2020 pandemic we could highlight that:

More than a 56% of people selected the living room as the space-room in which they felt more comfortable during the lockdown and this was the same lounge in which they stayed the longest

More than a 60% of people believes the COVID-19 quarantine affected their health and we underline that this last question is the most varied one in terms of results.

architects determined that their psychological and physical health were affected, El Pardo citizens confirmed it was their psychological health that was affected the most and finally Carabanchel citizens suffered a physical impact more than a psychological impact. This last appreciations makes us stablish some reflexions about the different indoor and outdoor factors thar could impact in our life.

As architects and researchers of the natural and urban environment, we are concerned about our health. We need to intervene by understanding people behavior and social responses to critical situations such as the current COVID-19 pandemic that is affecting the entire society. An international problem that not only concerns doctors but also all the intervening actors involved in helping to improve the citizen's situation in terms of global well-being.

New technologies have helped to facilitate the continuity of work activity inside the home. However, other mobility factors have seriously damaged the physical and psychological health of the citizen.

Although we had advanced in the implementation and development of the *Smart City* concept, we have realized that there is still a lot to do in the field of health and human well-being linked to the city itself. *Smart cities* continue to be projected as an ideal that needs to be met. In other words, the goal is to meet the desires of a changing and sometimes chaotic society by trying to submit to an artificial planimetric order that plays against the unforeseen and creates anxiety about what is to come, which when looked at through the positive eye of a human, will always be better.

Technologies help but there are other factors that go unnoticed and that are still there. We do not pay enough attention to them and we do not give them the importance they could have when projecting, but this study shows that if we inquire and consult citizens and architects, we are all interested in the analysis of the placement, the soil and the terrain in which we live as well as the geometry of our home. A low percentage of people has been reluctant or negative when it comes to stating that these concepts (discussed in here) can affect health.

ACKNOWLEDGMENT

This research is part of the financed project, "El paisaje periurbano de Madrid: visiones desde la memoria hacia la nueva ciudad", translated into English as "The Peri-Urban Landscape in Madrid: Visions from Memory to the New City" (financed by "el Ministerio de Ciencia e Innovación en la convocatoria 2019 Proyectos de I+D+i - RTI Tipo B." Translated into English as, "Ministry of Science and Innovation of Spain, code PID2019-110693RB-100)."

For the part of the study related to Universal Accessibility, we had the participation of students from international COIL.[18] This was a teaching innovation project from October to December 2020. Students studying for a degree in Universal Accessibility taught at the Universidad San Pablo CEU Madrid have also participated in this project.

This research has been translated by Diana Claveria (Architect from the University of Westminster, London, RIBA member and translator: www.dyfconsultants.com)

REFERENCES

Arnheim, R. (1954). Art and visual perception, second edition: A psychology of the creative eye. Arte y percepción visual. Psicología del ojo creador. Editorial Eudeba.

Moya Blanco, L. (1978). Artistas españoles contemporáneos. In *Artistas Españoles Contemporáneos*. Centro de Publicaciones. Ministerio de Educación y Ciencia.

Cantarero-García, G. (2018). Reflexiones urbanísticas. Referencias del pasado y situación actual de Madrid como ciudad inteligente potencial. In Gestión inteligente y sostenible de las ciudades. Gobernanza, smart cities y turismo. Valencia: Ed Tirant lo Blanch.

García, Á., Luis, J., Marquina, J. E., & Sanz, R. (1993). La esfera y el círculo en la historia. Ciencias, 30, 2-9.

Ghyka, M. (1983). *Esthétique des proportions dans la natue et dans les arts. Estética de las proporciones en la naturaleza y en las artes*. Editorial Poseidón.

Gombrich, E. (1982) *The Image and the eye. Furher studies in the Psichology of Pictorical representation.* Phaidon Press Limited.

González Capitel, A., & García-Gutiérrez Mosteiro, J. (2000). *Luis Moya Blanco. Arquitecto 1904-1990.* Ministerio de Fomento y Editorial Electa.

Heller, H., & Schiele, E. (1913). *Proportionstafeln der menschlichen gestalt: für kunstwerkstätten und fachschulen*. Editorial Kunstverlag Anton Schroll & Co.

Rasmussen, S. E. (1957). Om at opleve arkitektur. GEC Gads Forlag.

Ware, D., & Beatty, B. (1998). *Diccionario manual ilustrado de arquitectura*. Editorial Gustavo Gili.

ADDITIONAL READING

Boesiger, W. (1992). *Le Corbusier works and projects*. Editorial Gustavo Gili.

Coca, J., & Fernández, F. (2011). La Renovación del Manzanares: Transformaciones y Reciclajes Urbanos. *Proyecto, Progreso, Arquitectura*, *4*, 88–105.

KEY TERMS AND DEFINITIONS

Accessibility: The ability to access and benefit from a system or entity. The concept focuses on enabling access for people with disabilities or special needs.

Architecture: Knowledge of art, science, technology, and humanity. A general term used to describe buildings and other physical structures. The design activity performed by an architect.

Sacred Geometry: Refers to the geometric shapes that are present in the design of certain sites considered sacred.

Smart City: An urban area that uses different types of electronic Internet of things (IoT) such as sensors to collect data and use of insights gained from that data to efficiently manage assets, resources and services.

Social Intelligence: The capacity to know oneself and to know others. Social intelligence develops from experience with people and learning from successes and failures in social settings. It is more commonly referred to as "tact," "common sense," or "street smarts."

Tellurism: Refers to the earth and how it behaves above and below the surface.

Urban Landscape: Everything you can see when you look across an area of land, including buildings, bridges, and structures.

Urbanism: The study of how inhabitants use urban areas, such as towns and cities, and how they interact with the built environment. It is a direct component of disciplines, such as urban planning, which is a profession that focuses on the physical design and management of urban structures and urban sociology or the academic field of the study of urban life and culture.

ENDNOTES

1 A project financed by FONCE and the European Social Fund

2 A theory of everything (TOE or ToE), *final theory*, *ultimate theory* or *master theory* is a hypothetical, single, all-encompassing, coherent theoretical framework of physics that fully explains and links together all physical aspects of the universe. In: https://en.wikipedia.org/wiki/Theory_of_everything.

3 Aristóteles, De Motu, citado en I. Düring, 1987, Aristóteles. Exposición e interpretación de su pensamiento, UNAM, México, p. 571.

4 Nine vases were framed by static rectangles and the fluctuation range was 1 mm maximum.

5 Tellurium is a chemical element with the symbol Te and atomic number 52. It is a brittle, mildly toxic, rare, silver-white metalloid. Tellurium is chemically related to selenium and sulfur, all three of which are chalcogens. https://en.wikipedia.org/wiki/Tellurium

6 The supposed influence of emanations from the soil in producing disease en: https://en.wiktionary.org/wiki/tellurism

7 Dowsing is a pseudoscientific activity based on the claim that electrical, electromagnetic, magnetism and radiation stimuli from an emitting body can be perceived and sometimes handled by a person by means of simple artifacts held in unstable suspension such as a pendulum, L-shaped or Y-shaped rods that supposedly amplify the magnetoreception capacity of the human being. https://es.wikipedia.org/wiki/Radiestesia

8 A dowser is someone who claims to be able to detect changes in electromagnetism through the spontaneous movement of simple devices held in their hands, usually a Y-shaped or L-shaped wooden or metal rod or a pendulum. Dowsers claim to be able to detect the existence of magnetic fluxes or ley lines. https://es.wikipedia.org/wiki/Radiestesia

9 In Archivo Histórico Nacional. *Inq. Leg. 3735/394*

10 With the reference ZEPA ES0000011.

11 It is associated with the belief that a God is the geometer of the world. The geometry used in the design and construction of religious structures such as churches, temples, mosques, religious monuments, altars, and tabernacles has sometimes been considered sacred. The concept applies also to sacred spaces such as temenoi, sacred groves, village greens, pagodas and holy wells, and the creation of religious art. https://en.wikipedia.org/wiki/Sacred_geometry

12 Rafael Leoz's HELE Module is only one of the first phases of a theoretical system of division and arrangement of architectural space through geometric principles. In: López Díaz, Jesús: https://revistas.unav.edu/index.php/revista-de-arquitectura/article/view/1916/1783 3

13 EIDD. Declaration of Stockholm, 2004. El Diseño para Todos: http://www.xn--diseoparatodos-tnb.es/Documentacion/bibliografia/Paginas/urbanos.aspx

14 San Pablo CEU University in Madrid (Spain)

15 A project financed by FONCE and the European Social Fund

16 The lockdown took place between March and May, 2020 in Spain and throughout the autumn in Mexico.

17 Smart Citizen EPS CEU Projects. PhD. Guadalupe Cantarero-García (Director)

18 Monterrey University (México) and San Pablo CEU University Madrid (España)

Chapter 11
Sustainable Design for a Functional Reeducation of Senior Citizens About the Basic Activities of Daily Living

Omar Eduardo Omar Sánchez Estrada
Universidad Autónoma del Estado de México, Mexico

ABSTRACT

Developing useful objects for a functional reeducation of senior citizens persons about the basic activities of daily living must be conceptualized considering theories, techniques, and approaches in methodology, based on ecologically bearable structures, economically viable, and socially equitable. Consequently, the present chapter has the objective to state the criteria and strategies of a sustainable design, from a detailed study of applicability of 1) user-product interaction, observation, understanding, dimensional relationship, and evaluation; 2) creative process, identification, ideation, definition, prototypes, evaluation, and structuration; 3) technical specifications, structure, sustainability, ergonomics, aesthetics, and evaluation; 4) manufacture method, sustainability, production method, life cycle, capital assets, official norms, and optimization. A contextual and conceptual analysis is proposed for the beginning, development, and conclusion of the projects so as to reestablish the relationship between natural processes and human activity.

INTRODUCTION

The world contingency derived from Covid-19 has an important number of people around the planet worried, which means a loss of energy, focus and time in the activities carried out daily. The World Health Organization (WHO) states that it is normal to feel sad, stressed, confused, scared or angry throughout a crisis; so it is necessary to keep a healthy lifestyle. In the other hand, the Pan American Health Organization (PAHO) recommends to keep active at home, with correct postures and standing up constantly from the working area; likewise to join virtual classes of physical exercises or muscle force training and

DOI: 10.4018/978-1-7998-7279-5.ch011

balance. Therefore, the activities of daily living are those that are necessary and have a specific purpose for one person, which are important in order to have autonomy and physical and mental health.

At the end of the sixties, the activities of daily living (ADL) concept arose. These activities are one part of the assessment instruments of functional capacity, which can be identified for being all the tasks a person must carry out in order to live comfortably: mobility, feeding, personal hygiene and clothing. For Cipriani, Danti, Picchi, Nuti and Fiorino (2020), performing basic activities depends on the integrity of different functions: cognitive such as reasoning, planning; motor function, balance, skills; and perceptive, including sensorial functions. In 1984, the WHO established the term *senior citizen* in order to make reference to 60-year-old people or older; also in 1996, the UN names this part of the population as a group of older persons according to the WHO's statistics. This group of people is rapidly growing and it is estimated that by year 2050 there will be 2000 million senior citizens, which means that one out of every four people will be older than 60 years; therefore, a senior citizen is not necessarily followed by limitations in terms of mobility and social isolation.

Equally important for developing new products with a sustainable design, it is significant to analyze the relationship among material, energy and human resources as they have been progressively transformed by the prevailing economic system. Industrial production and its impact on the ecosystem increase in a disproportionate manner. Thus it is essential to reconsider methods that validate growth and development from environmental issues derived from them. It is important to mention that in the nineties, a significant link between environmental topic and industrial production arouse after controversies and agreements with a political and normative nature during the eighties; and after the experience during that time, it was shown that the environmental impact products could have once they are introduced to the market require to be conceived and projected based on sustainability (Barbero and Cozzo, 2009). Design as a discipline plays an important role within the development of new processes and creative products, it is a strategical area that promotes and creates scenarios under a determined environment, where users carry out their activities. Design is focused on planning and creating objects that integrate knowledge from many areas and different disciplines in such a way that processes, methods, techniques or objects fulfill their primary role (why they were created for) within a system of psychological, aesthetics, economic and productive values, among others that improve human life, through natural energy flows and understanding of the design's limitations and effects, always insisting on human rights and coexistence in healthy, supportive, diverse and sustainable conditions.

BACKGROUND

Nowadays, sustainability is an imperative issue when doing a research. Studies on the subject of humanity's global path show that resources equivalent to a planet and a half, have been overexploited (WWF, 2016). Johan Rockstrom and his research team have concluded that sustainable and safe life in the world is in danger, as the four planetary limits have been surpassed (climate change, nitrogen and phosphorus cycles, biodiversity and land-use change) and two more are getting close to their limits (Rockstrom et al., 2009; Steffen et al., 2015). It is important to highlight that for six decades now, when the "sustainable development" concept was recognized (Carson,1992; Hardin,1968), established measures and efforts have not been enough in order to achieve a favorable balance among environmental, economic, political, cultural and social issues. Therefore, the United Nations developed an agenda based on specific objectives that integrate actions for social development, environmental care and economic growth among others

(United Nations, 2015). In light of this global situation, design must reconsider any possible proposal to develop products and businesses from the first stages.

The sustainable design theory promotes rethinking organizational and productive development for any specific need. However, it has been shown that implementing new procedures based on sustainability deliver different problems that require concrete actions. Creating new products drawn from design and their purest conceptual structure must rethink productive processes, and even more how their businesses are created (Dobers and Strannegard, 2005). According to Simon (1968) "sustainable design" is a structured process to create something new based on rational design. For Sroufe and Curkovic (2000), developing products by means of a special attention to environmental aspects is a core subject, the same way in which the disassembling design must appear from the beginning of the project (Das and Naik, 2002).

Also, the design's life cycle analysis and useful life optimization are part of the objective (Heidrich and Tiwary, 2013). Under such terms, a product's sustainability is generally approached by possible reachable economic factors or characteristics that will allow positioning it before its competition. In view of this, it is necessary for corporations to authentically adopt a productive philosophy based on endurable structures in ecological terms, as well as being socially equitable so as to balance shared attributes and values for interested parties. Businessmen affirm that sustainable products prevent and reduce risks related to their development. From a social approach, they support sustainable development and improve social conditions (Dyllick and Rost, 2017). For Wang, Modi and Schoenherr (2021), teamwork with experienced suppliers guarantees profitability and enables environmental management of new products. In the other hand, the 2017 International Conference on Engineering Design (ICED) carried out at the University of British Columbia gathered different researchers in order to discuss challenges, opportunities and directions of sustainable design, and the community concluded the following: a) to create solid databases to support future research; b) to reach a consensus about the most favorable methods for developing products; c) to determine and improve easiness when using and applying tools; and d) to publish case studies and strategies in popular and open access media. Thus, sustainable design for functional reeducation in the "*Basic Activities of Daily Living*" (BADL) must start with authenticity and ethical compromise of its procedures.

Functional reeducation in the BADLs has a favorable impact in life quality, functions and independence of senior citizens. Some studies relate disability when carrying out the BADLs to biological, psychological and social factors (Liu et al. 2014). It is worth noting that *multimorbidity,* which is defined with more frequency as a coexistence of at least three chronic affections over a period of approximately one year, significantly increases with aging (Moussavi et al. 2007). Therefore, around 10% of senior citizens who live independently develop a new dependency in more than one BADL (Katz et al. 1983), functional dependency derives from cardiac illnesses, nervous system illnesses, chronic musculoskeletal injuries, low income and minimal education among others (Mor et al. 1989). Also, simple tests on physical performance deliver a direct association to functional dependency (Gill et al. 1995).

METHOD

This current research has a descriptive nature and it considers implementing sustainable design must depart from: general process necessities being identified, the current state of research and practice, in order to closely integrate conventional products design and their development according to functional reeducation in the BADLs; and then, developing the ergonomic intervention with a global approach on natural resources conservation, strengthening a balanced social evolution and long-lasting and sustainable procedures. This research was based on interviews and a questionnaire given to teachers at the Autonomous University of Chapingo (UACH) in Mexico (ages 60 -75). The origins were mainly from Mexico (95%), but also some from other countries such as Germany and Chile (5%). The main objective was focused on determining criteria and objectives from the ergonomic intervention stages, using sequences and parameters of sustainable design, so as to create an improved environment and to adapt products according to physical, cognitive and functional reeducation needs.

Ergonomics, Functional Reeducation for BADL

Functional reeducation of the BADLs requires design contributions, evaluations aimed at tasks, compatibility analysis and ergonomic studies in order to find an answer to the needs, abilities and limitations of senior citizens. Application of ergonomics allows to define factors that take place in the user-device interrelation, affected by the environment, through reciprocity in order to reach better performance, adapting the object to qualities for its management and communication.

Security, comfort and efficiency are requirements for the main space in senior citizens' lives. From and architectural point of view, physical space has a direct relationship with dimensions and movements that take place; general standards are the basis to comply with minimal admissible regulations, and initial

Figure 1. Ergonomic intervention phases
Source: Own elaboration

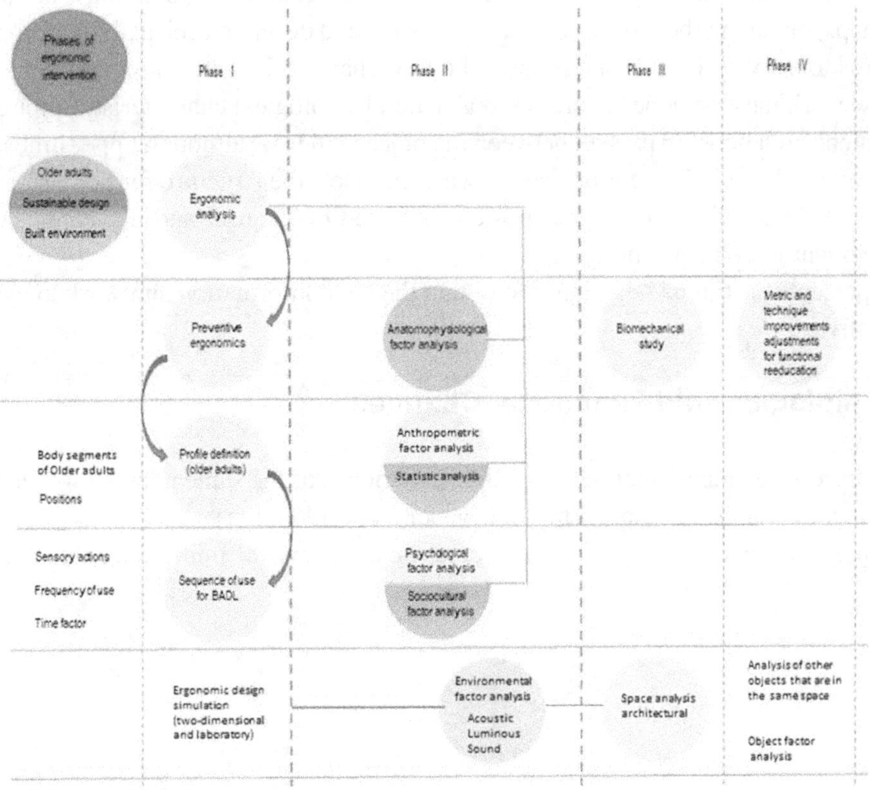

attention of such basic criteria allows the designer to project with coherence, pertinence and objectivity in subjects of applied biomechanics to the BADLs; likewise, working towards a built environment, joining physical material components and surrounding furniture (beds, chairs, support objects, toilets, etc.) in order to improve a specific area of functional mobility in the BADLs and not just to make it adequate. Another condition previous to sustainability and interactive adaptation with products is the one established with useful objects appropriation as experienced by senior citizens (Borjesson, 2008). Meanwhile, in order to identify problems with interactions it is necessary for the object that works as a simulator to be precise in its general structure, the reason is to avoid falling into mistakes previously experienced, besides establishing functional alteration points to know exactly what elements are affecting the use sequences. Therefore, applied ergonomics determine the understanding and development of different interactions that take place in a built environment, both physically and psychologically, which work as a tool to understand physical and emotional reactions. Figure 1 presents the ergonomic intervention components.

Once the activity concluded, a critical and objective evaluation of different BADLs is carried out in order to locate any incorrect interface among senior citizens, object and environmental factors. In table 1, concepts and how they can be structured are proposed so as to make a sequence of use.

Analysis of the Anatomophysiological Factor of Senior Citizens

In a biological aspect, molecular and cellular damages are associated to aging, gradually reducing physiological strength and increasing the risk for illnesses and their functional capacity (WHO, 2016). In this stage a body segment is identified and it intervenes in every sequence of use, a graphic report (photographs) facilitates an analysis of postures and movements, the photos must be taken using the three body maps, obtaining the most information possible and defining each activity according to cycles and work turns, observing if each one is carried out or characterized by strength, precision, repetition or mixed. The work must be done according to general physiological characteristics, for example when there is a sequence relationship present between the object and legs, although upper limbs are important they are secondary. In table 2, the proposal shown comprises: the structure for body segments analysis that intervene in the activity is proposed, postures adopted by the user and movements carried out by each body segment in every position.

Figure 2 presents the three body planes to obtain the most information and work in cycles and work shifts each activity.

Body, Physiological and Functional Changes

Aging is a progressive process that not all people experience at the same pace; however, physiological and body changes do not stop. Table 3 presents general considerations.

Figure 3 presents the frequency analysis to determine the level of importance that older adults gave to BADLs.

Table 1. Proposal for the development of ergonomic intervention in the sequence of use

Sequence of use			
Observation of the basic activities of daily life	**Description of the activity**	**Time / activity**	**Photographic evidence**
Functional mobility			
Ability to move from one position to another			
Care of assistive devices			
Eat and feed			
Sit up			
Handling objects for eating			
Elementary personal care			
Take a shower			
Dress			
Self care- (evacuation)			
Personal hygiene			
Personal cleanliness			
Daily rest			
Sleep			
Hygiene in the toilet			
Basic activities			
Intimate activities			
Individual activity			
Couple activity			
Total No.		Total time.	

Source: Own elaboration

Table 2. Activity by cycles and by work shift

Anatomophysiological factor				
Step	**Body Segment**	**Position**	**Movement**	**Method application**
1				RULA, OWAS ETC.
2				

Source: Own elaboration

Importance level

1. Functional mobility
2. Eat and feed
3. Daily rest
4. Hygiene in the toilet

5. Personal higiene
6. Elementary personal care
7. Intimate activities

Figure 2.
Source: Three body planes based on applied ergonomics (Cruz and Garnica, 2011)

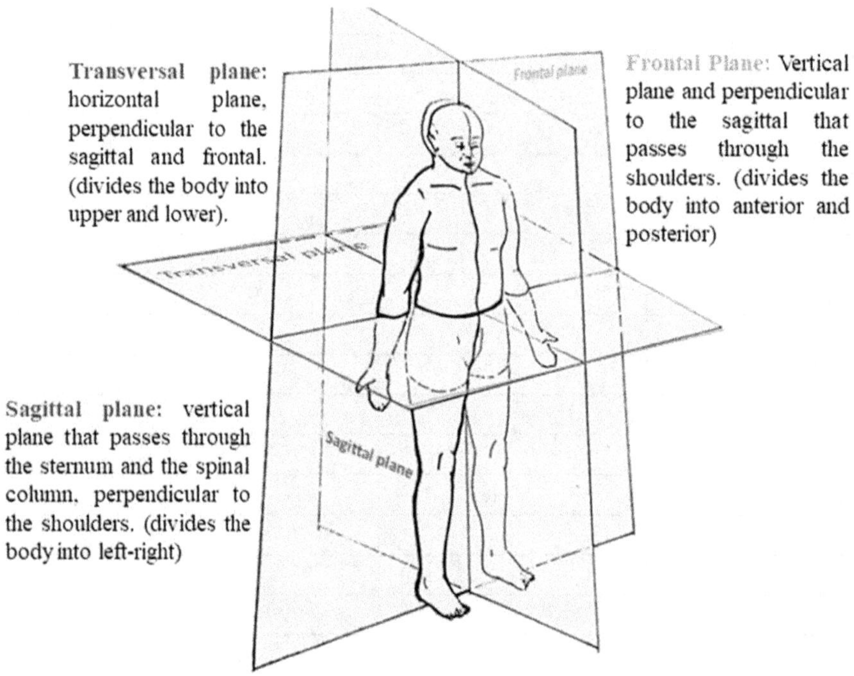

Table 3. Changes in body composition

Body composition			
Reduction of muscle mass	Affectation	Men	Woman
	Increase in fat mass (kidneys, liver, etc.) compared to the adult stage	18% adult male 36% in the elderly	33% adult women 45% in the elderly
	Decrease in total body water; increases the tendency or risk of dehydration		
	Decrease in bone mass; increased risk of fractures and osteoporosis, especially in women		
Physiological and functional modifications	Loss of jaw muscle strength and chewing power; less power to grind food		
Partial loss of sensory abilities: smell, taste, vision and hearing			

Source: Physiological characteristics of aging, based on (Eroski Consumer, 2021)

Figure 3. Frequency analysis
Source: Own elaboration

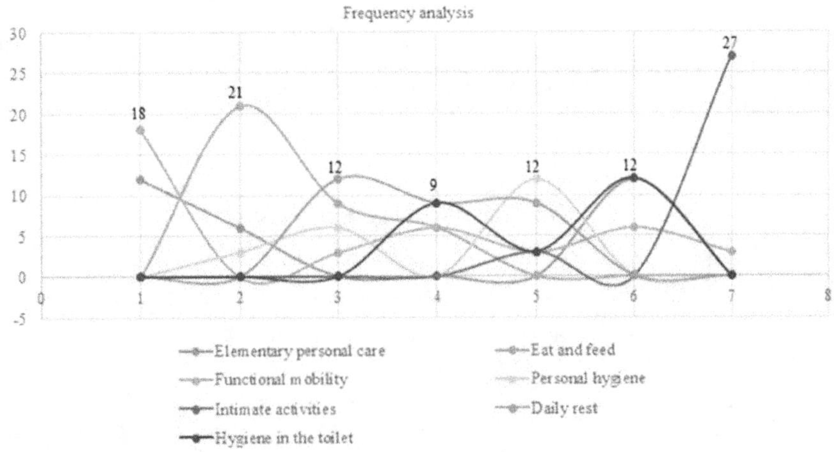

Figure 4. The level of importance for the attention of the BADLs
Source: Own elaboration

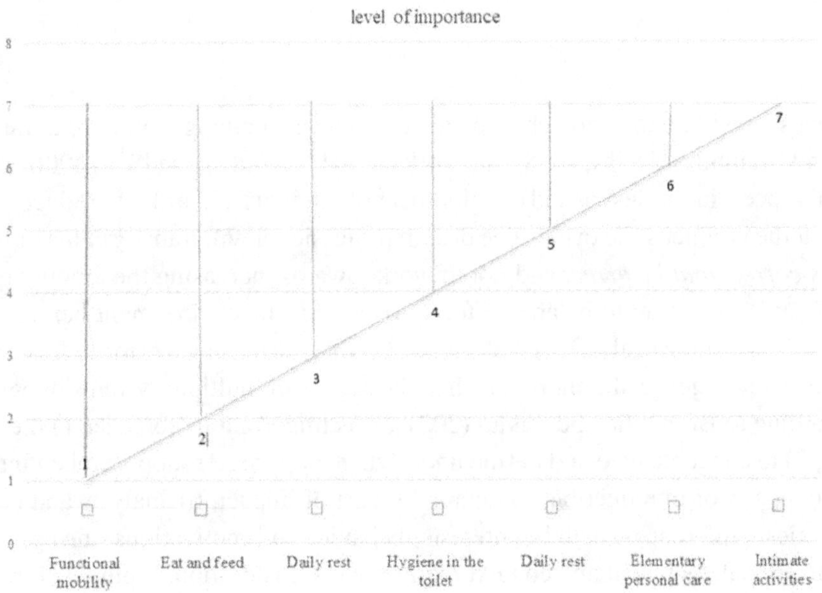

For Sustainable Design

Reassessment of production lines and all technical, normative and environmental factors are required in order to interpret and apply the four approaches of a sustainable design: eco-design, product service system design, sustainable business model design and collaborative business design. Figure 5 presents the interrelation.

Figure 5. Design approaches for sustainable innovation
Source: Design approaches to sustainable innovation based on the work of (Adams, Jeanrenaud, Bessant, Denyer y Overy, 2016; Ceschin y Gaziulusoy, 2016)

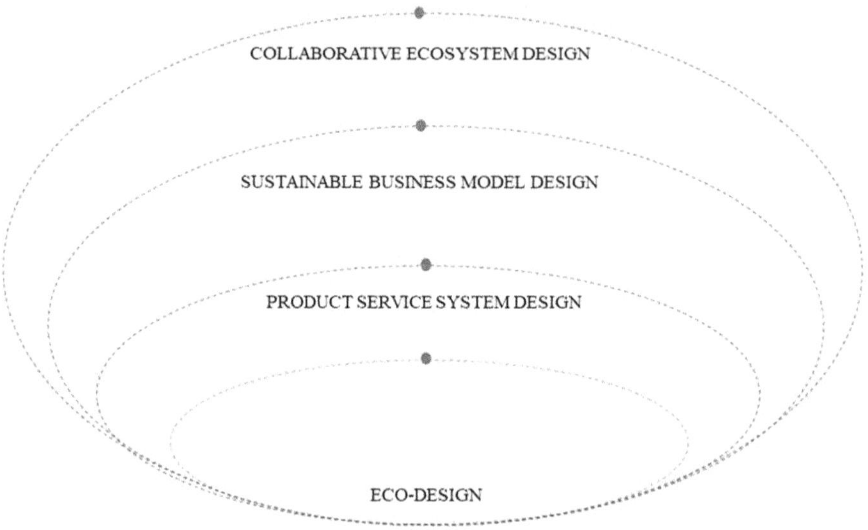

Eco-Design

The designer's first step will be to approach a social challenge, something similar to a transdisciplinary research (Sakao and Brambila-Macias, 2018), the work has to be based on the ISO 14006 norm "integrating environmental aspects in the design and development of products", in order to reduce environmental impacts throughout the product's life cycle. The design professional will transform his or her practice to understand *what's correct and incorrect* and not to work towards increasing the amount of tools (Boks and Stevels, 2007), it is important to balance efforts, to care for the environment before security, cost, quality and legality (Poulikidou et al. 2014), besides others that are usually a priority for developers such as a product's built-in intelligence, the short launch to the market or multiple systems integration (Albers et al. 2017). According to Brambilla and Sakao (2021), it is important to consider 1) the specific need of senior citizens, 2) to conceptualize and define underlying supports, 3) support taken into practice, 4) theoretical-practical basis of introduction, 5) detailed report of impact, 6) analysis and comparative of efficiency, 7) abilities, preferences, beliefs, interests, behavior and motivations during user's use, and 8) previous organizational, technical and context requirements. In addition, Figure 3 shows the support system proposal when making decisions in an eco-design process, based on the ISO 14062 norm.

Product-Service-System-Design

In this section, the objective is based on reaching a balanced development among tangible products and intangible services; this focus opens up the possibility to generate new strategies and market opportunities, increase competitiveness, consolidate the relationship with different clients and to promote obstacles for the entry of new competitors (Emili et al., 2016). Likewise, it is possible to reduce resource consumption and material use, leading to more efficiency in the use and longevity of a product (Kristensen and Remmen, 2019); moreover a network is created (co-production of value) among parties in order to provide with solutions for clients (Vezzoli et al. 2015). It must be added that it is necessary to strengthen the commercial perspective, including suppliers, changing the organization's mission and vision and accelerating implication with clients (Baines et al. 2007).

Sustainable Business Model Design

The objective is to lead and interconnect business products, services and strategies to redefine the established business model, presenting financial, environmental and social results; as the designer is considered to be a creating mind, he or she can make the clients connect their needs and dreams to new opportunities, science, technology and businesses (Esslinger, 2011). In the other hand, circular economy works as a business model, based on three principles: reduce, recycle and reuse materials (Pearce and Turner, 1990) considering a circular system where materials are recycled, applied energies are renewable, activities have a support character and rebuilding human needs and resources is used to create value (Zhu and Qiu, 2007).

Collaborative Ecosystem Design

Generating collaborations among companies in order to promote remodeling the market towards a sustainable global structure, working in favor of a systemic transformation in all economic, technological, institutional, organizational and sociocultural levels (Gaziulusoy et al. 2013), interdependency among diverse collaborating networks, as well as group participation among successful organizations for business models and those that have critical problems to be successful. Macro-model initiatives have been put to the test to show their viability according to environmental benefits, besides designing principles for circular ecosystems innovation, which reveal a timelessness problem when a structured trial and error process is carried out, it only reveals that the sustainable design theory connects with business models concepts, beyond companies' historic economic background and decontextualized models (Konietzko et al. 2020).

Therefore, projects can consider the following:

- Manufacture of support products for BADLs must start with a wide knowledge of the product's life-cycle, eco-design, energy efficiency and materials.
- Any producible design concept for functional reeducation must be tackled initially from environmental, economic, social and cultural sustainability throughout the product's life-cycle.
- Defining BADLs to implement sustainable manufacturing in every main phase of the life-cycle, considering multiple decisions that must be made during the design process and product development.
- Considering functional similarities of the BADLs from the project's first stages to include ecological suppliers, clients and consumers.
- To apply eco-design techniques and life-cycle analysis in order to predict evolution patterns of environments built in the conceptualization stage of support products for functional reeducation of senior citizens in their BADLs.
- Implementing support systems for decision making, based on sustainable manufacture concepts in order to make quantitative comparisons.

Figure 6 proposes a development based on the points set out above.

Figure 6. Comprehensive method, eco-design of products for functional reeducation in the BADLs
Source: Method developed based on the International Organization for Standardization. (2002). ISO / TR 14062.

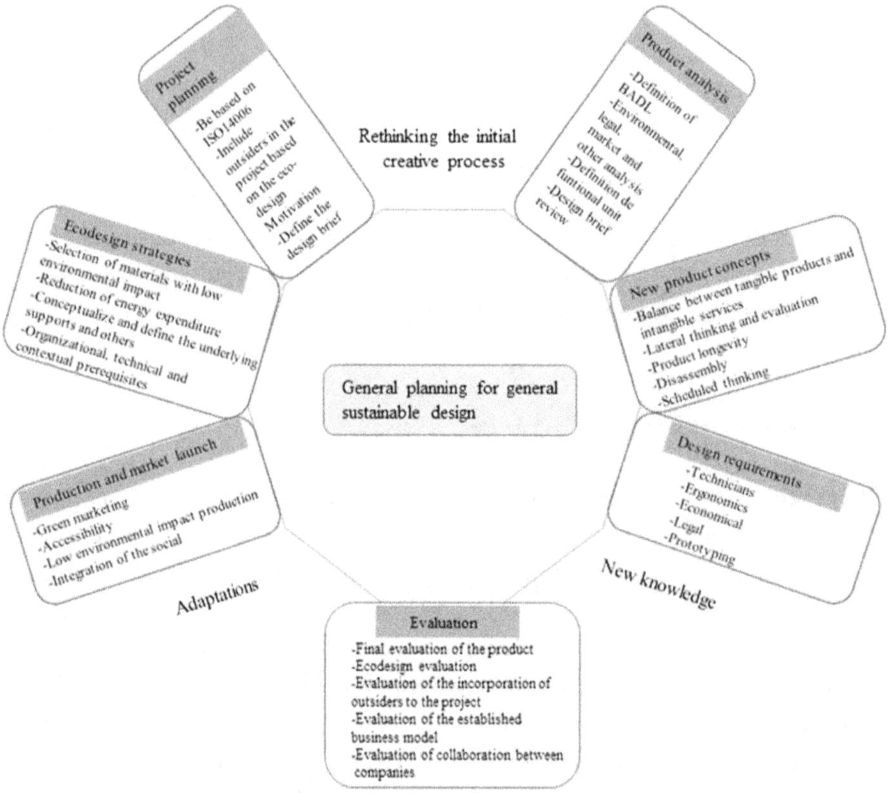

CONCLUSION

The BADLs among senior citizens are carried out according to cultural development, purchase power, history of physical care and activities that have strengthen their psychological balance. Most of the criteria and strategies to apply a sustainable design must be interpret according to the study group. Results obtained from the field research carried out with senior citizens, teachers at the Autonomous University of Chapingo, revealed interesting data, for example: 95% of professors had a clear idea that the most important aspect for any person is to have functional mobility, the other 5% had doubts about the importance between eating, personal hygiene and functional mobility. In the other hand, the BADLs related to intimacy and personal hygiene were less important to be attended; professors, regardless of their continuous education and their great knowledge about specific subjects, consider that they should not go through this situation. In relation to functional reeducation, application of ergonomic intervention allowed to redefine the steps that are usually applied to workstations at the companies, the phases facilitate creating use-sequence analysis schemes, therefore allowing the designer to anticipate design requirements that at some point will impact favorably the interconnections among the company, suppliers, clients and users. Finally, different criteria for sustainable design are not indisputable; however, combining different initiatives and the study of literature are about to find different answers, although partial, but without a doubt they will feed new knowledge and its application in favor of sustainability.

REFERENCES

Adams, R., Jeanrenaud, S., Bessant, J., Denyer, D., & Overy, P. (2016). Sustainability-oriented innovation: A systematic review. *International Journal of Management Reviews*, *18*(2), 180–205.

Albers, A., Behrendt, M., Klingler, S., Reiß, N., & Bursac, N. (2017). Agile product engineering through continuous validation in PGE–Product Generation Engineering. *Design Science, 3*.

Baines, T. S., Lightfoot, H. W., Evans, S., Neely, A., Greenough, R., Peppard, J., ... Wilson, H. (2007). State-of-the-art in product-service systems. *Proceedings of the Institution of Mechanical Engineers. Part B, Journal of Engineering Manufacture*, *221*(10), 1543–1552.

Barbero, S., & Cozzo, B. (2009). *Ecodesign*. Ullmann.

Boks, C., & Stevels, A. (2007). Essential perspectives for design for environment. Experiences from the electronics industry. *International Journal of Production Research*, *45*(18-19), 4021–4039.

Borjesson, K. (2008). *Affective Sustainability. Is this what timelessness really means?* Academic Press.

Brambila-Macias, S. A., & Sakao, T. (2021). Effective ecodesign implementation with the support of a lifecycle engineer. *Journal of Cleaner Production*, *279*, 123520.

Carson, R. (1962). *Silent spring*. Crest Book.

Ceschin, F., & Gaziulusoy, I. (2016). Evolution of design for sustainability: From product design to design for system innovations and transitions. *Design Studies*, *47*, 118–163.

Cipriani, G., Danti, S., Picchi, L., Nuti, A., & Fiorino, M. D. (2020). Daily functioning and dementia. *Dementia & Neuropsychologia*, *14*(2), 93–102. PMID:32595877

Cruz, A., & Garnica, A. (2011). *Applied ergonomics*. Ecoe Editions.

Das, S. K., & Naik, S. (2002). Process planning for product disassembly. *International Journal of Production Research*, *40*(6), 1335–1355.

Dobers, P., & Strannegård, L. (2005). Sustainability and Design. *Business Strategy and the Environment*, *14*(5), 269–271.

Dyllick, T., & Rost, Z. (2017). Towards true product sustainability. *Journal of Cleaner Production*, *162*, 346–360.

Emili, S., Ceschin, F., & Harrison, D. (2016). Product–Service System applied to Distributed Renewable Energy: A classification system, 15 archetypal models and a strategic design tool. *Energy for Sustainable Development*, *32*, 71–98.

Eroski Consumer. (2021) Physiological characteristics of aging. *Eroski Consumer,* (36). https://revista.consumer.es

Esslinger, H. (2011). Sustainable design: Beyond the innovation-driven business model. *Journal of Product Innovation Management, 28*(3), 401–404.

Gaziulusoy, A. I., Boyle, C., & McDowall, R. (2013). System innovation for sustainability: A systemic double-flow scenario method for companies. *Journal of Cleaner Production, 45*, 104–116.

Gill, T. M., Williams, C. S., & Tinetti, M. E. (1995). Assessing risk for the onset of functional dependence among older adults: The role of physical performance. *Journal of the American Geriatrics Society, 43*(6), 603–609. PMID:7775716

Hardin, G. (1968). The Tragedy of the Commons. *Science*. PMID:5699198

Heidrich, O., & Tiwary, A. (2013). Environmental appraisal of green production systems: Challenges faced by small companies using life cycle assessment. *International Journal of Production Research, 51*(19), 5884–5896.

International Organization for Standardization. (2002). *ISO/TR 14062: Environmental Management-Integrating Environmental Aspects Into Product Design and Development*. ISO.

ISO. (2011). 14006: 2011: Environmental management systems–Guidelines for incorporating ecodesign. Geneva: International Organization for Standardization.

Katz, S., Branch, L. G., Branson, M. H., Papsidero, J. A., Beck, J. C., & Greer, D. S. (1983). Active life expectancy. *The New England Journal of Medicine, 309*(20), 1218–1224. PMID:6633571

Konietzko, J., Bocken, N., & Hultink, E. J. (2020). Circular ecosystem innovation: An initial set of principles. *Journal of Cleaner Production, 253*, 119942.

Kristensen, H. S., & Remmen, A. (2019). A framework for sustainable value propositions in product-service systems. *Journal of Cleaner Production, 223*, 25–35.

Liu, C. J., Shiroy, D. M., Jones, L. Y., & Clark, D. O. (2014). Systematic review of functional training on muscle strength, physical functioning, and activities of daily living in older adults. *European Review of Aging and Physical Activity, 11*(2), 95–106.

Mor, V., Murphy, J., Masterson-Allen, S., Willey, C., Razmpour, A., Jackson, M. E., ... Katz, S. (1989). Risk of functional decline among well elders. *Journal of Clinical Epidemiology, 42*(9), 895–904. PMID:2778468

Moussavi, S., Chatterji, S., Verdes, E., Tandon, A., Patel, V., & Ustun, B. (2007). Depression, chronic diseases, and decrements in health: Results from the World Health Surveys. *Lancet, 370*(9590), 851–858. PMID:17826170

PAHO. (2021). *Weekly Breifing on the COVID-19 Situation in the Americas*. PAHO.

Pearce, D. W., & Turner, R. K. (1990). *Economics of natural resources and the environment*. JHU press.

Poulikidou, S., Björklund, A., & Tyskeng, S. (2014). Empirical study on integration of environmental aspects into product development: Processes, requirements and the use of tools in vehicle manufacturing companies in Sweden. *Journal of Cleaner Production, 81*, 34–45.

Rockström, J., Steffen, W., Noone, K., Persson, Å., Chapin, F. S., Lambin, E. F., ... & Foley, J. A. (2009). A safe operating space for humanity. *Nature, 461*(7263), 472-475.

Sakao, T., & Brambila-Macias, S. A. (2018). Do we share an understanding of transdisciplinarity in environmental sustainability research? *Journal of Cleaner Production, 170*, 1399–1403.

Simon, H. (1968). The Sciences of the Artificial. doi:10.2307/3102825

Sroufe, R., Curkovic, S., Montabon, F., & Melnyk, S. A. (2000). The new product design process and design for environment. *International Journal of Operations & Production Management*.

Steffen, W., Richardson, K., Rockström, J., Cornell, S. E., Fetzer, I., Bennett, E. M., ... Sörlin, S. (2015). Planetary boundaries: Guiding human development on a changing planet. *Science, 347*(6223). PMID:25592418

UN. (2015). *Transforming our world: The 2030 agenda for sustainable development*. United Nations, Department of Economic and Social Affairs.

UN. (2021). *Aging*. https://www.un.org/es/sections/issues-depth/ageing/index.htm

Vezzoli, C., Ceschin, F., Diehl, J. C., & Kohtala, C. (2015). New design challenges to widely implement 'Sustainable Product–Service Systems'. *Journal of Cleaner Production, 97*, 1–12.

Wang, Y., Modi, S. B., & Schoenherr, T. (2020). Leveraging sustainable design practices through supplier involvement in new product development: The role of the suppliers' environmental management capability. *International Journal of Production Economics*.

WHO. (2016). *Multisectoral Action for Healthy Aging Based on the Life Cycle: Draft Global Strategy and Plan of Action on Aging and Health: Report of the Secretariat (No. A69/17)*. World Health Organization.

WHO. (2020). *New coronavirus*. https://www.who.int/es/

WHO. (2021). *Aging*. http:www.who.int/topic/ageing/es/

WWF. (2016) *Living Planet Report 2016. Risk and resilience in a new era*. WWF International. http://awsassets.panda.org/downloads/lpr_living_planet_report_2016.pdf

Zhu, D. J., & Qiu, S. F. (2007). Analytical tool for urban circular economy planning and its preliminary application: A case of Shanghai. *City Planning Review, 31*(3), 64–69.

KEY TERMS AND DEFINITIONS

Anthropometry: Scientific tool that sizes the different segments of the human body for the design and adaptation of the physical environment that surrounds man's activity and with which he interacts directly.

Circumference: It is a closed measurement that follows the contour of the body. Therefore, this measure is not necessarily circular.

Curvature: It is a measurement from one point to another, following a contour, which is not usually closed or circular.

Distance: A straight line that measures from one point to another, between two marks on the body.

Endurance: Relate the two above. In the worker it depends to a great extent on his cardio-respiratory and metabolic capacity to cope with the demands and, on the other hand, on the integrity of the musculoskeletal system.

Force: Any cause capable of producing or modifying movement. It is defined as F = m x a (mass x acceleration). The moment of force is a measure of the rotational action of a force on a body.

Job: This result of applying a force on a point that moves in space and a formula is defined by T = F x e (force x space). According to the formula, if not movement there is no work; However, if we do a static work, there will be fatigue that requires contraction - permanent and imperceptible relaxation to the human eye, which in the strict sense makes it a dynamic work.

Mechanics: it can be divided into two parts: static and dynamic. Statics studies bodies in equilibrium, at rest or in uniform rectilinear motion (this state results from the cancellation of the forces and moments that act on bodies), WHILE Dynamics is interested in bodies in motion and understands kinetics and kinematics. The object of kinetics is to study bodies in motion, and the forces that produce it, while kinematics studies the relationships between displacements, speeds and accelerations in translational and rotational movements; therefore, it describes the movements themselves without taking into account the forces that cause them. We could typify it as the science of movement.

Power: It is defined as P = T X T (work X time ò F X V (force / velocity).

Pressure: It is the force applied per unit area (P = fxs). Thus, it will increase as the surface area decreases.

Scope: It is a measure from point to point, following along the axis of the arm or leg.

Speed: Ability to move from one side to another in the shortest possible time and is expressed as: V = e / t (space / time).

Thickness: Straight line that measures from one point to another horizontally, from front to back of the body.

Width: Straight line that measures from one point to another horizontally, crossing the body or a segment of it from side to side.

Chapter 12
Indoor Lighting Workplaces:
Towards New Indoor Lighting

David Baeza Moyano
Universidad CEU San Pablo, Spain

Roberto Alonso González Lezcano
https://orcid.org/0000-0002-6185-4929
Universidad CEU San Pablo, Spain

ABSTRACT

Office work has so far been carried out in company buildings and was largely based on the use of paper on a horizontal surface. Due to multiple reasons, more workers are working in their homes with electronic devices. As a result, both the working environment and personal tools are changing. Since the discovery about 20 years ago of the non-visual ways of light absorption, it was known that apart from the image forming effects (IF) of light from which the criteria for correct lighting have been developed, non-image forming effects (NIF) of light exist. The discovery of NIF has enhanced researcher belief in the importance of daylighting and has raised new criteria to be taken into account for proper interior lighting. Due to all the factors mentioned above, the parameters to be met by a luminaire and its environment for proper lighting of the workstation have been modified and expanded. The rapid advance in the development of new light-emitting diode (LED) luminaires with which the spectral power distribution (SPD) can be practically created opens the door to a genuine technological revolution comparable to the invention of electric lighting around 150 years ago. The authors of this study will review the latest published studies on the importance of light in our lives, IF and NIF effects of light, the parameters which from these effects are suggested to be taken into account for a correct indoor lighting, the regulations in force on indoor lighting workplaces, and proposals to improve indoor lighting and therefore the quality of life of workers.

DOI: 10.4018/978-1-7998-7279-5.ch012

When I was invited to write a chapter in this book about interior lighting, I thought at first I would call it Towards new Indoor lighting workplaces but when I was collecting information for its development, I was surprised because without realizing the Abstract I sent had simply titled Towards new Indoor lighting. I realized that my subconscious had made me put the title that comes closer and closer to the reality that we are living.

Cuttle asks himself at the beginning of one of his articles these questions, what is the situation of professionals working in lighting? Can we see the stages of our development, and are we at the beginning of a new and innovative stage? (Cuttle, 2010) I think the answer to the first question is that this is an exciting ongoing process of study and innovation. This article is a search for an affirmative answer to the second question you pose.

THE EFFECTS OF THE LIGHT

Humans are diurnal hunting mammals so their visual system is genetically designed to look and focus preferably at distant distances and their biorhythms are synchronized to live day and night.

Because the sun has been our source of natural light and for millions of years has shaped mammals endogenous circadian rhythms including when to wake up, body temperature, metabolism, oscillations of gene expression and hormone production throughout our bodies. (Edwards & Torcellini, 2002)

This change was radical since it was invented about 150 years ago electric light to be from that time much of our time indoors where the intensity of the lighting does not correspond to that of the outside and due to the characteristics of the luminaires, the spectral distribution we receive from such indoor lighting sources does not reproduce incompletely that of the sun. (Edwards & Torcellini, 2002)

Endogenous timekeepers are present in human beings. The suprachiasmatic nucleus (SCN) of the anterior hypothalamus is our master clock which coordinates individual oscillators in multicellular organisms. SCN is capable of maintaining rhythmicity in the absence of environmental inputs, but cues like sunrise increase its temporal fidelity. (Dibner et al., 2010) The expression of various genes and associated protein products vary throughout the day in the SCN and these variations are associated with changes in the synthesis, sensitivity, efficacy, and concentrations of various neurotransmitters, neuropeptides, and hormones throughout the brain and body. (Hirota & Fukada, 2004) The SCN exhibits cyclical patterns of electrical activity and responsiveness to input over an approximate 24 h cycle. (Edwards & Torcellini, 2002) The internal period of the human circadian rhythm can range between 23.5 and 24.7 h, with an average of 24.2 h among healthy adults and relies on a resetting response driven by light received at the retina to maintain entrainment with the local 24-h light/dark cycle. (Konis, 2017) These rhythmic patterns of activity, are called circadian oscillations (from Latin: “circa” = approximately and “diem” = day). Of the inputs received by the SCN, light, arriving at the SCN via the retino hypothalamic tract (RHT) from intrinsically photosensitive melanopsin expressing intrinsically photosensitive Retinal Ganglion Cells (ipRGCs) elicits the most robust effects within the SCN. When combined, these multimodal inputs inform daily cycles of SCN activity which then feed into the transcriptional and translational machinery of each neuron. Photic stimulation is an example of an environmental input that targets the core region of the SCN. Thus, the neurons within the core can be described as environmentally responsive, particularly to photic inputs. (Zelinski et al., 2014)

Melatonin circulates in the blood stream and is easily absorbed by individual cells, serving as a coordinating time-of-day (specifically, night time) signal throughout the body. At night, light absorbed by retinal photopigments signal the biological clock in the SCN of the hypothalamus to suppress nocturnal melatonin production by the pineal gland. (Rea & Figueiro, 2016)

Light is a powerful stimulus for the regulation of circadian, hormonal and behavioral systems. Retinal exposure to light stimulates three types of photoreceptors: rods, cones, and the melanopsin containing (ipRGC). Rods and cones transduce light into neural signals that carry IF information through ganglion cells. These are sent to the thalamus and the visual cortex in the brain where images are being processed. (Lucas et al., 2014)

The ipRGCs constitute a small fraction of the total number of ganglion cells that not only receive the input from rods and cones, but also are intrinsically photosensitive. They convert light into NIF neural signals that are transmitted via retino hypothalamic tract (RHT) to the SCN of the hypothalamus in the brain. The SCN, or biological clock, generates and regulates a set of endogenous rhythms of the human body through its connection to the central nervous system. Endogenous biological rhythms can be grouped according to their duration in Ultradian rhythms (<24 h), e.g., pupillary diameter, REM sleep; circadian rhythms (24 h), e.g., sleep awake, melatonin, alertness; infradian rhythms (>24 h), e.g., menstrual and circannual rhythms (approximately one year), e.g., seasonal changes in hormone secretion. (Khademagha et al., 2016)

NIF effects of light on pupil light reflex, performance and attention, sleep quality in young and older adults and hormone production. Circadian rhythms orchestrated by the SCN are fundamental to all biological life on earth, controlling such diverse cycles as DNA repair, insulin production, performance and the sleep/wake cycle. Given the importance of circadian rhythms to human health and wellbeing, lighting practice must begin to formally consider this NIF effect of light. It is now well established that the spectral, spatial, temporal and absolute sensitivities of the human circadian system are very different from those of the human visual system. (Rea et al., 2011)

The lighting features that affect the human circadian system are quantity, spectral power distribution of the light source, timing and duration of exposure, spatial distribution, and light history. (Figueiro, 2013) Photoreceptors in the human eye are sensitive to wavelengths from 380 to 780 nm. (##NO_NAME##, 1931) In terms of amount of light, the recommended levels for built environment are only based on the needs of the visual system (IF). The amount of polychromatic white needed to activate the circadian system is at least two orders of magnitude larger than necessary for the visual system. In spectral terms the circadian system has the peak of maximum sensitivity around 460 nm while that of the visual system is around 555 nm. (Brainard et al., 2001) (Thapan et al., 2001) From a temporal point of view, the operation of the visual system does not depend significantly on the moment when light is received, responding to a luminous stimulus at any time of day and night. The light can overtake or delay the master clock depending on when it is received. The visual system responds in less than a second to a luminous stimulus while minutes of light exposure may be needed to affect the circadian system. The spatial light distribution is important for the visual system and not for the circadian system. (Figueiro, 2013)

There are studies suggesting that artificial blue-enriched light competes with natural light as a zeitgeber to be the action-spectrum for non-visual light responses among human peaks in the blue range between 420–480 nm (Vetter et al., 2011). The maximum sensitivity peak would be 490 nm. (CIE TN 003:2015, 2013; Konis, 2017)

Lack of an effective light stimulus at the appropriate time during the day can disrupt the circadian system. Most individuals who exhibit total blindness and consequently lack access to a daily resetting response from light suffer from "non 24-h sleep wake disorder"(Lockley et al., 1999). If the presence of circadian rhythmicityis advantageous, the absence of circadian rhythmicity should be detrimental. Shift work, jetlag, obesity, diabetes, affective disorders, dementia, and cardiovascular diseases have all been linked to circadian rhythmicity or the disruption thereof in epidemiological studies and in experimental animal models(Edwards & Torcellini, 2002; Zelinski et al., 2014) the most severe health risks, such as cancer, diabetes, and coronary problems are identified from studies of populations engaged in shift work or employment on a rotating schedule, where an individual is required to deviate his/her sleep/ wake pattern from the local 24-h light/dark cycle. (Konis, 2017)

New evidence implicates circadian rhythms in eye growth and refractive error development. They suggest that this pathology is associated with an endogenous increase in young human adults in melatonin production due to a delay in melatonin circadian timing and a lower melatonin output compared to non myopes melatonin production. The retina also has an endogenous circadian clock related to dopamine, an important neurotransmitter found in the retina that not only modifies rhythms of the retina to light, cycle of darkness but also modulates refractive development. (Lin et al., 2016) Some authors claim that the part of the visible less wavelength than blue has a preponderant role in these processes. Violet light is abundant in sunlight while rarely detected in indoor ambient ligh. (Jiang et al., 2018)

Light that is applied before the minimum core body temperature* (4 am), which is reached approximately 1.5–2.5 hours before one naturally awakens, will delay the clock, resulting in later bedtimes and wake times the following day. Light applied after minimum core body temperature is reached will advance the clock, resulting in earlier bedtimes and wake times the following day. (Acosta et al., 2015)

Sleep disturbance in dermatological disorders can significantly affect the quality of mental and physical health of patients. Increased levels of cortisol in the afternoon in patients with inflammatory dermatosis and increased pruritus in the afternoon and evening (CIE, 2016)

It is currently unknown which is the optimal exposure to light that can be considered healthy for daily activity for both adults such as the ederly and children. The reasons are manifold. The variables to consider for light exposure or light dose are illminance level (ideally measured vertically to the eye at the glare angle; luminous exposure (expressed in lx:h) ;photon density (expressed in photons per square centimetre and second); duration of light exposure above a thershold. (CIE, 2016)

INDOOR LIGHTING

Concern about the possible risk to the human retina of light emitted by electronic devices and LED luminaires, specifically in the blue range, may have been overcome due to the small intensity that is radiated from these sources of artificial light but that does not mean that the light of electronic devices and luminaires that enters through our eyes does not influence our body independently of its function for vision. (Dain, 2020; Moyano, Mónica, & Roberto, 2020; Moyano et al., ; Moyano, Sola, & Roberto, 2020; Possible risks of LED lighting, 2018)

Lighting emerged as a profession in 1898 when at a meeting of gas engineers in Paris the foundations of the international photometry system were laid (Zelinski et al., 2014) The lighting criteria have been evolving and along with those based on IF, new factors have to be taken into account. After the discovery of the NIF of light, the optimization of the daylighting and the search for a correct circadian lighting have been incorporated into the factors to be taken into account.

Although climate-based daylight modeling is over a decade old, building guidelines and recommendations worldwide are still founded on idealized, static sky conditions such as the CIE standard overcast sky. Daylight metrics founded on climate-based simulations have begun to be considered as the basis for the next generation of building guidelines. (Andersen et al., 2012)

Natural light is highly dynamic and varies significantly with time, place, and weather conditions, rendering it difficult for designers to grasp that. Meanwhile, the design of natural daylighting must be combined with the form, lighting and shading of buildings, necessitating complex influencing factors. If an architect designs based on only experience or conventional analysis methods, not only will a significant amount of time be incurred, but also result quantification will be difficult; therefore, the expected and final environmental lighting effects will deviate significantly. In addition, it is difficult to accurately control the amount of daylighting as well as evaluate the daylighting effect accurately. (Khademagha et al., 2016)

The **daylight factor** is the ratio of the internal illuminance at a point in a building to the unshaded, external horizontal illuminance under a CIE overcast sky. It varies for different building designs and accordingly have the capacity to influence design choices. Building geometry, surrounding landscape and buildings, as well as surface properties (color, diffuseness, specularity, transmittance, reflectance) have an impact on the daylight factor. It is the reference overcast sky because is the worst case sky condition and therefore any other sky will lead to more daylight in the space. The movable shading devices – such as venetian blinds – are operated by occupants to avoid glare but usually provide sufficient daylight to avoid electric lighting. High windows, high reflective ceiling and wall finishes and skylight openings with high transmittance glazings are generally associated with good daylighting are indeed promoted by daylight factor. Para determinar whether the daylight situation at a sensor is '*adequate*' at a particular point in time, several criteria have been suggested:

Daylight Autonomy (DA) uses work plane illuminance as an indicator of whether there is sufficient daylight in a space so that an occupant can work by daylight alone.

Useful Daylight Illuminances (UDI), it aims to determine when daylight levels are 'useful' for the occupant. UDI results in three metrics, that is, the percentages of the occupied times of the year when the UDI was achieved (100–2000 lx), fell-short (<100 lx), or was exceeded (>2000 lx). The last bin is meant to detect the likely appearance of glare.

Annual Light Exposure is defined as the cumulative amount of visible light incident on a point of interest over the course of a year. Annual light exposure is measured in lux hours per year. (Reinhart et al., 2006)

Daily light-dark patterns incident on human eyes play an important role in maintaining a healthy circadian rhythm. Circadian lighting could be especially useful in spaces where daylight is insufficient, such as high-latitude regions, underground spaces, and city areas with high building density. Currently, there is no consensus on the exact amount of light dose required for daily circadian entrainment, however, a few emerging criteria for this threshold can be considered. (Dai et al., 2018)

The Lighting Research Center (LRC) at Rensselaer Polytechnic Institute has developed two metrics to characterize light as a stimulus to the biological clock circadian light and circadian stimulus, (Rea et al., 2005)

Circadian Light (CLA) is irradiance weighted by the spectral sensitivity of the retinal phototransduction mechanisms stimulating the biological clock,

Circadian Stimulus (CS), it is the percentage of melatonin supression under light exposure. (Dai et al., 2017; Figueiro et al., 2019) CS is a transformation of CLA into relative units from 0, the threshold for circadian system activation, to 0.7, response saturation, and is directly proportional to nocturnal melatonin suppression after 1-hour exposure (0–70%) assuming a fixed, 2.3mm diameter pupilis). (Dai et al., 2017; Figueiro et al., 2019)

Equivalent Melanopic Lux (EML) is proposed by the WELL Building Standard (International WELL Building Institute, 2018) recommends levels for "circadian lighting design. The suggested minimal EML threshold levels are 250 EML for break rooms, 200 EML for work areas and living environments, and 150 EML for learning areas.

The equivalent α-opic illuminance model proposed by Lucas et al. Each α-opic illuminance is found by convolving the spectral irradiance, for each wavelength, with the α-opic spectral efficiency function, and multiplying by the non-visual spectral efficacy constant, (Lucas et al., 2014) (Dai et al., 2018)

Otros investigadores mencionan otros parámetros a tener en cuenta para poder cuantificar los efectos no visuales de la luz como:

Circadian Action Factor (CAF)$\mathbf{a_{cv}}$ is proposed to represent the ratio of circadian and visual stimulus, (Dai et al., 2017; Figueiro et al., 2019) (Hunt & Pointer, 2006) which represents the impact of light on the hormones and biorhythm of an observer. (Kim et al., 2017)

Circadian Efficacy of Radiation (CER) the ratio of the circadian luminous flux to the radian flux

Circadian Illuminance (CIL) the product of VIL (v illuminance level) and CAF, is considered as a threshold for the relative melatonin suppression regardless of the type of optical sources (Lin et al., 2016)

The big difference between outdoor natural light and indoor artificial light sources is the distribution of wavelengths. Sunlight has a smooth spectral distribution along a wide band of wavelengths. Typical indoor light sources such as fluorescent or LED lamps emit in some wavelength regions while not in others. (Jiang et al., 2018)

It is well-known that building occupants almost without exception will prefer a workstation with a view of the outdoor environment to a windowless office. (Andersen et al., 2012) Window design is the key element for allowing daylight inside buildings and a proper design can improve thermal comfort and save electric lighting energy. Research efforts have investigated how windows provide daylight in a space in terms of the light distribution and potential lighting energy savings. Other studies have evaluated shading devices, defining the effect of blinds or overhangs on daylight availability inside buildings, as well as the relationship of these shading devices with electric lighting. Recent studies have also examined the relationship between daylighting and health outcomes. (Acosta et al., 2015)

Evening lighting in bedroom requires a low circadian stimulus for a good night's sleep, while morning lighting in bedroom may prefer a much higher circadian stimulus to easily awake; workplace lighting in general requires a brighter visual appearance compared to residential lighting, but a night-time working scenario may prefer a low CS for not disrupting the sleep rhythm after work indoor electric lighting that could mimic its time-dependent CS and visual brightness appearance is potentially beneficial and favorable, especially for those building occupants who rarely have chance to access daylight. For general illumination applications, the constraints on lighting spectra, such as requirements on white color coordinates, correlated color temperature (CCT), and color rendering index (CRI) or Ra, must be considered in the technical solution. (Dai et al., 2017; Figueiro et al., 2019)

Currently, indoor lighting design generally focuses on visual characteristics, for example, visual task performance, color rendition, reduction of glare, lit appearance (Dai et al., 2018) and illumination for task, as to ensure that 500 lux falls on the horizontal work plane. (Andersen et al., 2012) Luminous environment studies have focused on the development of luminaires with high efficiency and high colour rendering to achieve observer visual satisfaction. The brightness of an indoor luminous environment influences work efficiency, and excessive glare caused by luminaires can lead to observer discomfort or visual impairment. In addition, an indoor luminous environment can provide psychological stability and stimulation depending on the colour (wavelength), intensity and exposure time, which can also affect the hormones and biorhythms of occupants. The colour of indoor luminous environments affects the circadian rhythm and awakening of humans. To design an appropriate indoor luminous environment, the final colour of a space perceived by an observer must be accurately predicted and its effects on the observer must be considered. **Colour Quality Assessment Tool (CQAT)** is a parameter that utilizes the spectral reflectance factor of interior finishes and the spectral power distribution (SPD) data of luminaires to accurately calculate the luminous exitance radiated by interior finishes and the colour quality components of the SPD, luminance, CAF, colour coordinates, and CCT based on the colours of the interior finishes and light sources. (Kim et al., 2017)

All zones within a building that do not regularly achieve the lighting conditions necessary for effective circadian stimulus can be labeled as biologically dark, and considered as zones where sustained occupancy over extended time periods (e.g. regular workday schedules) may present a risk for disruption of the circadian system in the absence of supplemental electrical lighting capable of effective circadian stimulus. (Konis, 2017) More commonly used lighting metrics related to visual task performance (e.g. horizontal workplane illuminance and illuminance uniformity) (Dai et al., 2017; Figueiro et al., 2019) (International Well Building Institute, 2016), visual discomfort (e.g. probability of glare), lighting energy savings (e.g. electrical lighting energy reduction from photocontrols), and **Indoor Environmental Quality (IEQ)** (e.g. compliance with the U.S. Green Building Council's LEED Daylighting Environmental Quality (EQ) credit) International WELL Building Institute has recently developed a building certification system with the stated objective of measuring, certifying and monitoring the performance of building features that impact health and well-being". (International Well Building Institute, 2016)

Para la the provision of sufficient melanopic light intensity for work areas es impotente tener en cuenta the age of the occupants debido a que the relative level of light reaching the retina decreases due to age. Given that buildings should be expected to effectively accommodate a range of ages. The 65-year-old observer model requires a 6% greater stimulus intensity relative to a 32-year-old to achieve an equivalent effect, or a 11% greater intensity relative to a 10-year-old observer. At present, there is no consensus for the appropriate minimum light exposure threshold to ensure effective circadian stimulus in buildings, or for the duration at which the effects of light exposure saturate. As almost all interior lighting standards recommend illuminance levels on horizontal planes, but very few suggest vertical illuminance values, and with a growing push toward energy-efficient buildings, a typical lighting strategy would be directing most of the luminaire flux directly toward workplanes, which is indeed ubiquitous in practice. (Dai et al., 2017; Figueiro et al., 2019)

INDOOR LIGHTING STANDARDS

EN 12464-1:2019 specifies lighting requirements for humans in indoor workplaces, which meet the needs for visual comfort and performance of people. All usual visual tasks are considered, including Display Screen Equipment (DSE) and requirements for lighting solutions for most indoor workplaces and their associated areas in terms of quantity and quality of illumination. In addition, recommendations are given for good lighting practice including IF and NIF lighting needs. (EN 12464-1, 2019)

Lighting requirements are determined by the satisfaction of visual comfort, where the workers have a feeling of well-being; visual performance, where the workers are able to perform their visual tasks and safety. The main parameters determining the luminous environment with respect to artificial light and daylight are luminance distribution, illuminance, directionality of light, lighting in the interior space, variability of light (levels and colour of light); colour rendering and colour appearance of the light, glare and flicker.

The recommended scale of illuminance (in lx) according EN 12665 is:

20 - 30 - 50 - 75 - 100 - 150 - 200 - 300 - 500 - 750 - 1000 - 1500 - 2000 - 3000 – 5000. (EN 12665, n.d.)

The values are valid for normal visual conditions and take into account the psycho-physiological aspects such as visual comfort and well-being; requirements for visual tasks; visual ergonomics; practical experience; contribution to functional safety and economy.

The lighting for DSE work stations shall be appropriate for all tasks performed at the work station, e.g. reading from the screen, reading printed text, writing on paper, keyboard work. For these areas the lighting criteria and system shall be chosen in accordance with type of task or activity area, from the schedule in table 6.26 Offices:

Table 1.

Ref. no.	Type of task/activity area	$E_{m,r}$ lx	$E_{m,u}$ lx	E_z lx	$E_{m,wall}$ lx	$E_{m,ceiling}$ lx
6.26.1	Filing, copying, etc.	300	500	100	100	75
6.26.2	Writing, typing, reading, data processing	500	1 000	150	150	100
6.26.3	Technical drawing	750	1 500	150	150	100
6.26.4	CAD work stations	500	1 000	150	150	100
6.26.5.1	Conference and meeting rooms	500	1 000	150	150	100
6.26.5.2	Conference table	500	1 000	150	150	100
6.26.6	Reception desk	300	750	100	100	75
6.26.7	Archiving	200	300	75	75	50

$E_{m,r}$ lx: minimum maintained illuminance $\bar{E}_{m,r}$ on the reference surface for the interior (area) in which the task or activity from Column 2 is performed.

$E_{m,u}$ lx: upper maintained illuminance $\bar{E}_{m,u}$ on the reference surface for the interior (area) in which the task or activity from Column 2 is performed.

E_z lx: minimum cylindrical illuminance $\bar{E}_Z$ for the recognition of objects and people

$E_{m,wall}$ lx: minimum average illuminance on walls.

$E_{m,ceiling}$ lx: minimum average illuminance on ceilings. (EN 12464-1, 2019)

The specific requirements para el DSE-work son que se han de tener en cuenta the room brightness y que para el trabajo en conference and meeting rooms lighting should be controllable. Ranges of useful reflectances for the major interior surfaces are ceiling: 0,6 to 0,9; walls: 0,3 to 0,8; working planes: 0,2 to 0,6; floor: 0,1 to 0,5.(EN 12464-1, 2019)

The standard Lighting of indoor workplaces specifies lighting requirements for indoor workplaces and for people to perform the visual tasks efficiently, in comfort and safety throughout the whole work period. This standard does not explain how lighting systems or techniques should. (ISO 8995-1, 2002)

4.3 Illuminance level.

4.3.1 Visual task area. For the office area, the visual task area is defined. Recommended values of illuminance are specified separately for the visual task area and the surrounding areas. When a desk light is used for task lighting, the visual task area is defined as a 1/3 sector of a 50 cmn circle front of the desk light. When a desk light is not used for task lighting, in general, the visual task area is defined as a rectangle of 50 cm × 80 cm.

4.3.2 Horizontal illuminance. This document specifies illuminance on a horizontal work plane regardless of types of work. For each type of room in each area, the average value of horizontal illuminance is given with a recommended value of the maintenance factor.

- When the work plane is not specified, an imaginary horizontal plane of 0.8 m above the floor shall be the reference surface.
- Recommended value shall be an average illuminance along the center line within 0.1 m above the floor for passages and corridors.

Task area, standar horizontal illuminance para task areas e illumination de all indoor areas está entre 500, 750 (office and boardrooms) and 1500 lx (design and drafting rooms) (EN 12464-1, 2019)

High surface reflectances contribute to energy savings and may lead to better visual comfort. For choice of materials, recommended reflectances are ceiling: 0,7 to 0,9; walls: 0,5 to 0,8; floor: 0,2 to 0,6. The reflectance of major objects (like furniture, machinery, etc.) should be in the range of 0,2 to 0,7. (ISO 8995-1, 2002)

Warm colour appearance the correlated colour temperature is below 3.300 K, intermediate colour appearance the correlated colour temperature is below 3.300-5300 K, cool colour appearance the correlated colour temperature is above 5.300 K. (EN 12464-1, 2019) (ISO 8995-1, 2002)

The International Well Building Institute desarrolla la WELL Building Standard. La última versión se ha publicado en 2019. (Illuminating Engineering Society of North America (IESNA), n.d.)

The goal of this standard is an integrated and cost-effective adoption of green design and construction strategies, with human health care being a priority when evaluating building design, construction and operational strategies. Within this document on Indoor environmental quality (EQ) are the sections on how to be the interior lighting and daylight debtor requirements for new construction (nc), core and shell (cs), schools, retail, data centers, warehouses & distribution centers, hospitality and healthcare.

Interior lighting intent is to promote occupants productivity, comfort, and well-being by providing high-quality lighting. It shows how has to be Lighting Control and lighting quality.

Daylight intent is to connect building occupants with the outdoors, reinforce circadian rhythms, and reduce the use of electrical lighting by introducing daylight into the space. Provide manual or automatic (with manual override) glare-control devices for all regularly occupied spaces. It gives spatial simulation options Daylight Autonomy and Annual Sunlight Exposure, simulation illuminance calculations and measurement illuminance levels the floor area. (U.S. Green Building Council, 2019)

The 10th edition of the Illuminating Engineering Society North America (IESNA) Lighting Handbook of 2000 contain illuminance recommendations. Although the transmittance reduction varies considerably with wavelength, between the ages of 15 and 75, the intra ocular transmittance for optical radiation between 500 nm and 600 nm decreases by a factor of 6. It is neither practical nor appropriate to apply this factor directly to recommended illuminances, since habit and experience are known to mitigate some of the effects of reduced retinal irradiance. To account for these effects in a practical manner, the following has been adopted. It is reasonable to assume that legacy values of recommended illuminances were considered to apply to a population age of between 25 and 65 years. If it is known that at least half of the observers are at least 65 years old, then the legacy recommended illuminance (if one exists) is doubled. If it is known that at least half of the observers are less than 25 years old, then the value is halved. Visual perfomance description: visual performance is tipically daily life (and work) related, including much reading and writing of handcopies and electronic media consecutively and/or simultaneously. Recommended target illuminances (lux) are made based on visual ages of observers (years) for some indoor education situations showing horizontal and vertical illuminance recommendations. (Illuminating Engineering Society of North America (IESNA), n.d.) (David, 2011)

The purpose of lighting should be redefined in terms of the visual experience of illuminated surroundings, and two criteria are proposed for this purpose, both of which represent significant departures from conventional practice. The first assesses the adequacy of illumination for an activity in terms of the density of reflected light from surrounding room surfaces, and the second is concerned with how the luminaire luminous flux is directed onto selected target surfaces. Taken together, these criteria offer a quite new approach for designing lighting installations for general practice. the IESNA's 'Guide to designing quality lighting for people and buildings' (2008), which opens with "Task visibility is essential to lighting design; lighting exists to enable vision." The SLL Lighting Handbook (2009) states in relation to office lighting, "Unless specified otherwise, the recommended maintained illuminance is measured on a horizontal working plane at desk height." Again, the Handbook, and also the latest European workplace standard, EN 12464-1: 2011, prescribe a 'modelling index' defined as the ratio of mean cylindrical illuminance to the horizontal illuminance. (Carrier et al., 2002)

PROPOSALS FORNEW INDOOR LIGHTING

Light increase alertness and well-being of nightshift workers (Andersen et al., 2012) Exposures to both short-wavelength (blue) and long wavelength (red) lights in the middle of the night increased beta and reduced alpha power relative to preceding dark conditions, although only blue light significantly suppressed melatonin relative to darkness. Exposures to high (i.e., 40 lux at the cornea), but not low (i.e., 10 lux at the cornea), levels of red and of blue light significantly increased heart rate relative to darkness. Both blue and red lights can significantly increase nighttime cortisol levels and performance, as measured by short-term reaction times and matching-to-sample tests. The melatonin pathway does not seem to be the only light-sensitive pathway that can affect alertness and performance at night. A light source that can increase alertness without suppressing melatonin may be an optimal solution for maintaining alertness in shift workers. (Figueiro, 2013) The red lighting intervention in the afternoon around the time of the post-lunch dip (i.e. 15:00) significantly reduced subjective sleepiness and, although not statistically significant, increased subjective vitality. These field results are the first demonstrating that red light in combination with ambient white light provides an effective alerting stimulus in the middle of the afternoon. (Dai et al., 2017; Figueiro et al., 2019)

Office worker participants were recruited para un study para to evaluate whether a 'non-visual layer of light' in the vertical plane from a custom-built, desktop luminaire would support office occupants' entrainment and alertness during the daytime. Objective measures of sleep and circadian phase as well as subjective measures of sleepiness, alertness and vitality/energy were measured. Specifically, the research addressed three primary hypotheses:

1. Morning (06:00–12:00) blue light (CS>0.4) will promote entrainment and advance circadian phase. Sleep onset at night and sleep offset in the morning will be advanced relative to baseline following this lighting intervention. Given that receiving high CS in the morning advances the circadian clock, activity acrophase will also be advanced.
2. Morning blue light (CS_>0.4) will also elicit an acute alerting response from participants, reducing subjective sleepiness and increasing subjective vitality/energy.
3. Afternoon (13:30–17:00) red light (CS=0) will elicit an acute alerting response, reducing subjective sleepiness and increasing subjective vitality/energy, especially at 15:00, close to the time of the post-lunch. The red lighting intervention was selected for the afternoon to provide an alerting stimulus while avoiding excessive circadian-effective light in the latter part of the day, thereby limiting a light-induced delay of circadian phase. (Carrier et al., 2002)

It has been shown that age advances the biological clock, and as such, a lighting intervention designed to advance the clock even further may not be recommended for older individuals. (Carrier et al., 2002) (Kripke et al., 2007)

Lighting in the built environment should provide high circadian light stimulation during the day and low circadian stimulation at night, good visual performance (e.g., reading) during waking hours, and low-level night-lights that enable safe movement through the space and minimize sleep disruption. High circadian stimulation during daytime waking hours can probably be achieved by about 600 lux at the cornea of a 6500 K light source. (Kripke et al., 2007)

The researchers Andersen & Mardaljevic divide the 24 h into three moments or phases in relation to the light-dark balance. These are 6:00-10:00 a.m. (circadian resetting),10:00-18:00 (alerting effects of daylight), and 18:00-6:00 (bright light avoidance, dim light only). Access to bright, circadian effective light in the morning is most critical for circadian resetting. However, it is important to note that exposure to bright light during the 10:00-18:00 period may be desirable (and preferred) by occupants for its potential to increase alertness. In the present example, the analysis focuses on the circadian-resetting period (6:00-10:00 a.m.) annually, and the hour 6:00-7:00 a.m. is removed from analysis on the basis that the space would be unoccupied during this hour. (Konis, 2017) (Andersen et al., 2012) The SPD and intensity of each part of the spectrum will depend on the latitude, the season, the position in front of the daylighting of the worker, the characteristics of the furniture. (Dai et al., 2017; Figueiro et al., 2019)

Simply boosting the power of luminaires to achieve a corneal illuminance of 300–450 lx would significantly increase lighting energy consumption. Therefore, developing energy-efficient solutions is critical for the potential adoption of circadian lighting. Furthermore, high-quality circadian lighting consists of more than just providing circadian stimulus; general lighting constraints should also apply. In particular, light directly from sources to the eyes should be avoided in spatial illumination consideration, and reasonably high color rendition is desired in spectral design. The benefit of directing luminaire flux to the highly reflective ceiling is more than just providing a high indirect corneal illuminance. Compared with downlight mode, uplight mode can provide a much more uniform distribution of corneal illuminance. It can be concluded that to achieve a high indirect corneal illuminance with a uniform spatial distribution, one needs to improve the average room-surface reflectance and direct the initial flux to a highly reflective surface to benefit from a high value. (Dai et al., 2018)

A series of laboratory studies have shown that exposure to long wavelength (red) light can promote alertness during the mid-afternoon decline in performance known as the post-lunch dip. These findings are important for daytime applications in office environments because, unlike blue light, red light exposures in the mid-to-late afternoon and early evening can induce alertness without affecting circadian phase. Another series of studies have demonstrated that filtering out short-wavelength light at night reduced the suppression of melatonin while still maintaining alertness. These findings are important for night-shift work as the suppression of melatonin by light at night, especially short-wavelength light, has been linked to negative short-term and long-term health consequences. (Dai et al., 2017; Figueiro et al., 2019)

The great majority of indoor locations, including workplaces, the prime purpose of the lighting is to provide for surroundings that appear acceptably bright, at least to the extent of avoiding the appearance of being dull or gloomy. The convention of specifying illumination standards in terms of illuminance incident on workplanes is inappropriate for this purpose. Instead, a metric is needed that corresponds to reflected light arriving at the eye from surrounding room surfaces. in the context of three stages of the lighting profession, where the objective of the first stage was provision of uniform illuminance on a horizontal plane, and of the second stage, visual performance based lighting standards. The view is expressed that the second stage has failed, and that current practice remains dominated by the first stage objective. It is suggested that the third stage will have as its objective the provision of acceptably bright surroundings, and for this, lighting standards will be based on reflected light arriving at the eye. (Cuttle, 2010)

Illumination preferences vary between individuals Con unas condiciones de luminosidad semejantes muchos office occupants tend to work at lower daylight levels than the commonly referred 300 or 500 lx y varían los niveles de electric lighting. (Reinhart & Voss, 2003)

Lighting designers determine the electric-lighting design of spaces with or without taking daylight into account. Lamps and luminaires manufacturers determine the scope for development of electric lighting products from which lighting designers can choose. Six factors triggering the NIF light effects have been identified. Spectrum, quantity, spatial distribution (directionality), timing, duration, and history have to be taken into account on daylighting design in the built environment. (Khademagha et al., 2016)

Local authorities and city planners have profound influence on indoor daylight exposure as they decide on the overall height of buildings, width of streets, and urban design. Architects determine daylighting possibilities through designing the building's skin layer including facade and skylights. Glazing/window companies determine (luminous) characteristics of daylight entering the buildings. Interior designers and/or architects influence internal reflections of daylight via designing the shape and the spectral reflectance of interior walls, ceilings, floors, and furniture. (Khademagha et al., 2016)

CONCLUSION

Recent research ensures that both natural and electrical light can affect physiological and biological functioning through the IF and NIF pathways. Due to the benefits and risks that can occur on both routes, it is recommended that both effects should be taken into account in the design process of lighting installations.

It should be recommended to both public administrations responsible for the control of the construction and maintenance of public and private buildings and to private companies involved in this sector that lighting installations be included in an assessment project by a multidisciplinary team including occupational health experts, psychologists and others, regardless of whether the non-imaging effects were intentionally designed or a "conventional" lighting installation is used.

New studies highlight the importance of taking into account the inclination and composition of light entering through the cornea for proper lighting so it would be advisable to take into account in conjunction with daylighting, the new spectral distributions of the luminaires and the reflection of light on the surfaces of the rooms for proper lighting of the workstations. As a result, factors of reflection in the light of international norms would have to be reconsidered.

In a growing, progressive and seemingly no-turning-back way, For more and more workers, their basic tool of work is the electronic light-emitting devices that look at each other practically from the front instead of the paper resting on a horizontal surface in which the light has to be reflected and they carry out their work from their own house. As a result, the characteristics of the luminaires and the environment in which optimum work has to be carried out have to be adapted to this new reality outside the office buildings.

By simple evolutionary logic, the entire range of the visible electromagnetic spectrum to which the five types of photoreceptors of the human retina are sensitive must have a function, known or not by researchers. From the scientific discoveries of recent years, which we have tried to account for in our publication, We believe that the full range of the visible spectrum should be taken into account for the development of new luminaires for indoor lighting with a proportion and intensity that is as close as possible to the solar at every moment of the day. It would therefore be advisable for the light composition of the luminaires to vary throughout the day and to be taken into account according to the age of the person.

Faced with these new challenges, the first step is to bring new light sources and lighting systems to the market, which will facilitate the implementation of this "second kind of light" into the built environment. (Figueiro, 2013)

REFERENCES

Acosta, I., Leslie, R. P., & Figueiro, M. G. (2015). Analysis of circadian stimulus allowed by daylighting in hospital rooms. *Lighting Research & Technology*, *0*, 1–13.

Andersen, M., Mardaljevic, J., & Lockley, S. W. (2012). A framework for predicting the non-visual effects of daylight - Part I: Photobiology-based model. *Lighting Research & Technology*, *2012*(44), 37–53. doi:10.1177/1477153511435961

Brainard, Hanifin, Greeson, Byrne, Glickman, Gerner, & Rollag. (2001). Action spectrum for melatonin regulation in humans: Evidence for a novel circadian photoreceptor. *J. Neurosci.*, *21*, 6405-6412.

Carrier, J., Paquet, J., Morettini, J., & Touchette, E. (2002). Phase advance of sleep and temperature circadian rhythms in the middle years of life in humans. *Neuroscience Letters*, *320*(1-2), 1–4. doi:10.1016/S0304-3940(02)00038-1 PMID:11849749

CIE. (2016). Research Roadmap for healthful interior lighting applications. International Commission illumination. *CIE*, *218*.

CIE Commission Internationale de l'Eclairage Proceedings. (1931). Cambridge University Press.

CIE TN 003:2015 Report on the First International Workshop on Circadian and Neurophysiological Photometry, 2013.

Cuttle, C. (2010). Towards the third stage of the lighting profession. *Lighting Research & Technology*, *42*(1), 73–93. doi:10.1177/1477153509104013

Dai, Q., Cai, W., Shi, W., Hao, L., & Wei, M. (2017). A proposed lighting-design space: Circadian effect versus visual Illuminance. *Building and Environment*, *122*, 287–293. doi:10.1016/j.buildenv.2017.06.025

Dai, Q., Huang, Y., Hao, L., Lin, Y., & Chen, K. (2018). Luoxi Haoa, Yi Lin, Kaixuan Chen. Spatial and spectral illumination design for energy-efficient circadian lighting. *Building and Environment*, *146*, 216–225. doi:10.1016/j.buildenv.2018.10.004

Dain, S. (2020). The blue light dose from white light emitting diodes (LEDs) and other white light sources. *Ophthalmic & Physiological Optics*, *40*(5), 692–699. Advance online publication. doi:10.1111/opo.12713 PMID:32691888

David, L. (2011). A Procedure for Determining Target Illuminances, LEUKOS. *The Journal of the Illuminating Engineering Society of North America*, *7*(3), 145–158. doi:10.1582/LEUKOS.2011.07.03001

Dibner, C., Schibler, U., & Albrecht, U. (2010). The mammalian circadian timing sys-tem: Organization and coordination of central and peripheral clocks. *Annual Review of Physiology*, *72*(1), 517–549. doi:10.1146/annurev-physiol-021909-135821 PMID:20148687

Edwards, L., & Torcellini, P. (2002). Literature Review of the Effects of Natural Light on Building Occupants. *Lit. Rev. Eff. Nat. Light Build. Occup.*, *55*. Advance online publication. doi:10.2172/15000841

EN 12464-1 2019: Lighting of workplaces – Indoor workplaces. https://www.valosto.com/tiedostot/prEN%2012464-1.pdf

EN 12665, *Light and lighting — Basic terms and criteria for specifying lighting requirements*, n.d.

Figueiro, Steverson Heerwagen, Yucel, Roohan, Sahin, Kampschroer, & Rea. (2019). Light, entrainment and alertness: A case study in offices. *Lighting Research and Technology*.

Figueiro, M. G. (2013). An Overview of the Effects of Light on Human Circadian Rhythms: Implications for New Light Sources and Lighting Systems Design. *Journal of Light Visual Environment*, *37*(2 & 3), 51–61. doi:10.2150/jlve.IEIJ130000503

Hirota, T., & Fukada, Y. (2004). Resetting mechanism of central and peripheral circadianclocks in mammals. *Zoological Science*, *21*(4), 359–368. doi:10.2108/zsj.21.359 PMID:15118222

Hunt, R. W. G., & Pointer, M. R. (2006). *Measuring Colour* (4th ed.). Wiley.

Illuminating Engineering Society of North America (IESNA). (n.d.). https://www.ies.org/standards/ies-standards-cross-reference/

International Well Building Institute. (2016). *WELL Building Standard* (v1). Author.

ISO 8995-1 (2002): Lighting of indoor work places (CIE S008/2001)

Jiang, X., Kurihara, T., Torii, H., & Tsubota, K. (2018, September). Progress and Control of Myopia by Light Environments. *Eye & Contact Lens*, *44*(5), 273–278. doi:10.1097/ICL.0000000000000548 PMID:30048342

Khademagha, P., Aries, M. B. C., Rosemann, A. L. P., & van Loenen, E. J. (2016). Implementing non-image-forming effects of light in the built environment: A review on what we need. *Building and Environment*, *108*, 263–272. doi:10.1016/j.buildenv.2016.08.035

Kim, I. T., Choi, A. S., & Sung, M. K. (2017). Development of a Colour Quality Assessment Tool for indoor luminous environments affecting the circadian rhythm of occupants. *Building and Environment*, *126*, 252–265. doi:10.1016/j.buildenv.2017.10.009

Konis. (2017). A novel circadian daylight metric for building design and evaluation. *Building and Environment, 113*, 22-38.

Konis, K. (2017). A novel circadian daylight metric for building design and evaluation. *Building and Environment*, *113*, 22–38. doi:10.1016/j.buildenv.2016.11.025

Kripke, D. F., Elliott, J. A., Youngstedt, S. D., & Rex, K. M. (2007). Circadian phase response curves to lightin older and young women and men. *Journal of Circadian Rhythms*, *5*(0), 4. doi:10.1186/1740-3391-5-4 PMID:17623102

Lin, Zhu, Guo, Zheng, Lu, Shih, & Wu. (2016). Multi-function indoor light sources based on light-emitting diodes–a solution for healthy lighting. *Optics Express , 24(21).* doi:10.1364/OE.24.024401

Lockley, S. W., Skene, D. J., Butler, L. I., & Arendt, J. (1999). Sleep and activity rhythms related to circadian phase in the blind. *Sleep*, *22*(5), 616–623. doi:10.1093leep/22.5.616 PMID:10450596

Lucas, R. J., Peirson, S. N., Berson, D. M., Brown, T. M., Cooper, H. M., Czeisler, C. A., Figueiro, M. G., Gamlin, P. D., Lockley, S. W., O'Hagan, J. B., Price, L. L. A., Provencio, I., Skene, D. J., & Brainard, G. C. (2014, January). Measuring and using light in the melanopsin age. *Trends in Neurosciences*, *37*(1), 1–9. Advance online publication. doi:10.1016/j.tins.2013.10.004 PMID:24287308

Madhulika, A. (2013). Gupta. Aditya K.Gupta. Sleep-wake disorders and dermatology. *Clinics in Dermatology*, *31*(1), 118–126. doi:10.1016/j.clindermatol.2011.11.016 PMID:23245983

Moyano, D. B., Mónica, S. J. F., & Roberto, A. G. L. (2020). Towards a Sustainable Indoor Lighting Design: Effects of Artificial Light on the Emotional State of Adolescents in the Clasrroom. *Sustainability*, *12*(10), 4623. doi:10.3390u12104263

Moyano, D. B., Moyano, S. B., López, M. G., Aznal, A. S., & Roberto, A. G. L. Photometrics and colorimetric analysis of LED luminaires for interior lighting design. 2021. *Color Research and Application*. Advance online publication. doi:10.1002/COL.2216

Moyano, D. B., Sola, Y., & Roberto, A. G. L. (2020). Blue-light levels emitted from portable electronic devices compared to sunlight. *Energies*, *13*(16), 4276. doi:10.3390/en13164276

Possible risks of LED lighting. (2018). Conclusions of the Spanish Lighting Committee Working Group.

Rea, M. S., & Figueiro, M. G. (2016). Light as a circadian stimulus for architectural lighting. *Lighting Research & Technology*, *0*, 1–14.

Rea, M. S., Figueiro, M. G., Bierman, A., & Hamner, R. (2011). Modelling the spectral sensitivity of the human circadian system. *Lighting Research & Technology*. Advance online publication. doi:10.1177/1477153511430474

Rea, M. S., Figueiro, M. G., Bullough, J. D., & Bierman, A. (2005). A model of phototransduction by the human circadian system. *Brain Research. Brain Research Reviews*, *50*(2), 213–228. doi:10.1016/j.brainresrev.2005.07.002 PMID:16216333

Reinhart, C. F., Mardaljevic, J., & Rogers, Z. (2006). Dynamic daylight performance metrics for sustainable building design. *Leukos*, *3*(1), 7–31. doi:10.1582/LEUKOS.2006.03.01.001

Reinhart, C. F., & Voss, K. (2003). Monitoring manual control of electric lighting and blinds. *Lighting Research & Technology*, *35*(3), 243–260. doi:10.1191/1365782803li064oa

Thapan, K., Arendt, J., & Skene, D. J. (2001). An action spectrum for melatonin suppression:evidence for a novel non-rod, non-cone photoreceptor system in humans. *The Journal of Physiology*, *535*(1), 261–267. doi:10.1111/j.1469-7793.2001.t01-1-00261.x PMID:11507175

U.S. Green Building Council. (2019). LEED v4 for Building Design Construction. Author.

Vetter, C., Juda, M., Lang, D., Wojtysiak, A., & Roenneberg, T. (2011). Blue-enriched office light competes with natural light as a Zeitgeber. *Scandinavian Journal of Work, Environment & Health*, *37*(5), 437–445. doi:10.5271jweh.3144 PMID:21246176

Zelinski, Deibel, & McDonald. (2014). The trouble with circadian clock dysfunction: Multiple deleterious effects on the brain and body. *Neurosci. Biobehav. Rev.*, *40*, 80-101. https://www.ncbi.nlm.nih.gov/pubmed/24468109

Compilation of References

MODIS aerosol product information. (2019b). Retrieved from https://ladsweb.modaps.eosdis.nasa.gov/missions-and-measurements/productsMOD04_3K/

Rea, M. S., Figueiro, M. G., Bierman, A., & Hamner, R. (2011). Modelling the spectral sensitivity of the human circadian system. *Lighting Research & Technology*. Advance online publication. doi:10.1177/1477153511430474

Figueiro, M. G. (2013). An Overview of the Effects of Light on Human Circadian Rhythms: Implications for New Light Sources and Lighting Systems Design. *Journal of Light Visual Environment, 37*(2 & 3), 51–61. doi:10.2150/jlve.IEIJ130000503

Isaza, C., Mosquera, J. M., G6mez-Méndez, G. A., Zavala-De Paz, J. P., Anaya-Rivera, E. K., Rizzo-Sierra, J. A., & Palillero-Sandoval, O. (2019). Development of an acousto-optic system for hyperspectral image segmentation. *Metrology and Measurement Systems, 26*(3).

CIE Commission Internationale de l'Eclairage Proceedings. (1931). Cambridge University Press.

Rizzo Sierra, J. A., Isaza, C., Anaya Rivera, E. K., Zavala De Paz, J. P., & Mosquera, J. (2019). Acousto-Optic Dispersion Applicability to Plastic Auto-Part Color Characterization. In Progress in Optomechatronic Technologies (pp. 51-64). Springer. doi:10.1007/978-981-32-9632-9_7

Brainard, Hanifin, Greeson, Byrne, Glickman, Gerner, & Rollag. (2001). Action spectrum for melatonin regulation in humans: Evidence for a novel circadian photoreceptor. *J. Neurosci., 21*, 6405-6412.

Thapan, K., Arendt, J., & Skene, D. J. (2001). An action spectrum for melatonin suppression:evidence for a novel non-rod, non-cone photoreceptor system in humans. *The Journal of Physiology, 535*(1), 261–267. doi:10.1111/j.1469-7793.2001.t01-1-00261.x PMID:11507175

Vetter, C., Juda, M., Lang, D., Wojtysiak, A., & Roenneberg, T. (2011). Blue-enriched office light competes with natural light as a Zeitgeber. *Scandinavian Journal of Work, Environment & Health, 37*(5), 437–445. doi:10.5271jweh.3144 PMID:21246176

Konis, K. (2017). A novel circadian daylight metric for building design and evaluation. *Building and Environment, 113*, 22–38. doi:10.1016/j.buildenv.2016.11.025

CIE TN 003:2015 Report on the First International Workshop on Circadian and Neurophysiological Photometry, 2013.

Lockley, S. W., Skene, D. J., Butler, L. I., & Arendt, J. (1999). Sleep and activity rhythms related to circadian phase in the blind. *Sleep, 22*(5), 616–623. doi:10.1093leep/22.5.616 PMID:10450596

Lin, Zhu, Guo, Zheng, Lu, Shih, & Wu. (2016). Multi-function indoor light sources based on light-emitting diodes–a solution for healthy lighting. *Optics Express , 24(21).* doi:10.1364/OE.24.024401

Cuttle, C. (2010). Towards the third stage of the lighting profession. *Lighting Research & Technology*, *42*(1), 73–93. doi:10.1177/1477153509104013

Molina, L. T., Velasco, E., Retama, A., & Zavala, M. (2019). Experience from Integrated Air Quality Management in the Mexico City Metropolitan Area and Singapore. *Atmosphere*, *10*(9), 512. doi:10.3390/atmos10090512

Jiang, X., Kurihara, T., Torii, H., & Tsubota, K. (2018, September). Progress and Control of Myopia by Light Environments. *Eye & Contact Lens*, *44*(5), 273–278. doi:10.1097/ICL.0000000000000548 PMID:30048342

Acosta, I., Leslie, R. P., & Figueiro, M. G. (2015). Analysis of circadian stimulus allowed by daylighting in hospital rooms. *Lighting Research & Technology*, *0*, 1–13.

Madhulika, A. (2013). Gupta. Aditya K.Gupta. Sleep-wake disorders and dermatology. *Clinics in Dermatology*, *31*(1), 118–126. doi:10.1016/j.clindermatol.2011.11.016 PMID:23245983

CIE. (2016). Research Roadmap for healthful interior lighting applications. International Commission illumination. *CIE*, *218*.

Moyano, D. B., Moyano, S. B., López, M. G., Aznal, A. S., & Roberto, A. G. L. Photometrics and colorimetric analysis of LED luminaires for interior lighting design. 2021. *Color Research and Application*. Advance online publication. doi:10.1002/COL.2216

Moyano, D. B., Sola, Y., & Roberto, A. G. L. (2020). Blue-light levels emitted from portable electronic devices compared to sunlight. *Energies*, *13*(16), 4276. doi:10.3390/en13164276

Moyano, D. B., Mónica, S. J. F., & Roberto, A. G. L. (2020). Towards a Sustainable Indoor Lighting Design: Effects of Artificial Light on the Emotional State of Adolescents in the Clasrrom. *Sustainability*, *12*(10), 4623. doi:10.3390u12104263

Possible risks of LED lighting. (2018). Conclusions of the Spanish Lighting Committee Working Group.

Dain, S. (2020). The blue light dose from white light emitting diodes (LEDs) and other white light sources. *Ophthalmic & Physiological Optics*, *40*(5), 692–699. Advance online publication. doi:10.1111/opo.12713 PMID:32691888

Andersen, M., Mardaljevic, J., & Lockley, S. W. (2012). A framework for predicting the non-visual effects of daylight - Part I: Photobiology-based model. *Lighting Research & Technology*, *2012*(44), 37–53. doi:10.1177/1477153511435961

Edwards, L., & Torcellini, P. (2002). Literature Review of the Effects of Natural Light on Building Occupants. *Lit. Rev. Eff. Nat. Light Build. Occup.*, *55*. Advance online publication. doi:10.2172/15000841

Red Automática de Monitoreo Atmosférico de la ZMVT. (2019). *Técnicas de medición*. Retrieved from http://rama.edomex.gob.mx/tecnicas_medicion

Reinhart, C. F., Mardaljevic, J., & Rogers, Z. (2006). Dynamic daylight performance metrics for sustainable building design. *Leukos*, *3*(1), 7–31. doi:10.1582/LEUKOS.2006.03.01.001

Dai, Q., Huang, Y., Hao, L., Lin, Y., & Chen, K. (2018). Luoxi Haoa, Yi Lin, Kaixuan Chen. Spatial and spectral illumination design for energy-efficient circadian lighting. *Building and Environment*, *146*, 216–225. doi:10.1016/j.buildenv.2018.10.004

Rea, M. S., Figueiro, M. G., Bullough, J. D., & Bierman, A. (2005). A model of phototransduction by the human circadian system. *Brain Research. Brain Research Reviews*, *50*(2), 213–228. doi:10.1016/j.brainresrev.2005.07.002 PMID:16216333

Dai, Q., Cai, W., Shi, W., Hao, L., & Wei, M. (2017). A proposed lighting-design space: Circadian effect versus visual Illuminance. *Building and Environment*, *122*, 287–293. doi:10.1016/j.buildenv.2017.06.025

Figueiro, Steverson Heerwagen, Yucel, Roohan, Sahin, Kampschroer, & Rea. (2019). Light, entrainment and alertness: A case study in offices. *Lighting Research and Technology*.

Hunt, R. W. G., & Pointer, M. R. (2006). *Measuring Colour* (4th ed.). Wiley.

Kim, I. T., Choi, A. S., & Sung, M. K. (2017). Development of a Colour Quality Assessment Tool for indoor luminous environments affecting the circadian rhythm of occupants. *Building and Environment, 126*, 252–265. doi:10.1016/j.buildenv.2017.10.009

International Well Building Institute. (2016). *WELL Building Standard* (v1). Author.

EN 12464-1 2019: Lighting of workplaces – Indoor workplaces. https://www.valosto.com/tiedostot/prEN%2012464-1.pdf

EN 12665, *Light and lighting — Basic terms and criteria for specifying lighting requirements*, n.d.

ISO 8995-1 (2002): Lighting of indoor work places (CIE S008/2001)

Dibner, C., Schibler, U., & Albrecht, U. (2010). The mammalian circadian timing sys-tem: Organization and coordination of central and peripheral clocks. *Annual Review of Physiology, 72*(1), 517–549. doi:10.1146/annurev-physiol-021909-135821 PMID:20148687

Just, A. C., Wright, R. O., Schwartz, J., Coull, B. A., Baccarelli, A. A., Tellez-Rojo, M. M., Moody, E., Wang, Y., Lyapustin, A., & Kloog, I. (2015). Using high-resolution satellite aerosol optical depth to estimate daily PM2. 5 geographical distribution in Mexico City. *Environmental Science & Technology, 49*(14), 8576–8584. doi:10.1021/acs.est.5b00859 PMID:26061488

U.S. Green Building Council. (2019). LEED v4 for Building Design Construction. Author.

Illuminating Engineering Society of North America (IESNA). (n.d.). https://www.ies.org/standards/ies-standards-cross-reference/

David, L. (2011). A Procedure for Determining Target Illuminances, LEUKOS. *The Journal of the Illuminating Engineering Society of North America, 7*(3), 145–158. doi:10.1582/LEUKOS.2011.07.03001

Carrier, J., Paquet, J., Morettini, J., & Touchette, E. (2002). Phase advance of sleep and temperature circadian rhythms in the middle years of life in humans. *Neuroscience Letters, 320*(1-2), 1–4. doi:10.1016/S0304-3940(02)00038-1 PMID:11849749

Kripke, D. F., Elliott, J. A., Youngstedt, S. D., & Rex, K. M. (2007). Circadian phase response curves to lightin older and young women and men. *Journal of Circadian Rhythms, 5*(0), 4. doi:10.1186/1740-3391-5-4 PMID:17623102

Reinhart, C. F., & Voss, K. (2003). Monitoring manual control of electric lighting and blinds. *Lighting Research & Technology, 35*(3), 243–260. doi:10.1191/1365782803li064oa

Hirota, T., & Fukada, Y. (2004). Resetting mechanism of central and peripheral circadianclocks in mammals. *Zoological Science, 21*(4), 359–368. doi:10.2108/zsj.21.359 PMID:15118222

Volkova, K. A., Poberovsky, A. V., Timofeev, Y. M., Ionov, D. V., Holben, B. N., Smirnov, A., & Slutsker, I. (2018). Aerosol Optical Characteristics Retrieved from CIMEL Sun Photometer Measurements (AERONET) near St. Petersburg. *Atmospheric and Oceanic Optics, 31*(6), 635–641. doi:10.1134/S1024856018060180

Hair, J. W., Hostetler, C. A., Cook, A. L., Harper, D. B., Ferrare, R. A., Mack, T. L., Welch, W., Izquierdo, L. R., & Hovis, F. E. (2008). Airborne high spectral resolution lidar for profiling aerosol optical properties. *Applied Optics, 47*(36), 6734–6752. doi:10.1364/AO.47.006734 PMID:19104525

Konis. (2017). A novel circadian daylight metric for building design and evaluation. *Building and Environment, 113*, 22-38.

Van Donkelaar, A., Martin, R. V., Brauer, M., Kahn, R., Levy, R., Verduzco, C., & Villeneuve, P. J. (2010). Global estimates of ambient fine particulate matter concentrations from satellite-based aerosol optical depth: Development and application. *Environmental Health Perspectives*, *118*(6), 847–855. doi:10.1289/ehp.0901623 PMID:20519161

Zelinski, Deibel, & McDonald. (2014). The trouble with circadian clock dysfunction: Multiple deleterious effects on the brain and body. *Neurosci. Biobehav. Rev., 40*, 80-101. https://www.ncbi.nlm.nih.gov/pubmed/24468109

Holben, B. N., Tanre, D., Smirnov, A., Eck, T. F., Slutsker, I., Abuhassan, N., Newcomb, W. W., Schafer, J. S., Chatenet, B., Lavenu, F., Kaufman, Y. J., Castle, J. V., Setzer, A., Markham, B., Clark, D., Frouin, R., Halthore, R., Karneli, A., O'Neill, N. T., ... Zibordi, G. (2001, June 16). An emerging ground-based aerosol climatology: Aerosol optical depth from AERONET. *Journal of Geophysical Research, D, Atmospheres*, *106*(D11), 12067–12097. doi:10.1029/2001JD900014

Rea, M. S., & Figueiro, M. G. (2016). Light as a circadian stimulus for architectural lighting. *Lighting Research & Technology*, *0*, 1–14.

Lucas, R. J., Peirson, S. N., Berson, D. M., Brown, T. M., Cooper, H. M., Czeisler, C. A., Figueiro, M. G., Gamlin, P. D., Lockley, S. W., O'Hagan, J. B., Price, L. L. A., Provencio, I., Skene, D. J., & Brainard, G. C. (2014, January). Measuring and using light in the melanopsin age. *Trends in Neurosciences*, *37*(1), 1–9. Advance online publication. doi:10.1016/j.tins.2013.10.004 PMID:24287308

MODIS bands and spectral ranges. (2019). Retrieved from https://web.archive.org/web/20070715215437/http://edcdaac.usgs.gov/modis/table2.asp

Khademagha, P., Aries, M. B. C., Rosemann, A. L. P., & van Loenen, E. J. (2016). Implementing non-image-forming effects of light in the built environment: A review on what we need. *Building and Environment*, *108*, 263–272. doi:10.1016/j.buildenv.2016.08.035

MODIS aerosol product information. (2019a). Retrieved from https://ladsweb.modaps.eosdis.nasa.gov/missions-and-measurements/products/MOD04_L2/

Abalos, I., & Herreros, J. (2000). *Técnica y arquitectura en la ciudad contemporánea. 1950-2000*. Ed. Nerea.

Acks, K. (2006). A framework for cost-benefit analysis of green roofs: Initial estimates. *Green roofs in the New York metropolitan region: Research report.*

Adams, R., Jeanrenaud, S., Bessant, J., Denyer, D., & Overy, P. (2016). Sustainability-oriented innovation: A systematic review. *International Journal of Management Reviews*, *18*(2), 180–205.

ADEME. (2018). *Updated Energy-climate Scenario 2035-2050*. ADEME. https://www.ademe.fr/sites/default/files/assets/documents/energy-climate-scenario-ademe-2035-2050-010603.pdf

AFineLyne. (2019). https://gothamtogo.com/alica-kwade-selected-to-exhibit-on-met-roof-garden-spring-2019/

Ajuntament de Barcelona. (2018). *La Fàbrica del Sol enseña su interior*. https://ajuntament.barcelona.cat/ecologiaurbana/es/noticia/la-fabrica-del-sol-ensena-su-interior_636642

Akinlabi, E. T., Anane-Fenin, K., & Akwada, D. R. (2017). *Bamboo*. The Multipurpose Plant. doi:10.1007/978-3-319-56808-9

Albers, A., Behrendt, M., Klingler, S., Reiß, N., & Bursac, N. (2017). Agile product engineering through continuous validation in PGE–Product Generation Engineering. *Design Science, 3*.

Alnuman, N., & Altaweel, Z. (2020). Investigation of the Acoustical Environment in A Shopping Mall and Its Correlation to the Acoustic Comfort of the Workers. *Applied Sciences (Basel, Switzerland)*, *10*(3), 1170. doi:10.3390/app10031170

Anagal, V. (2010). *Sustainable urban solid waste management-a case study of Pune*. Academic Press.

Anderson, M. (2012). *Design And Development of A Roof Garden.* https://maintenance.transportation.org/Documents/10_Anderson_RoofGarden.pdf

Architecture, D. S. (2021). *Marmara Forum Commercial Complex.* http://www.dsmimarlik.com/project/Marmara-Forum-Commercial-Complex

Argiles & María. (1986). *Arquitectura de ladrillos del siglo XIX: técnica y forma.* Academic Press.

Arneborg, E. (n.d.). Altersschwerhörigkeit – Symptome, Ursachen, Folgen, Diagnostik, Therapie [Age-related hearing loss – symptoms, causes, consequences, diagnosis, therapy]. In *ASTM C423: Sound absorption and sound absorption coefficients by the reverberation room method.* American Society for Testing and Materials.

Arnheim, R. (1954). Art and visual perception, second edition: A psychology of the creative eye. Arte y percepción visual. Psicología del ojo creador. Editorial Eudeba.

Arroyo, G. A. (1973). Estudio analógico de la transmisión de calor en los muros tradicionales y ligeros. Instituto E. Torroja.

ASHRAE. (1992). *Thermal environment conditions for human occupancy*. American Society of Heating, Ventilating and Air Conditioning Engineers.

ASHRAE. (2005). *ASHRAE Handbook - Fundamentals. Refrigerating*. American Society of Heating and Air-Conditioning Engineers.

ASTM E 2400. (2006). *Standard Guide for Selection, Installation, and Maintenance of Plants for Green Roof Systems.* ASTM International.

ASTM E1110:2019: Standard Classification for Determination of Articulation Class. American Society for Testing and Materials. Pennsylvania, USA.

Atanda, J. (2015). Environmental impacts of bamboo as a substitute constructional material in Nigeria. *Case Studies in Construction Materials*, *3*, 33–39. doi:10.1016/j.cscm.2015.06.002

Austin, G. (2014). *Green infrastructure for landscape planning: integrating human and natural systems*. Routledge. doi:10.4324/9781315856780

Awalluddin, D., Ariffin, M. A. M., Osman, M. H., Hussin, M. W., Ismail, M. A., Lee, H.-S., & Lim, N. H. A. S. (2017). *Mechanical properties of different bamboo species.* Paper presented at the MATEC Web of Conferences.

Baines, T. S., Lightfoot, H. W., Evans, S., Neely, A., Greenough, R., Peppard, J., ... Wilson, H. (2007). State-of-the-art in product-service systems. *Proceedings of the Institution of Mechanical Engineers. Part B, Journal of Engineering Manufacture*, *221*(10), 1543–1552.

Balvers, J. R., Boxem, G., & de Wit, M. H. (2008). Indoor air quality in low-energy houses in the Netherlands, Does mechanical ventilation provide a healthy indoor Environment. Proceeding Indoor Air 2008.

Banbury, B., & Berry, D. C. (1998). The disruption office-related tasks by speech and office noise. *British Journal of Psychology*, *89*(3), 499–517. doi:10.1111/j.2044-8295.1998.tb02699.x

Banham, R. (1975). *La arquitectura del entorno bien climatizado*. Infinito.

Banik, R. L. (2015). Harvesting Techniques. In *Bamboo* (pp. 193–226). Springer. doi:10.1007/978-3-319-14133-6_7

Barbero, S., & Cozzo, B. (2009). *Ecodesign*. Ullmann.

Bass, B., & Baskaran, B. (2003). *Evaluating rooftop and vertical gardens as an adaptation strategy for urban areas*. Academic Press.

Basumatary, A., Middha, S. K., Usha, T., Brahma, B. K., & Goyal, A. K. (2015). Bamboo, as potential sources of food security, economic prosperity and ecological security in North-East India: An overview. *Research in Plant Biology*, *5*(2).

Baur. (2009). *Einfluss exogener Faktoren auf Altersschwerhörigkeit, HNO*. Springer Medizin Verlag.

Bayhan, B. (2015). *Dünyanın En Büyük Yeşil Çatısı Tasarlandı*. https://www.arkitera.com/haber/dunyanin-en-buyuk-yesil-catisi-tasarlandi/

Beldam, M.-B. (2019). Impact of acoustics on staff performance in operation rooms. Proceedings of Internoise.

Berglund, B., Lindvall, T., & Schwela, D. H. (1999). *Guidelines for community noise*. Technical Report World Health Organization.

Bian, F., Zhong, Z., Zhang, X., Yang, C., & Gai, X. (2020). Bamboo–An untapped plant resource for the phytoremediation of heavy metal contaminated soils. *Chemosphere*, *246*, 125750. doi:10.1016/j.chemosphere.2019.125750 PMID:31891850

Biondi, S. (2012, Noviembre 2). *Arquitectura Sostenible*. Retrieved from https://www.youtube.com/watch?v=wxIOK1V1joc&ab_channel=PUCPPUCP

Biswas, D., Lund, K., & Szocs, C. (2019). Sounds like a healthy retail atmospheric strategy: Effects of ambient music and background noise on food sales. *Journal of the Academy of Marketing Science*, *47*(1), 37–55. doi:10.100711747-018-0583-8

Boks, C., & Stevels, A. (2007). Essential perspectives for design for environment. Experiences from the electronics industry. *International Journal of Production Research*, *45*(18-19), 4021–4039.

Bordoloi, N., Sharma, A., Nautiyal, H., & Goel, V. (2018). An intense review on the latest advancements of Earth Air Heat Exchangers. *Renewable & Sustainable Energy Reviews*, *89*, 261–280. doi:10.1016/j.rser.2018.03.056

Borjesson, K. (2008). *Affective Sustainability. Is this what timelessness really means?* Academic Press.

Borooah, A., & Aster, D. (2009). *Toronto Green Roof Construction Standard: Supplementary Guidelines*. Academic Press.

Borrego, M., & Newswander, L. (2008). Characteristics of Successful Cross-disciplinary Engineering Education Collaborations. *Journal of Engineering Education*, *97*(2), 123–134. doi:10.1002/j.2168-9830.2008.tb00962.x

Boto-Álvarez, A., & García-Fernández, R. (2020). Implementation of the 2030 Agenda Sustainable Development Goals in Spain. *Sustainability*, *12*(6), 2546. doi:10.3390u12062546

Brambila-Macias, S. A., & Sakao, T. (2021). Effective ecodesign implementation with the support of a lifecycle engineer. *Journal of Cleaner Production*, *279*, 123520.

Brebbia, C. A., Longhurst, J., Marco, E., & Booth, C. (Eds.). (2017). *Sustainable development and planning IX* (Vol. 226). WIT press.

Breeam. (2011). *Manual BREEAM ES VIVIENDA®*. Galicia.

Brenneisen, S. (2003). *The Benefits of Biodiversity from Green Roofs œ Key Design Consequences* (Doctoral dissertation). Iowa State University.

Bribián, I. Z., Capilla, A. V., & Usón, A. A. (2011). Life cycle assessment of building materials: Comparative analysis of energy and environmental impacts and evaluation of the eco-efficiency improvement potential. *Building and Environment, 46*(5), 1133–1140. doi:10.1016/j.buildenv.2010.12.002

Brill, M., & Weidemann, S. (2001). *BOSTI: Disproving Widespread Myths about workplace design.* Kimball International.

Brown, G. (2009). NICU Noise and the Preterm Infant. *Neonatal Network, 28*(3), 165–173. doi:10.1891/0730-0832.28.3.165 PMID:19451078

Bunclark, L. (2020, Febrero 13). *Consideran al Perú en un nivel medio alto de estrés de agua.* Retrieved from https://rpp.pe/peru/actualidad/consideran-al-peru-en-un-nivel-medio-alto-de-estres-de-agua-noticia-1245508

Busch-Vishniac, I. J., West, J. E., Barnhill, C., Hunter, T., Orellana, D., & Chivukula, R. (2005). Noise Levels in John Hopkins Hospital. *The Journal of the Acoustical Society of America, 118*(6), 3629–3645. doi:10.1121/1.2118327 PMID:16419808

C40 Cities. (2018). *19 Global Cities Commit to Make New Buildings "Net-Zero Carbon" by 2030.* https://www.c40.org/press_releases/global-cities-commit-to-make-new-buildings-net-zero-carbon-by-2030

Cacciatore, F., Napoli, C., Abete, P., Marciano, E., Triassi, M., & Rengo, F. (1999). Quality of Life Derterminants and Hearing Function in an Elderly Population: Osservatorio Geriatrico Campano Study Group. *Gerontology, 45*(6), 323–328. doi:10.1159/000022113 PMID:10559650

Çalışkan, N. (2017). *Marmara Forum Shopping Center.* https://nilufercaliskan.info/projects/marmara-forum/

Campo Baeza, A. (1996). La Idea Construida; La arquitectura a la luz de las palabras. *Colegio oficial de arquitectos de Madrid,* 29.

Cantarero-García, G. (2018). Reflexiones urbanísticas. Referencias del pasado y situación actual de Madrid como ciudad inteligente potencial. In Gestión inteligente y sostenible de las ciudades. Gobernanza, smart cities y turismo. Valencia: Ed Tirant lo Blanch.

Cao, V. D., Pilehvar, S., Salas-Bringas, C., Szczotok, A. M., Rodriguez, J. F., Carmona, M., Al-Manasir, N., & Kjøniksen, A.-L. (2017). Microencapsulated phase change materials for enhancing the thermal performance of Portland cement concrete and geopolymer concrete for passive building applications. *Energy Conversion and Management, 133,* 56–66. doi:10.1016/j.enconman.2016.11.061

Caraiscos, C. (2009, August). Advanced control systems engineering for energy and comfort management in a building environment - a review. *Renewable & Sustainable Energy Reviews, 13*(6-7), 1246–1261. doi:10.1016/j.rser.2008.09.015

Carson, R. (1962). *Silent spring.* Crest Book.

Cavallo, A., Gatsby, K., & Reddy, T. (1991). Natural basement ventilation as a radon mitigation technique. *Proceedings of the 1991 International Symposium on Radon and Radon Reduction Technology, US Environmental Protection Agency, 2,* 1-24.

Cazzaniga, A., Furlanetto, L., & Molon, D. (1981). *Il Sistema di Raffrescamento Naturale delle Ville di Costozza* (Master's Thesis). Tesi di Laurea, Dipartimento di Architettura, Istituto Universitario di Architettura di Venezia, Venezia, Italy.

Çelikkol, U. (2015). *Alışveriş Merkezleri Değerlemesi Süreci Ve Yöntemleri, Marmara Forum Avm Değerleme Çalışması Örneği* (Doctoral dissertation). Fen Bilimleri Enstitüsü.

Ceschin, F., & Gaziulusoy, I. (2016). Evolution of design for sustainability: From product design to design for system innovations and transitions. *Design Studies, 47,* 118–163.

Chen, Y., Okudan, G. E., & Riley, D. R. (2010). Sustainable performance criteria for construction method selection in concrete buildings. *Automation in Construction, 19*(2), 235–244. doi:10.1016/j.autcon.2009.10.004

Cipriani, G., Danti, S., Picchi, L., Nuti, A., & Fiorino, M. D. (2020). Daily functioning and dementia. *Dementia & Neuropsychologia, 14*(2), 93–102. PMID:32595877

Clark, L., Londoño, X., & Ruiz-Sanchez, E. (2015). Bamboo taxonomy and habitat. In *Bamboo* (pp. 1–30). Springer. doi:10.1007/978-3-319-14133-6_1

Cliff, T. (1979). *Industria y paisaje*. Madrid I.E.A.L.

Código Técnico de la Edificación – Documento Básico de Protección Contra el Ruido (2009) – CTE DB HR [Spanish Building Regulations].

Corbusier, L. (1923). *Towards architecture*. Éditions Crès, Collection of "L'Esprit Nouveau", Paris. http://www.fondationlecorbusier.fr/corbuweb/morpheus.aspx?sysId=13&IrisObjectId=6463&sysLanguage=en-en&itemPos=46&itemSort=en-en_sort_string1%20&itemCount=47&sysParentName=&sysParentId=25

Correal, D. J. F., & Arbeláez, C. J. (2010). Influence of age and height position on Colombian Guadua angustifolia bamboo mechanical properties. *Maderas. Ciencia y Tecnología, 12*(2), 105–113. doi:10.4067/S0718-221X2010000200005

Costerdesign. (2021). *Foodcourt Marmara Forum Istanbul*. https://www.costerdesign.nl/post/food-court-marmara-forum-istanbul

Council of Europe. (2002). The European Higher Education Area. Joint Declaration of the European Ministers of Education (Bologna Declaration). Bologna, Italy, June 19, 1999. In *Compendium of Basic Documents in the Bologna Process: Steering Committee for Higher Education and Research (CD-ESR), 1st plenary session, Strasbourg, 3-4 October 2002, Item 7* (pp. 3-6). Academic Press.

Council, U. G. B. (1998). *US green building council*. US Green Building Council.

Crawford, R. H., & Pullen, S. (2011). Life cycle water analysis of a residential building and its occupants. *Building Research and Information, 39*(6), 589–602. doi:10.1080/09613218.2011.584212

Cruz, A., & Garnica, A. (2011). *Applied ergonomics*. Ecoe Editions.

CTE-DB HE-0. (2019). *Limitación del consumo energético*. Código técnico de la edificación. Ministerio de Transportes, Movilidad y Agenda Urbana, Gobierno de España.

CTE-DB HS-6. (2019). *Protección frente a la exposición al radón*. Código técnico de la edificación. Ministerio de Transportes, Movilidad y Agenda Urbana, Gobierno de España.

Dalton, D. S., Cruickshanks, K. J., Klein, B. E., Klein, R., Wiley, T. L., & Nondahl, D. M. (2003). The Impact of Hearing Loss on Quality of Life in Older Adults. *The Gerontologist, 43*(5), 661–668. doi:10.1093/geront/43.5.661 PMID:14570962

Darby, S., Hill, D., Deo, H., Auvinen, A., Barros-Dios, J.M., Baysson, H., Bochicchio, F., Falk, R., Farchi, S., Figueiras, A., Hakama, M., Heid, I., Hunter, N., Kreienbrock, L., Kreuzer, M., Lagarde, F., Mäkeläinen, I., Muirhead, C., Oberaigner, W., Pershagen, G., Ruosteenoja, E., & Schaffrath, A., Rosario, Tirmarche, M., Tomásek, L., Whitley, E., Wichmann, H-E., & Doll, R. (2006). Residential radon and lung cancer: Detailed results of a collaborative analysis of individual data on 7148 subjects with lung cancer and 14208 subjects without lung cancer from 13 epidemiologic studies in Europe. *Scandinavian Journal of Work, Environment & Health, 32*(Suppl 1), 1–83. PMID:16538937

Das, S. K., & Naik, S. (2002). Process planning for product disassembly. *International Journal of Production Research, 40*(6), 1335–1355.

Davidson, D., Castro-Delgado, S., Arias, J., & Mann, J. (2006). Unveiling a Ghost of Amazonian Rain Forests: Camponotus mirabilis, Engineer of Guadua Bamboo 1. *Biotropica, 38*(5), 653–660. doi:10.1111/j.1744-7429.2006.00194.x

Davis, B. E. (2011). Rooftop hospital gardens for physical therapy: A post-occupancy evaluation. *HERD: Health Environments Research & Design Journal, 4*(3), 14–43. doi:10.1177/193758671100400303 PMID:21866502

De Flander, K., & Rovers, R. (2009). One laminated bamboo-frame house per hectare per year. *Construction & Building Materials, 23*(1), 210–218. doi:10.1016/j.conbuildmat.2008.01.004

De Paepe, M., & Janssens, A. (2003). Thermo-hydraulic design of earth-air heat exchangers. *Energy and Building, 35*(4), 389–397. doi:10.1016/S0378-7788(02)00113-5

Delgado & Martín, E. (1892). La renta de tabacos. Academic Press.

Díaz, F. (1999). *Estrategias docentes para un aprendizaje significativo*. McGraw-Hill.

Dobers, P., & Strannegård, L. (2005). Sustainability and Design. *Business Strategy and the Environment, 14*(5), 269–271.

Dockrell, B., & Shield, J. (2008). *The effects of classroom and environmental noise on children's academic performance*. JASA.

Domínguez Amarillo, S. (2015). *Building envelopes and social housing in southern Europe energy assessment of the residential social stock of the city of Seville under the climate change scenario*. Academic Press.

Domínguez-Amarillo, S., Fernández-Agüera, J., Peacock, A., & Acosta, I. (2019). Energy related practices in Mediterranean low-income housing. *Building Research and Information*. Advance online publication. doi:10.1080/09613218.2019.1661764

Domínguez-Amarillo, S., Fernández-Agüera, J., Sendra, J. J., & Roaf, S. (2018). Rethinking User Behaviour Comfort Patterns in the South of Spain—What Users Really Do. *Sustainability, 10*(12), 4448. doi:10.3390u10124448

Domínguez-Amarillo, S., Fernández-Agüera, J., Sendra, J. J., & Roaf, S. (2019). The performance of Mediterranean low-income housing in scenarios involving climate change. *Energy and Building, 202*, 109374. doi:10.1016/j.enbuild.2019.109374

Dorr, E., Sanyé-Mengual, E., Gabrielle, B., Grard, B. J., & Aubry, C. (2017). Proper selection of substrates and crops enhances the sustainability of Paris rooftop garden. *Agronomy for Sustainable Development, 37*(5), 1–11. doi:10.100713593-017-0459-1

Dunnett, N. (2006). *Sheffield's Green Roof Forum: a multi-stranded programme of green roof infrastructure development for the UK's greenest city*. Academic Press.

Durup, N., Shield, B., Dance, S., Sullivan, R., & Gómez-Agustina, L. (2015). How classroom acoustics affect the vocal load of teachers. *Energy Procedia, 78*, 3084–3089. doi:10.1016/j.egypro.2015.11.761

Dyllick, T., & Rost, Z. (2017). Towards true product sustainability. *Journal of Cleaner Production, 162*, 346–360.

Eckert, H., & Koop, P. (2012). Roof Restoration With A Sunny Side. *ZinCo*. https://zinco.se/news/press_releases/press_release_details.php?id=76

Edge. (2021). *Guía del usuario de EDGE para todos los tipos de edificios Versión 3.0 BETA*. Recuperado el junio de 2021, de https://edgebuildings.com/wp-content/uploads/2021/02/201211-EDGE-User-Guide-for-All-Building-Types-Version-3.0.A-Beta.pdf

Edge. (n.d.). *Software EDGE*. Retrieved from https://edgebuildings.com/software/?lang=es

Emili, S., Ceschin, F., & Harrison, D. (2016). Product–Service System applied to Distributed Renewable Energy: A classification system, 15 archetypal models and a strategic design tool. *Energy for Sustainable Development*, *32*, 71–98.

EN 16487:2015: Acoustics - Test code for suspended ceilings - Sound absorption. European Standardization Organization.

Endalamaw, T. B., Lindner, A., & Pretzsch, J. (2013). Indicators and determinants of small-scale bamboo commercialization in Ethiopia. *Forests*, *4*(3), 710–729. doi:10.3390/f4030710

Eroski Consumer. (2021) Physiological characteristics of aging. *Eroski Consumer,* (36). https://revista.consumer.es

Espíndola, C., & Valderrama, J. O. (2012). Carbon Footprint. Part 1: Concepts, Estimation Methods and Methodological Complexities. *Información Tecnológica*, *23*(1), 163–176. doi:10.4067/S0718-07642012000100017

Esslinger, H. (2011). Sustainable design: Beyond the innovation-driven business model. *Journal of Product Innovation Management*, *28*(3), 401–404.

EU Commission. (2011). *Hoja de ruta hacia una economía hipocarbónica competitiva en 2050, Comunicación de la comisión al parlamento europeo, al consejo, al comité económico y social europeo y al comité de las regiones.* Author.

EU Council. (2014). *2030 climate and energy policy framework.* General Secretariat of the European Council.

Evans, G. W., & Johnson, D. (2000). Stress and open office noise. *The Journal of Applied Psychology*, *85*(5), 779–783. doi:10.1037/0021-9010.85.5.779 PMID:11055149

Fathy, H. (1986). *Natural energy and vernacular architecture. Principles and examples with reference to hot arid climates.* UNU.

Federal Emergency Management Agency-FEMA. (2007). *FEMA 430: Site and Urban Design for Security: Guidance-AgainstPotentialTerroristAttacks, ProvidingProtectionto People andBuildings.* Federal Emergency Management.

Fei, B., Liu, Z., Jiang, Z., Cai, Z., & Yu, Y. (2013). Mechanical properties of Moso bamboo treated with chemical agents. *Wood and Fiber Science*, *45*(1), 34–41.

Fernández, A. (n.d.). *Aguas residuaes en Perú, Problemática y uso en la agricultura.* Retrieved from https://www.ais.unwater.org/ais/pluginfile.php/356/mod_page/content/128/Peru%20INFORME%20DE%20PAIS.pdf

Fernández-Agüera, J., Domínguez-Amarillo, S., Alonso, C., & Martín-Consuegra, F. (2019). Thermal comfort and indoor air quality in low-income housing in Spain: The influence of airtightness and occupant behaviour. *Energy and Building*, *199*, 102–114. doi:10.1016/j.enbuild.2019.06.052

Fernandez-Cañero, R., Emilsson, T., Fernandez-Barba, C., & Machuca, M. Á. H. (2013). Green roof systems: A study of public attitudes and preferences in southern Spain. *Journal of Environmental Management*, *128*, 106–115. doi:10.1016/j.jenvman.2013.04.052 PMID:23722180

Fernandez, E. (2009). Aprendizaje experiencial, investigación-acción y creación organizacional de saber: La formación concebida como una zona de innovación profesional. *REIFOP*, *12*(3), 39–57.

Ferrucci, M., & Peron, F. (2018). Ancient Use of Natural Geothermal Resources: Analysis of Natural Cooling of 16th Century Villas in Costozza (Italy) as a Reference for Modern Buildings. *Sustainability*, *10*(12), 4340. doi:10.3390u10124340

Fiegel, A., Meullenet, J. F., Harrington, R. J., Humble, R., & Seo, H. S. (2014). Background music genre can modulate flavor pleasantness and overall impression of food stimuli. *Appetite*, *76*, 144–152. doi:10.1016/j.appet.2014.01.079 PMID:24530691

Florides, G. A., Tassou, S. A., Kalogirou, S. A., & Wrobel, L. C. (2002). Review of solar and low energy cooling technologies for buildings. *Renewable & Sustainable Energy Reviews*, *6*(6), 557–572. doi:10.1016/S1364-0321(02)00016-3

FMIC (Factory Mutual Insurance Company). (2007). *Green Roof Systems. FM Global Property Loss Prevention Data Sheets. 2007, 6 Temmuz 2011.* http://www.ci.berkeley.ca.us/uploadedFiles/Planning_and_Development/Level_3_Energy_and_Sustainable_Development/Factory%20Mutual%20Green%20Roof%2 0System.pdf

Fondo Mivivienda. (2020). *Procedimiento de Certificación de proyectos del Programa Mivienda Sostenible.* Retrieved from https://www.mivivienda.com.pe/PORTALCMS/archivos/documentos/8586096294727711719.PDF

Francis, R. A., & Lorimer, J. (2011). Urban reconciliation ecology: The potential of living roofs and walls. *Journal of Environmental Management*, *92*(6), 1429–1437.

Fried, & ... . (2002). The joint effects of noise, job complexity and gender on employee sickness absence, Journal of Occup and Organiz. *Psychology*, 75.

Future Green Studio. (2021). Empire Stores. *LANDEZİNE.* http://landezine.com/index.php/2021/01/empire-stores/

Gallardo Frías, L. (2013). Ser humano, lugar y eficiencia energética como fundamentos proyectuales en las estrategias arquitectónicas [The human being, place and energy efficiency as a projective basis in architectural strategies]. *Revista de Arquitectura*, *15*(1), 62–69. doi:10.14718/RevArq.2013.15.1.7

García de Paredes Andújar, J. (2008). *El cultivo del tabaco Virginia en España.* CETARSA

García Gener, P. (2016). *La docencia de la ETSAM en su contexto histórico.* TFG. Archivo digital UPM.

García, Á., Luis, J., Marquina, J. E., & Sanz, R. (1993). La esfera y el círculo en la historia. Ciencias, 30, 2-9.

Garner, W. W. (1951). *The production of tobacco.* Academic Press.

Gatóo, A., Sharma, B., Bock, M., Mulligan, H., & Ramage, M. H. (2014). Sustainable structures: bamboo standards and building codes. *Proceedings of the Institution of Civil Engineers-Engineering Sustainability.* 10.1680/ensu.14.00009

Gaziulusoy, A. I., Boyle, C., & McDowall, R. (2013). System innovation for sustainability: A systemic double-flow scenario method for companies. *Journal of Cleaner Production*, *45*, 104–116.

Gedge, D. (2003). From Rubble to Redstarts... Black Redstart Action Plan Working Group. *Proceedings from Greening Rooftops for Sustainable Communities, First North American Green Roof Infrastructure Conference.*

Getter, K. L., & Rowe, D. B. (2006). The role of extensive green roofs in sustainable development. *HortScience*, *41*(5), 1276–1285. doi:10.21273/HORTSCI.41.5.1276

Ghyka, M. (1983). *Esthétique des proportions dans la natue et dans les arts. Estética de las proporciones en la naturaleza y en las artes.* Editorial Poseidón.

Gill, T. M., Williams, C. S., & Tinetti, M. E. (1995). Assessing risk for the onset of functional dependence among older adults: The role of physical performance. *Journal of the American Geriatrics Society*, *43*(6), 603–609. PMID:7775716

Givoni, B. (1994). *Passive low energy Cooling of Buildings.* John Wiley & Sons, Inc.

Givoni, B. (1998). *Climate Considerations in Building and Urban Design.* John Wiley & Sons, Inc.

Gombrich, E. (1982) *The Image and the eye. Furher studies in the Psichology of Pictorical representation.* Phaidon Press Limited.

González Capitel, A., & García-Gutiérrez Mosteiro, J. (2000). *Luis Moya Blanco. Arquitecto 1904-1990.* Ministerio de Fomento y Editorial Electa.

Goodwin, J. (2001). *Otis: Giving rise to the modern City. Ivan R.* Dee Publisher.

Green Roof For Healthy Cities. (2021). https://greenroofs.org/

GRETA (Grupo de Estudios del Tabaco). (2002). *El consumo de tabaco en España en el siglo XVIII.* Cuadernos de Investigación Histórica nº 19.

Groundhog. (2021). *Keio University Roof Garden.* https://groundhog.la/projects/keio-university-roof-garden/

Guéguen, N., Hélène, L. G., & Jacob, C. (2004). Sound level of background music and alcohol consumption: An empirical evaluation. *Perceptual and Motor Skills, 99*(1), 34–38. doi:10.2466/pms.99.1.34-38 PMID:15446627

Guéguen, N., Jacob, N. C., Le Guellec, H., Morineau, T., & Lourel, M. (2008). Sound Level of Environmental Music and Drinking Behaviour: A Field Experiment with Beer Drinkers. *Clinical and Experimental Research, 32*(10), 1795–1798. doi:10.1111/j.1530-0277.2008.00764.x PMID:18647281

Guo, Z.-H., Chen, Y.-Y., Li, D.-Z., & Yang, J.-B. (2001). Genetic variation and evolution of the alpine bamboos (Poaceae: Bambusoideae) using DNA sequence data. *Journal of Plant Research, 114*(3), 315–322. doi:10.1007/PL00013993

GVL. (2021). *Yinian Rooftop Garden for Seniors.* https://landezine-award.com/yinian-rooftop-garden-for-seniors/

Hagerman, I., Rasmanis, G., Blomkvist, V., Ulrich, R., Eriksen, C. A., & Theorell, T. (2005). Influence of intensive coronary care acoustics on the quality of care and physiological state of patients. *International Journal of Cardiology, 98*(2), 267–270. doi:10.1016/j.ijcard.2003.11.006 PMID:15686777

Hai, C. (2014). *Building a community rooftop network: design prototypes for Taipei* (Doctoral dissertation).

Haq, G. (2016). *Win-win strategies to help older people face climate change.* https://www.sei.org/perspectives/older-people-climate-change/

Hardin, G. (1968). The Tragedy of the Commons. *Science.* PMID:5699198

Harper, S. (2006). *Climate Change and the Ageing Population – Oxford Programme for the Future of Cities.* Oxford Institute of Ageing, University of Oxford. http://www.futureofcities.ox.ac.uk/research/climate-change-and-the-ageing-population/

Harris Charles, W., & Dines Nicholas, T. (1998). *Time-saver standards for landscape architecture: design and construction data.* Academic Press.

Heidrich, O., & Tiwary, A. (2013). Environmental appraisal of green production systems: Challenges faced by small companies using life cycle assessment. *International Journal of Production Research, 51*(19), 5884–5896.

Heller, H., & Schiele, E. (1913). *Proportionstafeln der menschlichen gestalt: für kunstwerkstätten und fachschulen.* Editorial Kunstverlag Anton Schroll & Co.

Hernández, B. M. (1976). El cultivo del tabaco en la provincia de Cáceres: variedades de los tipos Burley y Flue-cured. Editorial Confederación Española de Cajas de Ahorros.

Hernández, S. (2008, October). El modelo constructivista con las nuevas tecnologías: Aplicado en el proceso de Aprendizaje. RUSC. *Universities and Knowledge Society Journal, 5*(2), 26–35.

Herzog & De Meuron. (1999). *AV Monographs Magazine, 77.*

Herzog, T. R., Maguire, P., & Nebel, M. B. (2003). Assessing the restorative components of environments. *Journal of Environmental Psychology*, *23*(2), 159–170.

Hirst, N. (2013). Buildings and climate change. In Design and Management of Sustainable Built Environments. doi:10.1007/978-1-4471-4781-7_2

Hopper, L. J. (Ed.). (2012). *Landscape architectural graphic standards* (Vol. 27). John Wiley & Sons.

HQE. (2014). *HQE™Scheme Environmental Performance Residential Building*. Retrieved from https://www.behqe.com/schemes-and-documents

HQE. (2014). User's Guide to the Tool for Target 5 – Water. Author.

Hu, S., Cabeza, L. F., & Yan, D. (2020). Review and estimation of global halocarbon emissions in the buildings sector. *Energy and Building*, *225*, 110311. doi:10.1016/j.enbuild.2020.110311

IDAE (Instituto para la Diversificación y Ahorro de la Energía). (2007). Guía técnica, Torres de refrigeración. Ahorro y eficiencia energética en Climatización. MITC.

IDAE (Instituto para la Diversificación y Ahorro de la Energía). (2008). Procedimientos para la determinación del rendimiento energético de plantas enfriadoras y equipos autónomos de tratamiento de aire. Instituto para la Diversificación y Ahorro de la Energía.

IEC 60268-16: Sound system equipment - Part 16: Objective rating of speech intelligibility by speech transmission index. International Electrotechnical Commission. Geneva, Switzerland.

IFC. (2018). *EDGE User Guide Versión 2.1*. IFC.

Inca, H. (n.d.). *Hidráulica Inca Camino- Inca del Agua*. Recuperado el 2021, de https://hidraulicainca.com/cusco/tipon/

INEI. (2020). *Nota de Prensa La población de Lima supera los nueve millones y medio de habitantes*. Retrieved from http://m.inei.gob.pe/media/MenuRecursivo/noticias/notadeprensa006.pdf

Instituto Nacional de Colonización. (1963). *Construye secaderos y mejorarás tu tabaco*. Publicaciones del Instituto Nacional de Colonización.

International Energy Agency and the United Nations Environment Programme. (2018). *Global Status Report: Towards a zero-emission, efficient and resilient buildings and construction sector*. Author.

International Organization for Standardization. (2002). *ISO/TR 14062: Environmental Management-Integrating Environmental Aspects Into Product Design and Development*. ISO.

ISN (Instituto de Seguridad Nuclear). (2021, February). *Mapa del potencial de radón de España*. https://www.arcgis.com/apps/SimpleViewer/index.html?appid=a3a435cfb6114e21ad03a5ac2961d8a8

ISO 10848-2:2017: Acoustics – Laboratory and field measurement of flanking transmission for airborne, impact and building service equipment sound between adjoining rooms – Part 2: Application to Type B elements when the junction has a small influence. Organization for Standardization, Geneva, Switzerland.

ISO 11654:1997. Acoustics – Sound absorbers for use in buildings–Rating of sound absorption, International Organization for Standardization, Geneva, Switzerland.

ISO 3382-1:2009. Acoustics – Measurement of room acoustic parameters – Part 1: Performance spaces, Organization for Standardization, Geneva, Switzerland.

ISO 3382-2:2008. Acoustics - Measurement of room acoustic parameters - Part 2: Reverberation time in ordinary rooms, Organization for Standardization, Geneva, Switzerland.

ISO 3382-3:2012. Acoustics – Measurement of room acoustic parameters – Part 3: Measurement of room acoustic parameters — Part 3: Open plan offices, Organization for Standardization, Geneva, Switzerland.

ISO 354:2013. Acoustics – Measurement of sound absorption in a reverberation room, International Organization for Standardization, Geneva, Switzerland.

ISO. (2011). 14006: 2011: Environmental management systems–Guidelines for incorporating ecodesign. Geneva: International Organization for Standardization.

ISO/FDIS 22955: Acoustic quality of open plan-offices. Organization for Standardization, Geneva, Switzerland.

Jack, J. (1931). Use of Bamboo in Subsoil Drainage. *Journal - Royal Sanitary Institute*, *52*(1).

Jafari, N., Utaberta, N., Yunos, M. Y. M., Ismail, N. A., Ismail, S., Ariffin, N. F. M., ... Valikhani, M. (2015). Benefits of roof garden in order to usage of urban agriculture at roof garden in high-rise building in Malaysia. *Advances in Environmental Biology*, *9*(24), 86–92.

Janssen, J. (2000). *Designing and building with bamboo. International Network for Bamboo and Rattan*. INBAR.

Jenkins, D. P. (2010). The value of retrofitting carbon-saving measures into fuel poor social housing. *Energy Policy*, *38*(2), 832–839. Advance online publication. doi:10.1016/j.enpol.2009.10.030

Jensen, K.L., Arens, E., & Zagreus, L. (2005). Acoustical quality in office workstations, as assessed by occupant's surveys. *Proceedings of Indoor Air*.

Johansson, L., Bergbom, I., Person-Waye, K., Ryherd, E., & Lindahl, B. (2012). The sound environment in an ICU patient room – A content analysis of sound levels and patient experiences. *Intensive & Critical Care Nursing*, *28*(5), 269–279. doi:10.1016/j.iccn.2012.03.004 PMID:22537478

Johnson, A. N. (2001). Neonatal response to control of noise inside the incubator. *Pediatric Nursing*, *27*(6), 600–605. PMID:12024534

Joint Commission. (2010). *Sentinel Event Data*. Root Causes by Event Type.

Jordan, G. (1994). *Tobacco in History: The cultures of dependence*. Academic Press.

Kaplan, R., & Kaplan, S. (1989). *The experience of nature: A psychological perspective*. Cambridge university press.

Katz, S., Branch, L. G., Branson, M. H., Papsidero, J. A., Beck, J. C., & Greer, D. S. (1983). Active life expectancy. *The New England Journal of Medicine*, *309*(20), 1218–1224. PMID:6633571

Kaur, P. J., Pant, K., Satya, S., & Naik, S. (2016). Bamboo: The material of future. *International Journal Series in Multidisciplinary Research*, *2*(2), 27–34.

Kaur, P. J., Satya, S., Pant, K. K., & Naik, S. N. (2016). Eco-friendly preservation of bamboo species: Traditional to modern techniques. *BioResources*, *11*(4), 10604–10624.

Kaushal, M. (2017). Geothermal cooling/heating using ground heat exchanger for various experimental and analytical studies. Comprehensive review. *Energy and Building*, *139*, 634–652. doi:10.1016/j.enbuild.2017.01.024

Kenda, B. (2006). Pneumatology in Architecture: The Ideal Villa. Proceedings of Healthy Buildings in Lissabon.

Kim, D. (2006). The natural environment control system of korean traditional architecture: Comparison with korean contemporary architecture. *Building and Environment*, *41*(12), 1905–1912. doi:10.1016/j.buildenv.2005.07.007

Klatte, M. & Lachmann, T. (2009). *A lot of noise about learning: acoustic conditions in classrooms and what they mean for teaching*. Academic Press.

Knaus, M., & Haase, D. (2020). Green roof effects on daytime heat in a prefabricated residential neighbourhood in Berlin, Germany. *Urban Forestry & Urban Greening*, *53*, 126738.

Köhler, M., Schmidt, M., Grimme, F. W., Laar, M., de Assunção Paiva, V. L., & Tavares, S. (2002). Green roofs in temperate climates and in the hot-humid tropics–far beyond the aesthetics. *Environmental Management and Health.*

Konietzko, J., Bocken, N., & Hultink, E. J. (2020). Circular ecosystem innovation: An initial set of principles. *Journal of Cleaner Production*, *253*, 119942.

Kristensen, H. S., & Remmen, A. (2019). A framework for sustainable value propositions in product-service systems. *Journal of Cleaner Production*, *223*, 25–35.

Kumar, S., Shukla, K., Dev, I., & Dobriyal, P. (1994). *Bamboo preservation techniques: a review*. Academic Press.

Kusuda, T., & Achenbach, P. H. (1965). Earth temperature and thermal diffusivity at selected stations in the United States. U.S. Department of Commerce. National Bureau of Standards, NBS doi:10.21236/AD0472916

Landschaftsentwicklung, F. (2008). *Guidelines for the planning, construction and maintenance of green roofing: Green roofing guideline*. Forschungsgesellschaft Landschaftsentwickung Landschaftsbau.

Lange, M. F. (2015). The sound of the intensive care unit - 3 weeks of continuous sound recording. *Proceedings of DASAIMs yearly meeting 2015*.

Larios-Meoño, J., González Taranco, C., & Morales Olivares, Y. (2015). Las aguas residuales y sus consecuencias en el Perú. *Saber y Hacer*, 21-23. Obtained from https://pre-www.usil.edu.pe/sites/default/files/revista-saber-y-hacer-v2n2.2-1-19set16-aguas-residuales.pdf

Latha, P., Darshana, Y., & Venugopal, V. (2015). Role of building material in thermal comfort in tropical climates–A review. *Journal of Building Engineering*, *3*, 104–113. doi:10.1016/j.jobe.2015.06.003

Laumann, K., Gärling, T., & Stormark, K. M. (2003). Selective attention and heart rate responses to natural and urban environments. *Journal of Environmental Psychology*, *23*(2), 125–134.

Lazzarin, R. M., Castellotti, F., & Busato, F. (2005). Experimental measurements and numerical modelling of a green roof. *Energy and Building*, *37*(12), 1260–1267.

Lee, T. (1982). *Rooftop landscape development: design implications for cool northern climates*. Academic Press.

Leed for Homes. (2011). *Guide to Green Building Rating Systems*. doi:10.1002/9781118259894.ch4

Liese, W. (1988). *Bamboo as an alternative material in the context of diminishing resources.* Paper presented at the International Bamboo Workshop, Cochin, India.

LIGHTDESIGN. (2021). *Seıbu Ike Bukuro Roof Garden.* https://lightdesign.jp/gallery/seibu-ikebukuro-roof-garden/

Liu, K., & Baskaran, B. (2003). *Thermal performance of green roofs through field evaluation.* Academic Press.

Liu, C. J., Shiroy, D. M., Jones, L. Y., & Clark, D. O. (2014). Systematic review of functional training on muscle strength, physical functioning, and activities of daily living in older adults. *European Review of Aging and Physical Activity*, *11*(2), 95–106.

Liu, W., Fox, J. E., & Xu, Z. (2000). Leaf litter decomposition of canopy trees, bamboo and moss in a montane moist evergreen broad-leaved forest on Ailao Mountain, Yunnan, south-west China. *Ecological Research, 15*(4), 435–447. doi:10.1046/j.1440-1703.2000.00366.x

Lloyd, N. (1925). *A History of English Brickwork*. The Antique Collectors' Club Ltd.

Lobovikov, M., Schoene, D., & Yping, L. (2012). Bamboo in climate change and rural livelihoods. *Mitigation and Adaptation Strategies for Global Change, 17*(3), 261–276. doi:10.100711027-011-9324-8

Luckett, K. (2009). *Green roof construction and maintenance*. McGraw-Hill Education.

Mackenzie, W. (1964). On the mechanical ventilation and warming of St. George's Hall, Liverpool. *Proceedings of the Institution of Mechanical Engineers Conference Proceedings.*

Madrid. (1948). *Cartilla para el cultivo y curado del tabaco en España*. Academic Press.

Mahdavi, M., Clouston, P., & Arwade, S. (2011). Development of laminated bamboo lumber: Review of processing, performance, and economical considerations. *Journal of Materials in Civil Engineering, 23*(7), 1036–1042. doi:10.1061/(ASCE)MT.1943-5533.0000253

Mairs, J. (2017). *Selgascano Adds Roof Extension With Pools And Plants To Second Home Offices İn London*. Academic Press.

Manandhar, R., Kim, J.-H., & Kim, J.-T. (2019). Environmental, social and economic sustainability of bamboo and bamboo-based construction materials in buildings. *Journal of Asian Architecture and Building Engineering, 18*(2), 49–59. doi:10.1080/13467581.2019.1595629

Mann, N. P., Haddow, R., Stokes, L., Goodley, S., & Rutter, N. (1986). Effect of Night and Day on Preterm Infants in a Newborn Nursery. *British Medical Journal, 293*(6557), 1265–1267. doi:10.1136/bmj.293.6557.1265 PMID:3096460

Mark, Gudith, & Klocke. (n.d.). *The Cost of Interrupted Work: More Speed and Stress*. University of California, Irvine.

Martínez, P., Luís, M., Serrano, G., & Patricio, Á. (1998). *Los secaderos de tabaco en la provincia de Granada*. Universidad EUAT de Granada.

Meteoblue. (2021). *İklim Bakırköy*. https://www.meteoblue.com/tr/hava/historyclimate/climatemodelled/bak%c4%b1rk%c3%b6y_t%c3%bcrkiye_751214

Minae, S. (1989). *Socio-economic issues in bamboo production and utilization in Kenya: present and future potentials*. Academic Press.

Minckley, B. B. (1968). A study of noise and its relationship to patient discomfort in the recovery room. *Nursing Research, 17*(3), 247–250. doi:10.1097/00006199-196805000-00018 PMID:5184904

Ministerio de Ambiente. (2015). *Regionalización y Caracterización de sequias en Perú*. Obtained from https://www.senamhi.gob.pe/pdf/estudios/hidro_2015_Reg_car_seq_Per.pdf

Ministerio de Fomento del Gobierno de España. (2017). Código técnico de la Edificación (CTE). Author.

Ministerio de Salud. (2011). *Reglamento de la calidad del agua para Consumo Humano*. Obtained from http://www.digesa.minsa.gob.pe/publicaciones/descargas/reglamento_calidad_agua.pdf

Miranda, A. L. (2018, mayo 28). *¿Agua o Energía?* (E. Samamé, Interviewer). Academic Press.

Moreira, L., & Ghavami, K. (2001). The influence of initial imperfections on the buckling of bamboo columns. *Proceedings of the International Workshop on the role of Bamboo in Disaster avoidance.*

Mor, V., Murphy, J., Masterson-Allen, S., Willey, C., Razmpour, A., Jackson, M. E., ... Katz, S. (1989). Risk of functional decline among well elders. *Journal of Clinical Epidemiology*, *42*(9), 895–904. PMID:2778468

Moussavi, S., Chatterji, S., Verdes, E., Tandon, A., Patel, V., & Ustun, B. (2007). Depression, chronic diseases, and decrements in health: Results from the World Health Surveys. *Lancet*, *370*(9590), 851–858. PMID:17826170

Moya Blanco, L. (1978). Artistas españoles contemporáneos. In *Artistas Españoles Contemporáneos*. Centro de Publicaciones. Ministerio de Educación y Ciencia.

National Park Board. (2017). *A handbook on developing sustainable highrise gardens, Bringing Greenery Skywards*. https://www.nparks.gov.sg/-/media/srg/files/handbook-1.pdf

National Park Service. (2021). *Green Roof Benefits*. https://www.nps.gov/tps/sustainability/new-technology/green-roofs/benefits.htm

Negreira, J., Svensson, C., Oseland, N., & Canto, R. (2019) Good acoustics as an extra source of income in restaurants – A case study. Proceedings of Internoise.

Neila, J. (2020). *Diferencias entre dos cabañas de madera: la isba rusa y la vivienda popular rumana*. http://sostenibilidadjavierneila.blogspot.com/

Neila, F. J. (2004). *Arquitectura Bioclimática en un entorno sostenible*. Munilla-Leira.

Nejat, P., Jomehzadeh, F., Taheri, M. M., Gohari, M., & Majid, M. Z. A. (2015). A global review of energy consumption, CO2 emissions and policy in the residential sector (with an overview of the top ten CO2 emitting countries). *Renewable & Sustainable Energy Reviews*, *43*, 843–862. doi:10.1016/j.rser.2014.11.066

Nightingale, F. (1859), *Notes on Nursing*. Academic Press.

Nurdiah, E. A. (2016a). *The potential of bamboo as building material in organic shaped buildings*. Petra Christian University.

Nurdiah, E. A. (2016b). The potential of bamboo as building material in organic shaped buildings. *Procedia: Social and Behavioral Sciences*, *216*, 30–38. doi:10.1016/j.sbspro.2015.12.004

Oberndorfer, E., Lundholm, J., Bass, B., Coffman, R. R., Doshi, H., Dunnett, N., Gaffin, S., Köhler, M., Liu, K. Y., & Rowe, B. (2007). Green Roofs as Urban Ecosystems: Ecological Structures, Functions and Services. *BioScience, 57*(10), 823-833. www.biosciencemag.org

Oetelaar, T., Johnston, C., Wood, D., Hughes, L., & Humphrey, J. (2013). A computational investigation of a room heated by subcutaneous convection – A case study of a replica Roman bath. *Energy and Building*, *63*, 59–66.

Ogunwusi, A. (2013). The impact of forest policy and land tenure system on bamboo development in Nigeria. *Public Policy and Administration Research*, *3*(5), 13–20.

Okokpujie, I., Akinlabi, E., & Fayomi, O. (2020). Assessing the policy issues relating to the use of bamboo in the construction industry in Nigeria. *Heliyon*, *6*(5), e04042. doi:10.1016/j.heliyon.2020.e04042 PMID:32478193

Olgyay, V. (1998). Arquitectura y Clima. Manual de diseño bioclimático para Arquitectos y Urbanistas. Gustavo Gili.

Oliveira, S., Olsen, L., Malki-Epshtein, L., Mumovic, D., & D'Ayala, D. (2021). Transcending disciplines in architecture, structural and building services engineering: A new multidisciplinary educational approach. *International Journal of Technology and Design Education*. Advance online publication. doi:10.100710798-020-09645-3

Olson Family Garden. (2021). *St. Louis Children's Hospital*. https://www.greenroofs.com/projects/olson-family-garden-st-louis-childrens-hospital/

Organización Mundial de la Salud. (2015). *OMS | Datos interesantes acerca del envejecimiento*. WHO. https://www.who.int/ageing/about/facts/es/

Oseland, N., & Hodsman, P. (2018). A psychoacoustical approach to resolving office noise distraction. *Journal of Corporate Real Estate*, *20*(4), 260–280. doi:10.1108/JCRE-08-2017-0021

Osmundson, T. (1999). *Roof gardens: history, design, and construction*. WW Norton & Company.

OXFAM. (n.d.). *OXFAM en Perú*. Retrieved from Entre 7 y 8 millones de peruanos no tienen acceso a agua potable: https://peru.oxfam.org/qu%C3%A9-hacemos-ayuda-humanitaria/entre-7-y-8-millones-de-peruanos-no-tienen-acceso-agua-potable

PAHO. (2021). *Weekly Breifing on the COVID-19 Situation in the Americas*. PAHO.

Palacio, B. (2016). La enseñanza integral de la Arquitectura, desde la perspectiva de la sostenibilidad ambiental. *Módulo Arquitectura CUC*, *16*(1), 35–58. doi:10.17981/moducuc.16.1.2016.02

Panagopoulos, T., Guimaraes, M., Barreira, A. P., & Pana, R. (2013). *aging population and climate change induced migration as causes of urban decline in Portugal*. Academic Press.

Panizzoni, L. (2001). La Villa che Respira. Technical Report. Istituto Regionale delle Ville Venete.

Parada & Tamar. (2015). *Tobacco industrial architecture in Peninsular Spain: dryers and factories*. E.T.S.A.M. Polytechnical University of Madrid.

Pearce, D. W., & Turner, R. K. (1990). *Economics of natural resources and the environment*. JHU press.

Peck, S. W., Callaghan, C., Kuhn, M. E., & Bass, B. (1999). *Greenbacks from green roofs: forging a new industry in Canada*. Academic Press.

Peck, S. W., & Kuhn, M. (2003). *Design guidelines for green roofs*. Ontario Association of Architects.

Peek, K. (2016). How to Survive in a Warmer World. *Scientific American*. https://www.scientificamerican.com/article/how-to-survive-in-a-warmer-world-interactive/

Peretti, C., Zarrella, A., Carli, M. D., & Zecchin, R. (2013). The design and environmental evaluation of earth-to-air heat exchangers (EAHE). A literature review. *Renewable & Sustainable Energy Reviews*, *28*, 107–116. doi:10.1016/j.rser.2013.07.057

PérezC. J. (2017). fromhttp://repositorio.senamhi.gob.pe/bitstream/handle/20.500.12542/246/Causa-sequ%C3%ADas-severas-sur-Per%C3%BA_2017.pdf?sequence=1&isAllowed=y

Pintos, P. (2021). *Marmara Forum Cloud Playground / Carv*. https://www.archdaily.com/939901/marmara-forum-cloud-playground-carve?ad_medium=gallery

Plumridge, A., & Meulenkamp, W. (1993). *Brickwork: Architecture and Design*. Harry N Abrams.

Poulikidou, S., Björklund, A., & Tyskeng, S. (2014). Empirical study on integration of environmental aspects into product development: Processes, requirements and the use of tools in vehicle manufacturing companies in Sweden. *Journal of Cleaner Production*, *81*, 34–45.

Pouya, S. (2019). Evaluation of Roof Gardens as Recreation Areas. *Türkiye Peyzaj Araştırmaları Dergisi*, *2*(1), 40–49.

Priority Zone. (2021). *Rooftop Garden Inner-City Greening & Beautification*. http://priorityzone.weebly.com/rooftop-garden.html#

Proxima (2021). Compherensive Green Roof in Mexico City (INFONAVIT). *Landezine*. https://landezine-award.com/comprehensive-green-roof-in-mexico-city-infonavit/

Puig-Pey Clavería, A. M. (2017). El Arquitecto: Formación, Competencias Y Práctica Profesional. *ACE: Architecture, City and Environment, 12*(34), 301–320. . http://hdl.handle.net/2117/106075 doi:10.5821/ace.12.34.5296

PUPC. (2018). *Informe Puntoedu sobre estrés hídrico en el Perú*. Retrieved from https://puntoedu.pucp.edu.pe/noticia/informe-puntoedu-sobre-estres-hidrico-en-el-peru/

Raj, A. D., & Agarwal, A. B. (2014). Bamboo as a Building Material. *J. Civ. Eng. and Env. Tech, 1*(3), 56–61.

Rasmussen, S. E. (1957). Om at opleve arkitektur. GEC Gads Forlag.

Reddy, B. V. (2004). Sustainable building technologies. *Current Science*, 899–907.

Revista peruana Geo-Atmosférica RPGA. (2010). *Recent droughts in the Peruvian Amazonas basin: Climate origins and.* Revista Peruana Geo-Atmosferica RPGA. Obtained fromhttps://web2.senamhi.gob.pe/rpga/pdf/2011_vol03/art5.pdf

Roaf, S., Nicol, F., & De Dear, R. (2013). The wicked problem of designing for comfort in a rapidly changing world. *Architectural Science Review, 56*(1), 1–3. Advance online publication. doi:10.1080/00038628.2012.753783

Roaf, S., Nicol, F., & Rijal, H. (2015). Designing for comfort at high temperatures. *Architectural Science Review, 58*(1), 35–38. doi:10.1080/00038628.2014.972069

Roberts, E., & Henwood, K. (2019). "It's an Old House and That's How It Works": Living Sufficiently Well in Inefficient Homes. *Housing Theory and Society, 36*(4), 1–20. doi:10.1080/14036096.2019.1568296

Rockström, J., Steffen, W., Noone, K., Persson, Å., Chapin, F. S., Lambin, E. F., ... & Foley, J. A. (2009). A safe operating space for humanity. *Nature, 461*(7263), 472-475.

Rojas, F., Lew, M., & Naeim, F. (2010). An overview of building codes and standards in Chile at the time of the 27 February 2010 Offshore Maule, Chile earthquake. *Structural Design of Tall and Special Buildings, 19*(8), 853–865. doi:10.1002/tal.676

S.N.C.F.T. (1952). *El secado de la hoja de tabaco*. Author.

S.N.C.F.T. (1962). *Construye secaderos y mejorarás tu tabaco*. Author.

Saikia, P., Dutta, D., Kalita, D., Bora, J. J., & Goswami, T. (2015). Improvement of mechano-chemical properties of bamboo by bio-chemical treatment. *Construction & Building Materials, 101*, 1031–1036. doi:10.1016/j.conbuildmat.2015.10.106

Sailor, D. J. (1995). Simulated urban climate response to modifications in surface albedo and vegetative cover. *Journal of Applied Meteorology and Climatology, 34*(7), 1694–1704.

Sakao, T., & Brambila-Macias, S. A. (2018). Do we share an understanding of transdisciplinarity in environmental sustainability research? *Journal of Cleaner Production, 170*, 1399–1403.

Sanchez-Guevara, C., Núñez Peiró, M., Taylor, J., Mavrogianni, A., & Neila González, J. (2019). Assessing population vulnerability towards summer energy poverty: Case studies of Madrid and London. *Energy and Building, 190*, 132–143. doi:10.1016/j.enbuild.2019.02.024

Sansone, C. (1999). Traditional Bio-Climate Building Techniques. *Proceedings Sharing Knowledge on Sustainable Buildings, Mediterranean Conference.*

Santamouris, M., Paravantis, J. A., Founda, D., Kolokotsa, D., Michalakakou, P., Papadopoulos, A. M., Kontoulis, N., Tzavali, A., Stigka, E. K., Ioannidis, Z., Mehilli, A., Matthiessen, A., & Servou, E. (2013). Financial crisis and energy consumption: A household survey in Greece. *Energy and Building*, *65*, 477–487. doi:10.1016/j.enbuild.2013.06.024

Sanyé-Mengual, E., Orsini, F., Oliver-Solà, J., Rieradevall, J., Montero, J. I., & Gianquinto, G. (2015). Techniques and crops for efficient rooftop gardens in Bologna, Italy. *Agronomy for Sustainable Development*, *35*(4), 1477–1488.

Schönwälder, H.-G., Ströver, F., & Tiesler, G. (2008). *Health promoting influences on performance ability in school education*. Academic Press.

Scurlock, J. M., Dayton, D. C., & Hames, B. (2000). Bamboo: An overlooked biomass resource? *Biomass and Bioenergy*, *19*(4), 229–244. doi:10.1016/S0961-9534(00)00038-6

Section 504. (2021). *Building And Rooftop Acces*. https://up.codes/s/building-and-rooftop-access

Seddigh, A., Berntson, E., Jönsson, F., Danielson, C. B., & Westerlund, H. (2015). The effect of noise absorption variation in open-plan offices: A field study with a cross-over design. *Journal of Environmental Psychology*, *44*, 34–44. doi:10.1016/j.jenvp.2015.08.004

Senamhi. (n.d.). *Eventos Climáticos - Fenómeno del Niño*. Retrieved from Senamhi: http://senamhi.gob.pe/?p=fenomeno-el-nino

Shah, A. U. M., Sultan, M. T. H., Jawaid, M., Cardona, F., & Talib, A. R. A. (2016). A review on the tensile properties of bamboo fiber reinforced polymer composites. *BioResources*, *11*(4), 10654–10676.

Sharma, B., Gatoo, A., Bock, M., Mulligan, H., & Ramage, M. (2015). Engineered bamboo: State of the art. *Proceedings of the Institution of Civil Engineers-Construction Materials*, *168*(2), 57–67. doi:10.1680/coma.14.00020

Sharma, P., Dhanwantri, K., & Mehta, S. (2014). Bamboo as a building material. *International Journal of Civil Engineering Research*, *5*(3), 249–254.

Shuang, H. (2021). *Pixeland / 100architects*. Https://www.Archdaily.Com/915563/Pixeland-100architects

Simon, H. (1968). The Sciences of the Artificial. doi:10.2307/3102825

Simon, M., Tackenberg, P., Hasselhorn, H.-M., Kümmerling, A., & Büscher, A. (2005). *Auswertung der ersten Befragung der NEXT-Studie in Deutschland*. Wuppertal University.

Slevin, M., Farrington, N., Duffy, G., Daly, L., & Murphy, J. F. (2000). Altering the NICU and measuring infants' responses. *Acta Paediatrica (Oslo, Norway)*, *89*(5), 577–581. doi:10.1111/j.1651-2227.2000.tb00342.x PMID:10852196

Snodgrass, E. C., & Snodgrass, L. L. (2006). Green roof plants: a resource and planting guide (No. 04; SB419. 5, S5.). Portland, OR: Timber Press.

Soltani, M., Kashkooli, F., Sanij, A. D., Kazemi, A., Bordbar, N., Farschini, M., Elmi, M., Gharali, K., & Dusseault, M. (2018). A comprehensive study of geothermal heating and cooling systems. *Sustainable Cities and Society*.

Srenco. (2007). *Looking at Rooftop Garden at St. Louis Childrens Hospital in St. Louis MO 63108*. http://www.srencoaerialphoto.com/srencobuildings/Pages/12.html

Sroufe, R., Curkovic, S., Montabon, F., & Melnyk, S. A. (2000). The new product design process and design for environment. *International Journal of Operations & Production Management*.

Stafford, L. D., Fernandes, M., & Agobiani, E. (2012). Effects of noise and distraction on alcohol perception. *Food Quality and Preference*, *24*(1), 218–224. doi:10.1016/j.foodqual.2011.10.012

Stang, M. & Møller, C. (2018). Between regulation mechanisms and professional essentials: Exploring current challenges in architectural education. *Artifact: Journal of Design Practice, 5*(1). doi:10.1386/art.5.1.3.1_1

Steffen, W., Richardson, K., Rockström, J., Cornell, S. E., Fetzer, I., Bennett, E. M., ... Sörlin, S. (2015). Planetary boundaries: Guiding human development on a changing planet. *Science, 347*(6223). PMID:25592418

Sturrock, N., & Lawson-Smith, P. (2006). The Work and Influence of David-Boswell Reid, Physician, Chemist, Engineer (1805-63). *Proceedings of the Second International Congress on Construction History*, 3, 2981-2998.

Syla, A. (2019). *Global Warming and role of Construction Materials in consume energy*. Academic Press.

Takahashi, J., & del Bambú–Perubambu, A. P. (2006). Bamboo in Latin America: Past, Present and the Future. *Bamboo for the Environment, Development and Trade*, 4.

Tan, T., Rahbar, N., Allameh, S., Kwofie, S., Dissmore, D., Ghavami, K., & Soboyejo, W. (2011). Mechanical properties of functionally graded hierarchical bamboo structures. *Acta Biomaterialia, 7*(10), 3796–3803. doi:10.1016/j.actbio.2011.06.008 PMID:21704742

Thomas, K. (1996). *Masonry walls: Specification and design.* Academic Press.

Tiesler, G. (2018). Communication behaviour and workload of students and teachers in highly absorbent classrooms. Proceedings of Euronoise 2018.

Tiesler, G., & Oberdöster, M. (2006). *Acoustic ergonomics of school.* Publication Series from the Federal Institute for Occupational Safety and Health - Research Report - Fb 1071.

Tolderlund, L. (2010). *Design guidelines and maintenance manual for green roofs in the semi-arid and arid west.* Green Roofs for Healthy Cities.

Tooke, T. R., Coops, N. C., Voogt, J. A., & Meitner, M. J. (2011). Tree structure influences on rooftop-received solar radiation. *Landscape and Urban Planning, 102*(2), 73–81.

Tripathi, Y. (2008). Bamboo entrepreneurship-Opportunities for rural employment. *Indian Forester, 134*(9), 1199–1210.

U.S. Green Building Council. (2017). *LEED v4 for Homes design and Construction.* LEED.

Ulrich, R. S. (1998). View through a window may influence recovery from surgery. *Science, 224*, 42M21.

Ulrich, R. S., Simons, R. F., Losito, B. D., Fiorito, E., Miles, M. A., & Zelson, M. (1991). Stress recovery during exposure to natural and urban environments. *Journal of Environmental Psychology, 11*(3), 201–230.

UN. (2015). *Transforming our world: The 2030 agenda for sustainable development.* United Nations, Department of Economic and Social Affairs.

UN. (2021). *Aging.* https://www.un.org/es/sections/issues-depth/ageing/index.htm

Unite Nations. (2012). *Enable. Accessibility for the disabled-A design manual for a barrier Free environment.* https://www.un.org/esa/socdev/enable/designm/AD4-01.htm

Van der Lugt, P., Van den Dobbelsteen, A., & Janssen, J. (2006). An environmental, economic and practical assessment of bamboo as a building material for supporting structures. *Construction & Building Materials, 20*(9), 648–656. doi:10.1016/j.conbuildmat.2005.02.023

Vanzolini. (n.d.). Obtained from https://vanzolini.org.br/aqua/certificacao-aqua-hqe/

Vargas Marcos, F., & Gallego Pulgarín, I. (2005, March-April). Environmental quality: Wellfare, confort and health. *Revista Espanola de Salud Publica, 79*(2), 243–251. doi:10.1590/S1135-57272005000200011 PMID:15913058

Velazquez, S. L. (2005). *Organic Greenroof Architecture: Sustainable Design for the New Millennium; Making the most of your building's fifth façade*. Wiley Periodicals, Inc.

Venkatarama Reddy, B. (2009). Sustainable materials for low carbon buildings. *The International Journal of Low Carbon Technologies, 4*(3), 175–181. doi:10.1093/ijlct/ctp025

Vezzoli, C., Ceschin, F., Diehl, J. C., & Kohtala, C. (2015). New design challenges to widely implement 'Sustainable Product–Service Systems'. *Journal of Cleaner Production, 97*, 1–12.

Vogtländer, J., Van der Lugt, P., & Brezet, H. (2010). The sustainability of bamboo products for local and Western European applications. LCAs and land-use. *Journal of Cleaner Production, 18*(13), 1260–1269. doi:10.1016/j.jclepro.2010.04.015

Wachenfeldt, B.J., & Bell, D. (2003). *Building Integrated Energy Systems in Smart Energy Efficient Buildings – A State-of-the-art.* SINTEL Project report, STF22 A04503.

Wang, T., & Pryor, M. (2019). *Social Value of Urban Rooftop Farming: A Hong Kong Case Study*. Agricultural Economics-Current Issues.

Wang, Y., Modi, S. B., & Schoenherr, T. (2020). Leveraging sustainable design practices through supplier involvement in new product development: The role of the suppliers' environmental management capability. *International Journal of Production Economics*.

Ware, D., & Beatty, B. (1998). *Diccionario manual ilustrado de arquitectura*. Editorial Gustavo Gili.

Weiler, S. K., & Scholz-Barth, K. (2009). Green Roof Systems – A Guide to the Planning, Design and Construction of Landscape Over Structure. Hoboken, NJ: John Wiley & Sons, Inc.

Weinstein, N. D. (1974). Effect of noise on intellectual performance. *The Journal of Applied Psychology, 59*(5), 548–554. doi:10.1037/h0037338

Weise, C. H. (2010). *Investigation of patient perception of hospital noise and sound level measurements: before, during and after renovations of a hospital wing.* Architectural engineering – Dissertations and Student Research (Master Thesis Report).

WELL. (2018). *Well V2 tm*. WELL.

WELL. (2021). *WELL Performance Verification Guidebook*. Obtained from https://a.storyblok.com/f/52232/x/29668f7afb/well-performance-verification-guidebook_q2-2021.pdf

Wells, E. M., Berges, M., Metcalf, M., Kinsella, A., Foreman, K., Dearborn, D. G., & Greenberg, S. (2015). Indoor air quality and occupant comfort in homes with deep versus conventional energy efficiency renovations. *Building and Environment, 93*(P2), 331–338. doi:10.1016/j.buildenv.2015.06.021

Werthmann, C. (2007). *Green Roof-A Case Study: Michael Van Valkenburgh Associates' Design for the Headquarters of the American Society of Landscape Architects*. Princeton Architectural Press.

WHO. (2016). *Multisectoral Action for Healthy Aging Based on the Life Cycle: Draft Global Strategy and Plan of Action on Aging and Health: Report of the Secretariat (No. A69 / 17)*. World Health Organization.

WHO. (2020). *New coronavirus*. https://www.who.int/es/

WHO. (2021). *Aging*. http:www.who.int/topic/ageing/es/

WHO. (2021). *More countries act against exposure to radon and associated cancer risks.* https://www.who.int/news/item/04-02-2021-more-countries-act-against-exposure-to-radon-and-associated-cancer-risks

Wilkinson, P., Smith, K. R., Joffe, M., & Haines, A. (2007). A global perspective on energy: health effects and injustices. Lancet. doi:10.1016/S0140-6736(07)61252-5

Wilkinson, S. J., Knott, J., Goddard, J. G., & Craft, L. (2016). *RICS Best Practice Guidance Note on Green Roofs and Green Walls.* RICS Best Practice Guidance Note on Green Roofs and Green Walls.

Willem, V. C. (2005, April). ROOFTOP GARDENING, a big step to the future. *Conference Paper, First International Summit for Aforestation Roof Gardens in China.*

Woloshynowych, M., Davis, R., Brown, R., & Vincent, C. (2007). Communication patterns in a UK emergency department. *Annals of Emergency Medicine, 50*(4), 407–413. doi:10.1016/j.annemergmed.2007.08.001 PMID:17881316

Wong, N. H., Chen, Y., Ong, C. L., & Sia, A. (2003). Investigation of thermal benefits of rooftop garden in the tropical environment. *Building and Environment, 38*(2), 261–270.

Woods, A. T., Poliakoff, E., Lloyd, D. M., Kuenzel, J., Hodson, R., Gonda, H., Batchelor, J., Dijksterhuis, G. B., & Thomas, A. (2011). Effect of background noise on food perception. *Food Quality and Preference, 22*(1), 43–47. doi:10.1016/j.foodqual.2010.07.003

WorldPress. (2021). *Roof Garden of The Metropolitan Museum of Art.* http://wirednewyork.com/museums/met-museum/roof-garden/

WWF. (2016) *Living Planet Report 2016. Risk and resilience in a new era.* WWF International. http://awsassets.panda.org/downloads/lpr_living_planet_report_2016.pdf

Xiao, Y., Yang, R., & Shan, B. (2013). Production, environmental impact and mechanical properties of glubam. *Construction & Building Materials, 44*, 765–773. doi:10.1016/j.conbuildmat.2013.03.087

You Stop the Music: How Sounds in Retail Stores Divide Shoppers. (n.d.). Available here: https://bit.ly/2PTo22F

Yudodibroto, H. (1985). Bamboo research in Indonesia. *Proceeding from the International Bamboo Workshop.*

Yuen, B., & Hien, W. N. (2005). Resident perceptions and expectations of rooftop gardens in Singapore. *Landscape and Urban Planning, 73*(4), 263–276.

Zahr, L. K., & de Traversay, J. (1995). Premature infant responses to noise reduction by earmuffs: Effects on behavioral and physiologic measures. *Journal of Perinatology, 15*(6), 448–555. PMID:8648453

Zakikhani, P., Zahari, R., Sultan, M. T. H. H., & Majid, D. L. A. A. (2017). Morphological, mechanical, and physical properties of four bamboo species. *BioResources, 12*(2), 2479–2495. doi:10.15376/biores.12.2.2479-2495

Zeiler, W., & Boxem, G. (2009). Geothermal Active Building Concept. In R. J. Howlett, L. C. Jain, & S. H. Lee (Eds.), *Sustainability in Energy and Buildings.* Springer. doi:10.1007/978-3-642-03454-1_32

Zhou, A., Huang, D., Li, H., & Su, Y. (2012). Hybrid approach to determine the mechanical parameters of fibers and matrixes of bamboo. *Construction & Building Materials, 35*, 191–196. doi:10.1016/j.conbuildmat.2012.03.011

Zhu, D. J., & Qiu, S. F. (2007). Analytical tool for urban circular economy planning and its preliminary application: A case of Shanghai. *City Planning Review, 31*(3), 64–69.

ZinCo. (2020). *Planning Guide Walkways and Driveways on Roofs and Decks.* https://docs.google.com/viewerng/viewer?url=https%3A%2F%2Fzinco-greenroof.com%2Fsites%2Fdefault%2Ffiles%2F2020-

About the Contributors

Roberto A. González-Lezcano is a PhD in Industrial Engineering, Postgraduate Diploma in Plant Engineering, Postgraduate Diploma in University Didactics, Master in Mathematical Engineering Extraordinary Doctorate Award. Assistant Professor of the Department of Architecture and Design, in the area of Facilities at the Higher Polytechnic School of the CEU San Pablo University. He has been teaching at Building Installations, Electromechanics and Materials, Physics, Mathematics, Mechanical Engineering and Mechanics of Continuous Media and Theory of Structures. Accredited Professor by the ACAP in the figures of Professor Hired Doctor, Professor Doctor of Private University and Tenured Professor. A six-year research period recognized by the CNEAI. He has taught in undergraduate and master's degrees at the Carlos III University of Madrid, Camilo José Cela University, European University of Madrid, Antonio de Nebrija University, Technical University of Madrid and Alfonso X El Sabio University. He has published several books and articles concerning the areas of Energy, Installations and Continuous Media Mechanics.

* * *

Tamar Awad has a PhD in Architecture by Polytechnic University of Madrid.

David Baeza has a Ph.D by Universidad San Pablo CEU (CEU), degree in Pharmacy and Optics and Optometry by the Universidad Complutense de Madrid (UCM). Master's degree in renewable energies and Master's degree in higher education and professional training. Adjunct Professor of Optics of the Faculty of Pharmacy of CEU Biosanitary trainer both in the university and in-company, and researcher of new sources of light useful for health and aesthetics. Expert in Photobiology. His studies focus on the analysis of the form of absorption and possible effects of the energy to which the human body is sensitive. Technical director of laboratory Futuro Tecnológico Español SL for the measurement of UV tanning devices irradiance.

Guadalupe Cantarero-García has a PhD in Architecture (ETSAM) Degree in Architecture Coordinator- Institute of Technology Senior Lecturer San Pablo CEU University Smart Cities Lab. (Dir.) - San Pablo CEU University Universal Accessibility Title (Dir.) - San Pablo CEU University.

Samuel Dominguez-Amarillo is Sr. Lecturer in Architectural Engineering at the College of Architecture of the University of Seville. He is sr. researcher in the R&D TEP-130: Architecture, Heritage and Sustainability group with extensive scientific publication and participation in international forums and committees. In his professional career is an Expert Consultant on Hi-performance building Systems. He has extensive background as adviser on environmental control for Cultural Heritage, Environmental Quality of Buildings, Energy Efficiency and Smart Buildings Management with a wide portfolio of national and international projects.

Jesica Fernandez-Agüera is a Researcher in Architectural Engineering at the College of Architecture of the University of Seville. She is researcher in the R&D TEP-130: Architecture, Heritage and Sustainability group with extensive scientific publication and participation in international forums and committees. She has extensive background on Indoor Air Quality, Energy Efficiency and Health in Buildings.

Nerea García Cortés is an Architect and researcher at the University of Seville. She currently live in Seville and is dedicating her professional life to the study and understanding of a sustainable, accessible, and inclusive architecture for all.

Selim Gündüz was born in İstanbul in 1987. He completed undergraduate education at Istanbul Aydin University, Faculty of Architecture and Design, in Department of Architecture. And he was graduated master's degree at Istanbul Aydin University, Institute of Science and Technology, Department of Architectural Design. He began his working life in İstanbul and Kastamonu cities of opening his own architectural office, and still designing different projects in his own office.

Carlos Miguel Iglesias Sanz is a PhD Architect. SAN PABLO CEU professor. Pathology and Conservation of Buildings specialist.

Juan Negreira holds a PhD in vibro-acoustic engineering from the University of Lund (Sweden) and an industrial engineer master degree from the University of Vigo (Spain). He was a full-time professor and researcher for 10 years at Lund University, with which he still collaborates today as an associate professor. He currently works at Ecophon (a company that develops, manufactures and markets room acoustic solutions) as Concept Developer. Likewise, he belongs to the Spanish acoustic standardisation group, is a board member of AECOR (Spanish association for acoustic quality) and is part-time professor at La Salle University (Barcelona).

David Palomar Aguilar is a PhD Architect. ETSAM professor. Energy Efficiency Advisor.

Omar Sánchez is an industrial designer with a postgraduate degree in industrial design from the National Autonomous University of Mexico (UNAM) and a doctorate in education from the International Postgraduate Center. Member of the national system of researchers (NSR level 1) in Mexico by the National Council of Science and Technology (CONACYT), full-time professor of the degree in industrial design, coordinator of the master's degree in sustainable design and business management studies and leader from the academic body of research at the Autonomous University of the State of Mexico UAEMex.

Gökçen Firdevs Yücel received her BArch from Istanbul University, Landscape Architecture Department (1995) and MSc in Landscape Planning Program from Istanbul Technical University (1998). She earned her PhD degree in Landscape Planning Program from Istanbul Technical University (2006). She worked İstanbul Commerce University Interior Architecture & Environmental Design Department (2008-2009) and Cyprus International University Architecture Department (2009-2010). Currently, she works as an Assistant Professor at Istanbul Aydın University Architecture and Design Faculty (2013-). Her major research interests include landscape architecture and design. Dr. Yücel has published in her areas of expertise in national and international congresses, national journals, and international book chapters.

Index

www.ingramcontent.com/pod-product-compliance
Lightning Source LLC
LaVergne TN
LVHW080525300926
849162LV00007B/1542